Neglected Tropical Diseases

Neglected Tropical Diseases

Neglected Tropical Diseases

Editor: Cyrus Hank

AMERICAN
MEDICAL PUBLISHERS
www.americanmedicalpublishers.com

AMERICAN
MEDICAL PUBLISHERS
www.americanmedicalpublishers.com

Cataloging-in-Publication Data

Neglected tropical diseases / edited by Cyrus Hank.
p. cm.
Includes bibliographical references and index.
ISBN 979-8-88740-296-3
1. Tropical medicine. 2. Medical climatology. 3. Communicable diseases--Prevention. I. Hank, Cyrus.
RC961 .N44 2023
616.988 3--dc23

American Medical Publishers,
41 Flatbush Avenue,
1st Floor, New York,
NY 11217, USA

ISBN 979-8-88740-296-3 (Hardback)

Contents

Preface

Neglected tropical diseases (NTDs) are a diverse group of tropical infections that are prevalent in developing regions of Africa, Asia, and the Americas. These diseases are caused by various types of pathogens that include parasitic worms like helminthes, protozoa, viruses and bacteria. There are several types of NTDs including buruli ulcer, chagas disease, cysticercosis, dengue fever, echinococcosis, fascioliasis, etc. These diseases are most common in tropical areas, where people do not have access to clean water or safe ways to dispose human waste. There are several preventive measures to control and eradicate NTDs, such as by controlling the vectors like mosquitoes and black flies. Some other highly effective strategies against NTDs are improvements in basic sanitation and hygiene. The topics included in this book on neglected tropical diseases are of utmost significance and bound to provide incredible insights to readers. It will explore all the important aspects of these diseases in the present day scenario. This book will serve as a valuable source of reference for graduate and post graduate students.

This book is a result of research of several months to collate the most relevant data in the field.

When I was approached with the idea of this book and the proposal to edit it, I was overwhelmed. It gave me an opportunity to reach out to all those who share a common interest with me in this field. I had 3 main parameters for editing this text:

1. Accuracy - The data and information provided in this book should be up-to-date and valuable to the readers.

2. Structure - The data must be presented in a structured format for easy understanding and better grasping of the readers.

3. Universal Approach - This book not only targets students but also experts and innovators in the field, thus my aim was to present topics which are of use to all.

Thus, it took me a couple of months to finish the editing of this book.

I would like to make a special mention of my publisher who considered me worthy of this opportunity and also supported me throughout the editing process. I would also like to thank the editing team at the back-end who extended their help whenever required.

Editor

1

Relative Performance and Predictive Values of Plasma and Dried Blood Spots with Filter Paper Sampling Techniques and Dilutions of the Lymphatic Filariasis Og4C3 Antigen ELISA for Samples from Myanmar

Jesse Masson [1,*], Jan Douglass [1], Maureen Roineau [1], Khin Saw Aye [2], Kyi May Htwe [2], Jeffrey Warner [1] and Patricia M. Graves [1]

1 College of Public Health, Medical and Veterinary Sciences, James Cook University, Cairns, QLD 4870, Australia; jan.douglass@my.jcu.edu.au (J.D.); Maureenroineau@wanadoo.fr (M.R.); jeffrey.warner@jcu.edu.au (J.W.); patricia.graves@jcu.edu.au (P.M.G.)

2 Department of Medical Research, Myanmar Ministry of Health and Sports, Nay Pyi Taw, Myanmar; ksadmr@gmail.com (K.S.A.); Kyimaywin31@gmail.com (K.M.H.)

* Correspondence: Jesse.masson@my.jcu.edu.au;

Academic Editors: Thewarach Laha and Peter A. Leggat

Abstract: Diagnostic testing of blood samples for parasite antigen Og4C3 is used to assess *Wuchereria bancrofti* in endemic populations. However, the Tropbio ELISA recommends that plasma and dried blood spots (DBS) prepared using filter paper be used at different dilutions, making it uncertain whether these two methods and dilutions give similar results, especially at low levels of residual infection or resurgence during the post-program phase. We compared results obtained using samples of plasma and DBS taken simultaneously from 104 young adults in Myanmar in 2014, of whom 50 (48.1%) were positive for filariasis antigen by rapid antigen test. Results from DBS tests at recommended dilution were significantly lower than results from plasma tested at recommended dilution, with comparisons between plasma and DBS at unmatched dilutions yielding low sensitivity and negative predictive values of 60.0% and 70.6% respectively. While collection of capillary blood on DBS is cheaper and easier to perform than collecting plasma or serum, and does not need to be stored frozen, dilutions between different versions of the test must be reconciled or an adjustment factor applied.

Keywords: lymphatic filariasis; Og4C3; ELISA; filter paper; DBS; ICT; immunochromatographic test

1. Introduction

Accurate and reliable screening assays that can be performed in low-resource laboratory settings have become vital for the Global Program to Eliminate Lymphatic Filariasis (GPELF). Currently, the use of the parasite antigen Og4C3 ELISA is among several techniques used to identify infection with lymphatic filariasis (LF) in *Wuchereria bancrofti* endemic areas [1–3]. Along with rapid immunochromatographic testing (ICT), which generates positive/negative results, the Og4C3 ELISA is used in monitoring and evaluation of the mass drug administration (MDA)-led elimination programs among endemic populations, producing quantitative results based on antigen units derived from a standard curve [4–6].

The Og4C3 ELISA, originally developed under Tropbio Pty. Ltd. at James Cook University, has been commercially available since the 1990s. Since 2013, the Og4C3 ELISA has been manufactured and supplied by Cellabs Pty. Ltd., Australia. Using categorical positive/negative results generated by using a cut-off value for positivity, the test has previously demonstrated a high level of sensitivity for the detection of filarial antigen when compared with the ICT rapid test [7–9]. Typically, the Og4C3 ELISA is performed using serum or plasma, either immediately after the sample has been obtained, or more often, from frozen samples. However, the Og4C3 ELISA also offers an alternative application method through the use of dried blood spots (DBS) collected on filter paper, an inexpensive and convenient method that requires less space and less stringent refrigeration for transport and storage.

Both plasma and DBS can make an important contribution to the final stages of LF elimination and to ensuring that re-emergence of disease has not occurred, despite some differences in practicability. For example, plasma samples can be directly applied to ELISA, yielding final results within a few hours if onsite laboratory facilities are available. However, DBS may be more convenient for field work and cost-effectiveness, as laboratory conditions are not mandatory despite the required overnight elution. Limited sample variation due to fluctuations in temperature and detection of antigen even after 12 months has also been demonstrated [10].

Despite the convenience in having two methods of application, studies which have directly compared Og4C3 ELISA DBS results to those from serum or plasma have shown discordance. Reeve and Melrose [11] compared results for 354 individuals from Papua New Guinea and observed significantly higher proportions of samples classified as positive by Og4C3 ELISA for serum (48.2%) than for DBS (32.5%). They demonstrated that the DBS technique yielded high specificity (99.2%; N = 391) and positive predictive value (PPV) (98.8%), but that sensitivity (67.2%; N = 354) and negative predictive values (NPV) (77%) were low when comparing DBS to serum as the gold standard. Interestingly, Tropbio and Cellabs recommend the dilution for plasma at 1:4 [12], while filter paper is recommended at an estimated dilution of 1:13.3, suggesting that the difference in dilution could be an underlying factor for discordance.

A second study by Itoh et al. [10], compared Og4C3 results for serum and DBS using a sample of 60 people in Sri Lanka, 55% of whom were reported to be positive for microfilariae, 65% positive by Og4C3 using serum, and 63.3% positive when using DBS. While these proportions positive by DBS and serum were not significantly different, this study used serum at a 1:3 dilution, applied at 16.7 μL per well, while DBS samples at an estimated dilution of 1:5 were applied at 3.3 μL per well. The authors then employed a 5-fold upward correction to the DBS antigen unit results to correct this difference in dilution. It is not clear how the results would have aligned if both sample types had been tested at currently recommended dilutions, and not adjusted.

Given the routine use of the Og4C3 ELISA by either plasma or DBS worldwide, this study aims to validate the existing instructions regarding the different dilutions of sample collected, and to determine if DBS is appropriate and comparable to plasma at the recommended dilutions.

2. Materials and Methods

The study site was the Amarapura Township of the Mandalay Region in Central Myanmar, an area known to have a high prevalence of LF infection. Persons aged 10–21 years were invited to participate. Ethical approval for the study was obtained from the James Cook University Research Human Ethics Committee, approval number H5261, and the Myanmar Ministry of Health and Sports.

2.1. Study Population

All participants were screened for LF infection using BinaxNOW® filariasis ICT (Alere International Limited, Ireland). Participants who tested positive by ICT were age and gender matched to uninfected controls and invited to participate in the longitudinal study. Written consent was obtained from 18–21 year olds and from the parent or guardian of 10–17 year olds. Blood collection was conducted with the assistance of the Myanmar Ministry of Health and Sports.

2.2. Preparation of Plasma and DBS Samples

A 10 mL sample of venous blood was collected from each individual in cooled ethylenediaminetetraacetic acid (EDTA) anticoagulant vacutainers (BD Biosciences, Becton, Dickinson and Company, North Ryde, NSW, Australia). Ten microlitres of blood was blotted using a micropipette onto each of six protruding filter paper sections (TropBio filter papers), which were left to completely dry before being placed in individual plastic bags. The remaining whole blood was placed on crushed ice and delivered to the Public Health Laboratory in Mandalay within four hours of collection. Whole blood was spun for 15 min at $3000\times g$ so that plasma could be aliquoted into 2 mL tubes. Plasma samples and DBS were stored short term at −20 °C until transported to Yangon on dry ice for −80 °C storage at the Department of Medical Research. One vial of each plasma sample was further aliquoted and refrozen before being shipped to James Cook University in Cairns, Australia, for storage at −80 °C. Filter papers were sealed in plastic containers and kept in either 4 °C refrigeration or hand luggage during direct transport to Cairns where they were stored at −80 °C.

2.3. Application of the TropBio Og4C3 Filariasis ELISA

The Og4C3 antigen was detected in plasma using the commercially available TropBio Og4C3 kits (Cellabs Pty. Ltd., Manly, Australia) at 1:4 dilution (50 μL of plasma into 150 μL of sample diluent, rather than 100 μL of plasma into 300 μL of sample diluent as recommended by the TropBio kit, to conserve samples) and at 1:16 dilution (50 μL of the 1:4 dilution into 150 μL of sample diluent). DBS samples were not tested at 1:4, since the volume of the three DBS protrusions was too large to elute in a small enough volume to test at 1:4.

The DBS dilution used three filter paper protrusions per sample, representing 30 μL of whole blood. We diluted the DBS into 200 μL of diluent. If the haematocrit was 50%, this would give a dilution of 1:13, making the assumption that the dried blood occupies no volume. Given wide individual variation in haematocrit, we are not able to specify an exact dilution factor for DBS. The filter paper insert supplied by TropBio suggests that the DBS assay is approximately 4-fold less sensitive than plasma or serum tested at recommended dilution of 1:4. Therefore the dilution is likely in the range of 1:11 to 1:16. In this study all DBS were tested as per kit recommended dilution (three spots into 200 μL). DBS were eluted overnight at 4 °C.

Positive control samples of serum were created at identical dilutions to ensure plate-to-plate consistency using a pool of ten known positive sera from a LF endemic area of Papua New Guinea (PNG). Negative controls from Australian lab workers were also used. Diluted samples were boiled using a water bath for 10 min before centrifuging at $2000\times g$ for 15 min. Fifty μL of the supernatant from each diluted sample was added to each well of the plate for primary sample incubation at 37 °C for 1 h, with the remainder of the ELISA technique performed as described in the instructions provided with the Tropbio Og4C3 kit [12]. Following initial incubation, wells which contained DBS samples were emptied and treated with washing buffer before the addition of 50 μL of 1% hydrogen peroxide solution, made by diluting 400 μL of 30% hydrogen peroxide in 11.6 mL of prepared wash buffer, and incubated for 10 min before subsequent washing.

2.4. Statistical Analysis

A standard curve was constructed for each ELISA plate using the kit-supplied controls, assigning an arbitrary high value of 32,768 units with subsequent 4-fold dilutions. The Softmax Pro v5 software (Molecular Devices, Sunnyvale, CA, USA) was used to convert optical density readings of the test samples to units based on a four-parameter curve. A single cut off point of >32 units (representing the sixth point of the standard curve from subsequent dilutions) was used to determine positive readings. Differences in unit values, between sampling techniques and test variations, were examined using paired t-tests, odds ratio, chi-square and correlation analysis. All analyses were performed using the IBM statistical software SPSS Version 23.0 (IBM, Armonk, NY, USA). Sensitivity, specificity, positive predictive value (PPV), and negative predictive value (NPV) of comparisons were also analysed. Confidence intervals (CI) were reported at 95%.

3. Results

Individuals between 10 to 21 years of age, irrespective of gender, were tested by ICT using fingerprick blood collected during October 2014. For each ICT-positive participant, an age and sex matched ICT negative participant was identified. Both were invited to return for full participation in a study of physical characteristics and to give a sample of venous blood for serological testing. Not all selected individuals (cases and controls) returned for the second venous sample; therefore, a final collection of 48 positive and 56 negative samples were included in this study.

3.1. Analysis of Categorical Results Used to Compare the ICT and Og4C3 ELISA

To investigate how results classified as positive and negative varied between the ICT and the Og4C3 ELISA using plasma and DBS, categorical results were compared. Positive proportions of 46.2% obtained through the ICT were not significantly different to the proportion of 48.1% when using plasma at 1:4 dilution (Table 1). However, values became significantly different, dropping to 37.5% and 34.6% respectively, when plasma at 1:16 dilution or DBS was used (Table 1).

Table 1. Positive proportions and chi-square results of comparisons between the immunochromatographic test and the Og4C3 ELISA.

Standard	N Positive	% Positive (95% Confidence Interval (CI))	Comparative Test	N Positive	% Positive (95% CI)	McNemar Chi Sq	*P* Value
ICT	48	46.2 (36.9–55.7)	Plasma 1:4	50	48.1 (38.7–57.6)	0.3	$p = 0.8$
-	-	-	Plasma 1:16	39	37.5 (28.8–47.1)	6.2	$p = 0.02$
-	-	-	Dried blood spot (DBS)	36	34.6 (26.2–44.2)	8.00	$p = 0.008$

Holding the ICT as a relative standard, agreement with the Og4C3 ELISA using plasma and DBS was assessed. When ELISA using plasma at a 1:4 dilution was compared to ICT, sensitivity was 85.4% and specificity 83.9%, while PPV and NPV were 82.0% and 87.0%, respectively (Table 2). The use of a 1:16 dilution for plasma or use of DBS resulted in a decrease in sensitivity and NPV when compared to ICT, while specificity and PPV increased (Table 2). This suggests that the Og4C3 ELISA is significantly affected by dilution and application method when compared to ICT, with the 1:4 dilution yielding higher sensitivity and NPV, while the 1:16 plasma dilution or DBS yields higher specificity and PPV.

Table 2. Sensitivity, specificity, positive predictive value (PPV), negative predictive value (NPV) and odds ratio results from ICT and Og4C3 ELISA comparisons.

Standard	Comparative Test	Sensitivity (95% CI)	Specificity (95% CI)	PPV (95% CI)	NPV (95% CI)	Odds Ratio (95% CI)	*P* Value
ICT	Plasma 1:4	85.4% (72.2–93.9)	83.9% (71.7–92.4)	82.0% (71.2–89.3)	87.0% (77.0–93.1)	30.6 (10.5–89.4)	$p < 0.0001$
-	Plasma 1:16	77.1% (62.7–88.0)	96.4% (87.7–99.6)	94.9% (82.5–98.6)	83.1 (74.5–89.2)	90.8 (19.0–433.8)	$p < 0.0001$
-	DBS	68.8% (53.8–81.3)	94.5% (85.1–98.9)	91.7% (78.3–97.1)	77.9% (69.8–84.4)	38.9 (10.5–144.6)	$p < 0.0001$

Odds ratios were used to predict the likelihood of positive and negative results from comparative Og4C3 samples when compared to the ICT standard. Odds ratio was highest at 90.8 for comparison against plasma using a 1:16 dilution, but decreased to 30.6 when using plasma at 1:4 dilution, and to 38.9 when using DBS (Table 2). This suggests that agreement between the ICT and Og4C3 ELISA is best when using the Og4C3 with plasma at a 1:16 dilution.

3.2. Analysis of Categorical Results Used to Compare Plasma at 1:4 and 1:16 Dilutions and DBS

To assess results achieved by Og4C3 ELISA, plasma application at a 1:4 dilution was held as a standard for comparison. Again, we used chi-square tests to find a significant value of 7.5 ($p = 0.009$) when comparing plasma at 1:4 to DBS, which remained significant at 5.3 ($p = 0.04$) when plasma was compared using 1:4 and 1:16 dilutions (Table 3). Therefore, both plasma application at 1:16 and DBS give different results to plasma tested at the recommended 1:4 dilution.

Table 3. Positive proportions and chi-square results of comparisons between Og4C3 ELISA application method and dilution.

Standard	N Positive	% Positive (95% CI)	Comparative Test	N Positive	% Positive (95% CI)	McNemar Chi Sq	*P* Value
Plasma 1:4	50	48.1 (38.7–57.6)	DBS	36	34.6 (26.2–44.2)	7.5	$p = 0.009$
-	-	-	Plasma 1:16	39	37.5 (28.8–47.1)	5.3	$p = 0.04$

To investigate if matched dilutions might improve plasma and DBS concordance between proportions, both methods were compared using plasma at 1:16 as the new standard. The difference was not significant when comparing plasma at 1:16 and DBS, achieving a chi-square value of 0.7 (Table 4). This confirms high agreement of positive proportions when plasma and DBS are applied using similar dilutions.

Table 4. Positive proportions and chi-square results of comparisons between Og4C3 ELISA applications at 1:16 dilution.

Standard	N Positive	% Positive (95% CI)	Comparative Test	N Positive	% Positive (95% CI)	McNemar Chi Sq	*P* Value
Plasma 1:16	39	37.5 (28.8–47.1)	DBS	36	34.6 (26.2–44.2)	0.7	$p = 0.6$

To determine how application of plasma and DBS with recommended dilution affects final results of each test, sensitivity, specificity, PPV and NPV were calculated. Sensitivity and NPV were low at 60.0% and 70.6% when DBS was compared to plasma at 1:4 (Table 5). Higher values of 88.9% and 83.3% were recorded for specificity and PPV respectively (Table 5). Test performance remained relatively unchanged when plasma at 1:16 was compared to plasma at 1:4, with the exception of an increase in sensitivity to 66.0% over DBS when using a similar dilution (Table 5).

Table 5. Sensitivity, specificity, PPV, NPV and odds ratio results from Og4C3 method and dilution comparisons.

Standard	Comparative Test	Sensitivity (95% CI)	Specificity (95% CI)	PPV (95% CI)	NPV (95% CI)	Odds Ratio (95% CI)	*P* Value
Plasma 1:4	DBS	60.0% (45.2–73.6)	88.9% (77.4–95.8)	83.3% (67.2–93.6)	70.6% (58.3–81.0)	12.0 (4.3–33.3)	$p < 0.0001$
-	Plasma 1:16	66.0% (51.2–78.8)	88.9% (77.4–95.8)	84.6% (69.5–94.1)	73.9% (61.5–84.0)	15.5 (5.5–43.5)	$p < 0.0001$

Kappa agreement statistic was used to analyse concordance between comparisons against the 1:4 diluted plasma gold standard. Kappa values were relatively low at 0.55 and 0.49 for comparisons of plasma at 1:4 with plasma at 1:16 dilution and DBS respectively.

To assess if more closely-matched dilutions might improve positive and negative detection rates, plasma at 1:16 dilution was employed as a standard and compared against DBS. This resulted in relatively high sensitivity (79.5%), specificity (92.3%), PPV (86.1%), and NPV (88.2%), suggesting that both plasma and DBS yield highest concordance in positive and negative results when applied using similar dilutions (Table 6).

Table 6. Sensitivity, specificity, PPV, NPV and odds ratio results from Og4C3 ELISA applications of plasma at 1:16 dilution and DBS.

Standard	Comparative Test	Sensitivity (95% CI)	Specificity (95% CI)	PPV (95% CI)	NPV (95% CI)	Odds Ratio (95% CI)	*P* Value
Plasma 1:16	DBS	79.5% (63.5–90.7)	92.3% (83.0–97.5)	86.1% (70.5–95.3)	88.2% (78.1–94.8)	46.5 (14.0–154.2)	$p < 0.0001$

An odds ratio of 46.5 was also achieved when comparing plasma at a 1:16 dilution and DBS (Table 6) which was higher than odds ratio achieved when using plasma at 1:4 dilution as the standard (Table 5). This suggests a stronger association between plasma and DBS when dilutions are matched.

Concordance between the 1:16 diluted plasma sample and the DBS sample was also measured using kappa agreement statistic. Values were higher at 0.73 than observed with comparisons that used a 1:4 diluted gold standard. This suggests higher concordance between samples when dilutions are matched.

3.3. Analysis of Quantitative Mean Results Used to Compare Plasma at 1:4 and 1:16 Dilutions and DBS

Antigen unit values are shown for each sample type and dilution expressed as log (units+1) in Figure 1.

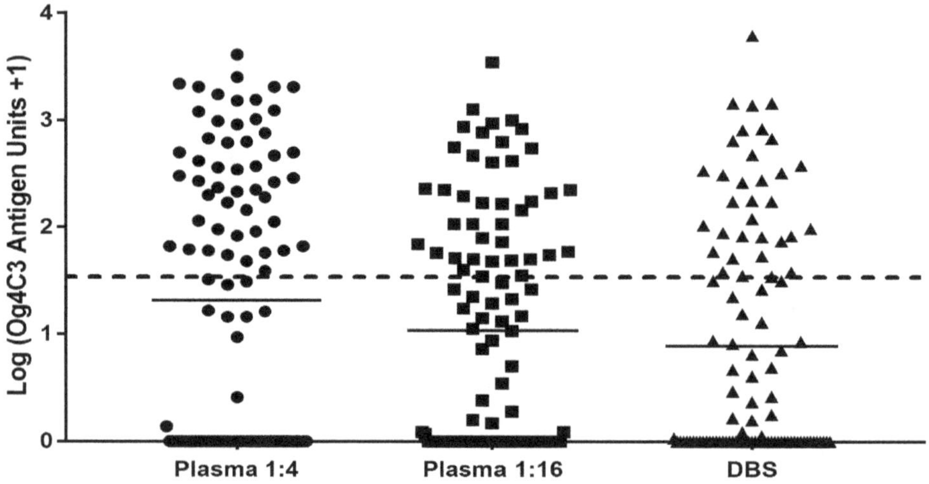

Figure 1. Filariasis Og4C3 ELISA antigen unit concentration comparisons of dilution, plasma and whole blood application. Horizontal black lines refer to mean log antigen unit concentration of each assay (Table 7). All antigen unit concentrations above the defined cut-off (log (32 antigen units + 1)), shown by the horizontal segregated line, are considered positive, while all readings below are considered negative.

Table 7. Comparison of mean Og4C3 antigen units between sample applications and dilutions.

Group 1			Group 2			*t*-Test			
Test	Mean Log (Antigen Unit +1)	Geometric Mean	Test	Mean Log (Antigen Unit +1)	Geometric Mean	N	Mean Log Difference	SD	*P* Value
Plasma 1:4	1.32	19.75	DBS	0.89	6.81	104	0.42	0.88	$p < 0.0001$
Plasma 1:4	1.32	19.75	Plasma 1:16	1.03	9.83	104	0.28	0.74	$p < 0.001$
Plasma 1:16	1.03	9.83	DBS	0.89	6.81	104	0.14	0.67	$p = 0.03$

Analysis of log unit values + 1 was used to approximate a normal distribution for comparisons. From these units, the mean log value for plasma at 1:4 (1.32) was significantly higher than the mean log values achieved for DBS (0.89; $p < 0.0001$) (Table 7). The mean log for plasma at 1:4 was also significantly higher than for plasma at 1:16 dilution (Table 7). Despite a statistically significant p value when dilutions were similar for plasma and DBS, the mean difference was smaller than previous comparisons. These quantitative comparisons are consistent with the results described above.

3.4. Correlation Comparisons Analysis of Og4C3 Concentrations from Plasma and Eluates from DBS

To compare differences in antigen unit concentrations between tests, correlation coefficients were measured between sample types and dilutions. When comparing recommended dilutions of plasma at 1:4 against DBS, correlation was lowest at 0.7 (Figure 2A). Correlation increased to 0.8 when plasma at 1:4 and 1:16 dilutions were compared (Figure 2B), and when plasma at 1:16 and DBS were compared (Figure 2C). This suggests improved correlation is achieved through either matched sample application or dilution.

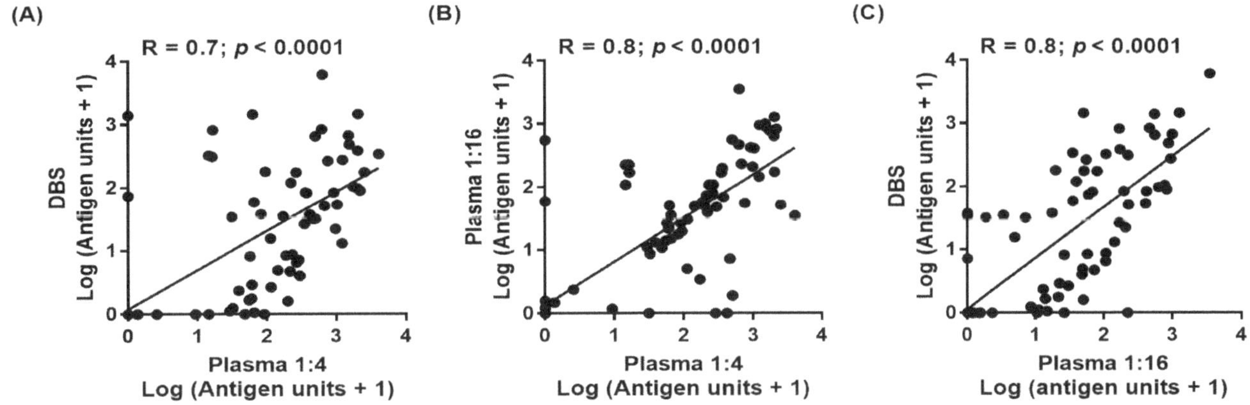

Figure 2. Filariasis Og4C3 ELISA antigen unit concentration correlation comparisons. (**A**) Plasma at recommended 1:4 dilution plotted against DBS samples. (**B**) Plasma at recommended 1:4 dilution plotted against 1:16 dilution. (**C**) Plasma at 1:16 dilution plotted against DBS samples.

4. Discussion

The major finding of this study is that the agreement of results between plasma and DBS samples is lowest when using recommended dilutions of 1:4 for plasma, and that better agreement between these tests is achieved when using plasma at 1:16 against DBS. However, significantly fewer samples are classed as positive when using the lower 1:16 dilution for plasma or using DBS.

We showed that the ICT had similar positive proportions and predictive values to the Og4C3 ELISA when using plasma at 1:4, but that sensitivity is reduced when using the 1:16 dilution. Previous literature has shown that the ICT is less sensitive than the Og4C3 ELISA at 1:4 dilution, detecting only 66.5% of known bancroftian filariasis cases with no microfilariae confirmed by microscopy [13], but that both tests yield identical detection rates when microfilariae were detectable [13–16]. Og4C3 has also been reported to detect significantly smaller titres of filarial antigen when compared to the ICT [13,17], although ICT and Og4C3 both showed an improved detection rate average of up to 25% over microfilariae detection[18]. The current study suggests that despite the higher sensitivity of Og4C3 at lower antigen dilutions, the dilution recommended for DBS application reduces the amount of antigens per sample to a titre that will not accurately yield a positive result when the disease is present.

When analysing positive proportions, results were similar at 46.15% and 48.08% for ICT and plasma at 1:4, and again at 37.50% and 34.62% for plasma at 1:16 and DBS. Positive proportion similarity between plasma and DBS has previously been discussed by Itoh and colleagues [10] as having a 97.4% concordance. However, these results were produced using a 5-fold upwards adjustment to the DBS antigen units.

Lack of concordance between plasma at 1:4 and DBS was supported by Chi-square analysis, which showed significant difference when recommended dilutions for plasma and DBS were used, but no significant difference with matched dilution comparisons. These data support the notion that it is not sample type per se but dilution factor that affects quantitative results, and lower positive proportions for plasma at 1:16 and DBS are detected when compared to ICT or plasma at 1:4 dilution.

Sensitivity and NPV was lowest when DBS was compared to plasma using recommended dilutions. This comparison also yielded an odds ratio of 12.00 and kappa of 0.49, the lowest value among each of these comparisons. These results are similar to those found by Reeve and Melrose [11], where sensitivity and NPV was 67.2% and 77.0% respectively using the dilutions recommended by the Og4C3 kit. As sensitivity and NPV increased to 79.49% and 88.24% respectively when comparing plasma at 1:16 and DBS samples, these results suggest that dilution directly affects how likely it is that the assay will detect the presence of *Wuchereria bancrofti* in someone with LF, as well as how likely it is to detect someone with a negative result when they do not have LF. These statistics were also supported by an odds ratio, which was highest at 45.50, and by the kappa agreement statistic, which was also highest at 0.73, when dilutions were matched.

There was a higher mean antigen concentration in plasma compared to DBS at recommended dilutions, but the difference in mean antigen units was greatly reduced when dilutions were more closely matched. While plasma samples were tested at 1:4 and 1:16 dilutions, equal to a 4-fold difference, geometric mean (antigen unit +1) values were 19.75 and 9.83 respectively. The difference in means is much less than 4-fold. The geometric means were 9.83 and 6.81 for plasma at 1:16 and DBS respectively. The non-linear antigen unit relationship to dilution factor may be attributed to high saturation of each ELISA well by a higher concentration of sample, which would be left with fewer spare antibodies bound to the plastic surface available for the free floating antigens to bind during the initial 1-h incubation period. It is possible that a lower concentration of sample antigen may bind fewer antibodies initially, but will not saturate the well as the higher concentration sample would, allowing a greater number of unbound antibodies on the plate to attach to free floating antigens during incubation [19,20].

Correlation was found to be highest when either dilutions or sample application methods were matched, but was low when plasma at 1:4 and DBS were compared. No previous study has compared matching low dilutions but it is not surprising that matched dilutions may result in higher agreeability between plasma and DBS. This is important as higher dilutions are less sensitive overall when compared with ICT and therefore must be used with caution.

The results of this study indicate that the currently recommended dilution for the Og4C3 ELISA using DBS is not as sensitive as for plasma, and that more than 25% of positive cases may be being missed when using DBS. Concordance between methods would improve if similar dilutions were used. Unfortunately, a 1:4 dilution is not possible with the current prescribed method of DBS preparation and amount of sample, since that would require eluting three filter paper discs in 60 μL of diluent, leaving insufficient supernatant for a single well after boiling and spinning. While high correlation can be achieved when the fold difference in antigens is matched [10], Lalitha and colleagues [21] show that correlation can drop to 0.83 when plasma and DBS are used at 1:4 and 1:20 dilutions respectively.

The outcomes of this research lead to a recommendation that further assessment be carried out to determine how both plasma and DBS perform at other matched dilutions, such as 1:8 or 1:10. Any such tests must accommodate the volume needed to fully saturate each dried blood spot, allow for boiling, precipitation and spinning, and yielding 50 μL to be applied to the well of an Og4C3 ELISA. Improved concordance between Og4C3 plasma and DBS application that also achieves a similar detection rate as the ICT would greatly support the reliability of the Og4C3 ELISA for field collection in non-laboratory locations, as DBS is a convenient method of collecting samples, requiring less in-depth training, and less storage space or refrigeration during transport.

A major limitation attributed to enzyme immunoassays, referred to as the 'hook' effect, is shown when a decrease in reactivity is seen as the concentration of free antigen or antibody increases [22–24]. As each plate will always give different readings, a reliable standard curve must be used to mitigate plate-to-plate variation and avoid error in classifications of positive or negative from test to test.

One strategy may be to perform each sample at two dilutions in order to obviate such occurrences and to ensure that antibody or antigen excess does not occur. A two-dilution application could also evaluate each individual plate by showing if any non-linearity between results has occurred.

In conclusion, the current recommended dilutions for plasma and DBS did not demonstrate adequate agreement. The data obtained shows that both plasma and DBS are capable of yielding similar results, but only when dilutions are more closely matched than is currently recommended. Definition of a single suitable dilution factor lower than 1:16 which can be applied to both DBS and plasma assays, and to compare specificity, sensitivity and predictive values between DBS and plasma upon application is required. Results achieved from antigen unit analysis using DBS assays need to be adjusted upwards to be comparable with plasma tests. We recommend that similar studies be repeated in other endemic situations, with different test predictive values, to confirm our results and to determine the adjustment factors required. In the longer term, the dilutions for the two test types need to be reconciled.

Acknowledgments: The authors would like to thank the Myanmar Ministry of Health and Sports and the Department of Medical Research (Lower Myanmar) for laboratory support and storage of the samples. We are grateful to Luke Becker of the Australian Institute for Tropical Health and Medicine and Ye Ye and Thi Thi Lwin of the Public Health Laboratory in Mandalay (Central Myanmar) for assistance with sample collection and separation. We would like to thank Diane Dogcio-Hall and Cellabs Pty. Ltd., New South Wales, Australia, for advice and discussions. We are very grateful to the NIH/NIAID Filariasis Reagent Resource Center (www.filariasiscenter.org) that provided positive controls for the ICT cards. Additional thanks must also be given to Mathew Hayes and Adam Bowen for their support and advice.

Author Contributions: P.M.G., J.D., J.M. and J.W. conceived of and designed the experiments; J.M., M.R., and K.M.H. performed the experiments; K.S.A. provided storage and lab facilities, J.M. and P.M.G. analysed the data; J.M., P.M.G. and J.D. wrote the paper with input from J.W.; all authors reviewed the final draft and provided input.

References

1. Lau, C.L.; Won, K.Y.; Becker, L.; Soares Magalhaes, R.J.; Fuimaono, S.; Melrose, W.; Lammie, P.J.; Graves, P.M. Seroprevalence and spatial epidemiology of lymphatic filariasis in American Samoa after successful mass drug administration. *PLoS Negl. Trop. Dis.* **2014**, *8*, e3297. [CrossRef] [PubMed]
2. Mwakitalu, M.E.; Malecela, M.N.; Pedersen, E.M.; Mosham, F.W.; Simonsen, P.E. Urban lymphatic filariasis in the metropolis of Dar es Salaam, Tanzania. *Parasites Vectors* **2013**, *6*, 286. [CrossRef] [PubMed]
3. Hamlin, K.L.; Moss, D.M.; Priest, J.W.; Roberts, J.; Kubofcik, J.; Gass, K.; Streit, T.G.; Nutman, T.B., Eberhard, M.L.; Lammie, P.J. Longitudinal monitoring of the development of antifilarial antibodies and acquisition of *Wuchereria bancrofti* in a highly endemic area of Haiti. *PLoS Negl. Trop. Dis.* **2012**, *6*, e1941. [CrossRef] [PubMed]
4. Harrington, H.; Asugeni, J.; Jimuru, C.; Gwalaa, J.; Ribeyro, E.; Bradbury, R.; Streit, T.G.; Nutman, T.B.; Eberhard, M.L.; Lammie, P.J. A practical strategy for responding to a case of lymphatic filariasis post-elimination in Pacific Islands. *Parasites Vectors* **2013**, *6*, 218. [CrossRef] [PubMed]
5. Weerasooriya, M.V.; Gunawardena, N.K.; Itoh, M.; Qiu, X.G.; Kimura, E. Prevalence and intensity of *Wuchereria bancrofti* antigenaemia in Sri Lanka by Og4C3 ELISA using filter paper-absorbed whole blood. *Trans. R. Soc. Trop. Med. Hyg.* **2002**, *96*, 41–45. [CrossRef]
6. World Health Organization. *Lymphatic Filariasis: A Manual for National Elimination Programmes*; WHO Press: Geneva, Switzerland, 2011; pp. 7–8.
7. Gass, K.; Beau de Rochars, M.V.; Boakye, D.; Bradley, M.; Fischer, P.U.; Gyapong, J.; Itoh, M.; Ituaso-Conway, N.; Joseph, H.; Kyelem, D.; et al. A multicenter evaluation of diagnostic tools to define endpoints for programs to eliminate bancroftian filariasis. *PLoS Negl. Trop. Dis.* **2012**, *6*, e1479. [CrossRef] [PubMed]
8. Rocha, A.; Braga, C.; Belém, M.; Carrera, A.; Aguiar-Santos, A.; Oliveira, P.; Texeira, M.G.; Furtado, A. Comparison of tests for the detection of circulating filarial antigen (Og4C3-ELISA and AD12-ICT) and ultrasound in diagnosis of lymphatic filariasis in individuals with microfilariae. *Mem. Inst. Oswaldo Cruz* **2009**, *104*, 621–625. [CrossRef] [PubMed]

9. Gounoue-Kamkumo, R.; Nana-Djeunga, H.C.; Bopda, J.; Akame, J.; Tarini, A.; Kamgno, J. Loss of sensitivity of immunochromatographic test (ICT) for lymphatic filariasis diagnosis in low prevalence settings: Consequence in the monitoring and evaluation procedures. *BMC Infect. Dis.* **2015**, *15*, 579. [CrossRef] [PubMed]
10. Itoh, M.; Gunawardena, N.K.; Qiu, X.G.; Weerasooriya, M.V.; Kimura, E. The use of whole blood absorbed on filter paper to detect *Wuchereria bancrofti* circulating antigen. *Trans. R. Soc. Trop. Med. Hyg.* **1998**, *92*, 513–515. [CrossRef]
11. Reeve, D.; Melrose, W. Evaluation of the Og34C filter paper technique in lymphatic filariasis prevalence studies. *Lymphology* **2014**, *47*, 65–72. [PubMed]
12. Tropbio Pty. Ltd. *ELISA Kit for Detecting and Quantifying Wuchereria bancrofti Antigen*; Cellabs Pty. Ltd.: Brookvale, NSW, Australia, 2014.
13. Nuchprayoon, S.; Porksakorn, C.; Junpee, A.; Sanprasere, V.; Poovorawan, Y. Comparative assessment of an Og4C3 ELISA and an ICT filariasis test: A study of Myanmar migrants in Thailand. *Asian Pac. J. Allergy Immunol.* **2003**, *21*, 253–257. [PubMed]
14. Freedman, D.O.; de Almeida, A.; Miranda, J.; Plier, D.A.; Braga, C. Field trial of a rapid card test for *Wuchereria bancrofti*. *Lancet* **1997**, *350*, 1681. [CrossRef]
15. Simonsen, P.E.; Dunyo, S.K. Comparative evaluation of three new tools for diagnosis of bancroftian filariasis based on detection of specific circulating antigens. *Trans. R. Soc. Trop. Med. Hyg.* **1999**, *93*, 278–282. [CrossRef]
16. Nuchprayoon, S.; Sanprasert, V.; Porksakorn, C.; Nuchprayoon, I. Prevalence of bancroftian filariasis on the Thai-Myanmar border. *Asian Pac. J. Allergy Immunol.* **2003**, *21*, 179–188. [PubMed]
17. Nguyen, N.L.; Plichart, C.; Esterre, P. Assessment of immunochromatographic test for rapid lymphatic filariasis diagnosis. *Parasite* **1999**, *6*, 355–358. [CrossRef] [PubMed]
18. Melrose, W.; Pisters, P.; Turner, P.; Kombati, Z.; Selve, B.P.; Hii, J.; Speare, R. Prevalence of filarial antigenaemia in Papua New Guinea: Results of surveys by the School of Public Health and Tropical Medicine, James Cook University, Townsville, Australia. *P. N. G. Med. J.* **2000**, *43*, 161–165. [PubMed]
19. Butler, J.E.; McGivern, P.L.; Swanson, P. Amplification of the enzyme-linked immunosorbent assay (ELISA) in the detection of class-specific antibodies. *J. Immunol. Methods* **1978**, *20*, 365–383. [CrossRef]
20. Winzor, D.J. Allowance for antibody bivalence in the characterization of interactions by ELISA. *J. Mol. Recognit.* **2011**, *24*, 139–148. [CrossRef] [PubMed]
21. Lalitha, P.; Ravichandran, M.; Suba, S.; Kaliraj, P.; Narayanan, R.B.; Jayaraman, K. Quantitative assessment of circulating antigens in human lymphatic filariasis: A field evaluation of monoclonal antibody-based ELISA using blood collected on filter strips. *Trop. Med. Int. Health* **1998**, *3*, 41–45. [CrossRef] [PubMed]
22. Pesce, A.J.; Michael, J.G. Artifacts and limitations of enzyme immunoassays. *J. Immunol. Methods* **1992**, *150*, 111–119. [CrossRef]
23. Rodbard, D.; Feldman, Y.; Jaffe, M.L.; Miles, L.E. Kinetics of two-site immunoradiometric (sandwich) assays—II. Studies on the nature of the 'high-dose hook-effect'. *Immunochemistry* **1978**, *15*, 77–82. [CrossRef]
24. Ryall, R.G.; Story, C.J.; Turner, D.R. Reappraisal of the causes of the 'hook-effect' in two-site immunoradiometric assays. *Anal. Biochem.* **1982**, *27*, 308–315. [CrossRef]

2

Investigation of a Scabies Outbreak in Drought-Affected Areas in Ethiopia

Wendemagegn Enbiale [1,*] and Ashenafi Ayalew [2]

[1] Dermatology and Venerology, Bahir Dar University, P.O. Box 1996, Bahir Dar, Ethiopia
[2] Amhara Regional Health Bureau, P.O. Box 744, Amhara, Ethiopia; ashunets@gmail.com
* Correspondence: wendaab@gmail.com;

Abstract: The impact of the severe drought in Ethiopia, attributed to El Niño weather conditions, has led to high levels of malnutrition that have, in turn, increased the potential for disease outbreaks. In 2015, Ethiopia faced a scabies outbreak in drought-affected areas where there was a shortage of safe water for drinking and personal hygiene. Following a house-to-house census to assess the prevalence of scabies, a detailed study was conducted looking at the disease burden. Following the outbreak report, training was provided on scabies identification and management for zonal and district health officials from administrative districts affected by the drought (nutritional hot-spot *woredas*). The training was cascaded down to the health extension workers in the affected areas. Screening and management guidelines and protocols were also distributed. House-to-house data collection was undertaken by 450 health extension workers (HEWs) to assess the prevalence of scabies. The HEWs used a simplified reporting tool. Subsequently, data were collected and validated in two zones and six *woredas* from 474 participants who had been diagnosed with scabies using a standardized questionnaire. This was designed to look at the specificity of the diagnosis of scabies, age distribution, severity, duration of illness, secondary infection and other sociodemographic variables as preparation for mass drug administration (MDA). The HEWs screened 1,125,770 people in the 68 districts in Amhara Region and a total of 379,000 confirmed cases of scabies was identified. The prevalence in the different districts ranged from 2% to 67% and the median was 33.5% [interquartile range (IQR) 19–48%]. 49% of cases were school-aged children. The detailed study of 474 individuals who were recorded as scabies cases revealed that the specificity of the diagnosis of scabies by the HEWs was 98.3%. The mean duration of illness was 5 months (SD of $\pm$ 2.8). One third of patients were recorded as having severe illness, 75.1% of cases had affected family members, and 30% of affected children were noted to have secondary bacterial infection. Eleven percent of the students had discontinued school due to scabies or/and drought and 85% of these had secondary bacterial infection. These community-based data serve as reliable proxy indicators for community-based burden assessment of the scabies epidemic. This study will also provide a good basis for advocating the use of a community-level clinical diagnostic scheme for scabies using an algorithm with a simple combination of signs and symptoms in resource-poor settings.

Keywords: scabies; outbreak; drought; emergency state

---

1. Background

Scabies is a common public health problem, globally affecting about 200 million people. It is a particular problem where there is social disruption, overcrowding, and where personal hygiene is poor. Immunosuppression, poor nutritional status, and dementia are also risk factors for scabies [1–3]. Natural disasters, war, and poverty lead to overcrowding and have been associated with increased rates of transmission [4].

Scabies is caused by an ecto-parasitic infestation of the skin by the human itch mite, *Sarcoptes scabiei* var. *hominis* [1]. It usually spreads by direct, prolonged, skin-to-skin contact with an infested individual. The main effect of scabies is debilitating itching, leading to scratching, which in turn is followed by breakdown of the barrier function of the skin and complications due to bacterial infection, ranging from impetigo, abscesses, and cellulitis, to more serious conditions such as septicemia and glomerulonephritis, leading to renal failure and rheumatic heart disease [1,4].

1.1. Drought

The data from The International Disaster Database indicate that in Africa more than 40 million people were affected by drought in 2015–2016. Following the 2015–2016 El-Niño event, which affected many countries globally, Ethiopia experienced drought and extreme water shortage across large parts of the country. This has further limited access to water for personal hygiene and basic sanitation for many individuals, especially those in rural communities, leading to a great increase in the risk of communicable diseases like scabies and diarrheal diseases [5].

Most definitions of drought describe it as a prolonged period of abnormally low rainfall, leading to a shortage of water. The effects of drought are critically dependent on both context and vulnerability of the underlying population. The development and severity of the drought depends on the background level of water use, which may also influence the timing of the onset, duration, and end of the drought, as well as the social, economic, and administrative infrastructures which address the consequences of water deficit. The impact on health is particularly dependent on the socio-economic environment that, in turn, has a direct impact on the resilience of the population. Poor health, poverty, and conflict are additional contributing factors that exacerbate the impact of drought [6,7].

1.2. Government Priorities/Political Setting

Following official acknowledgment by the Ethiopian government of a food crisis in July 2015, the Federal Ministry of Health established a command post spearheaded by the Public Health Emergency Management (PHEM) directorate. In September 2015, the Amhara Regional State PHEM announced the first report of a scabies epidemic [8]. To validate the diagnosis, a team of field epidemiologists and a dermatologist visited three of the areas where the claim had emerged. The experts collected data from three health centers and six health posts in addition to visiting households that had been previously diagnosed with scabies at local health facilities. The experts concluded that scabies was the major active public health problem affecting the community, with the status of an outbreak [9].

Prior to September 2015, the regular review of drought-related public health emergencies, in both federal and regional PHEM disease surveillance systems, focused solely on malnutrition, diarrheal diseases, measles, malaria, and meningitis; however, there was no consideration of skin-related conditions. A recent literature review by Anderson and Davies has shown that El Niño has been associated with increases in the occurrence of sun-related skin diseases and certain vector-borne and waterborne diseases [10]. Despite outbreak reports in some parts of the country [8], scabies was not included in either the list of reportable diseases or the weekly reports.

After the first visit to some of the affected zones and a review of information regarding the burden of the problem, the inspection team advocated the inclusion of scabies as a separate item on the weekly surveillance list for the Federal Ministry of Health and Regional Health Bureau. Since October 2015, scabies has been included as one of the reportable diseases in the drought affected areas. The weekly PHEM surveillance reports revealed that scabies was becoming significantly more extensive than its more usual occurrence as sporadic clinical cases, and was now a public health concern affecting wider geographic areas and population groups, especially in the *woredas* most severely affected by drought and malnutrition. Hence, it required public mobilization and public health emergency interventions. The report revealed that the Amhara, Tigray, and Oromia regions had the highest burdens of scabies in Ethiopia.

The extent of the drought and the increased number of water-scarce *woredas* with limited access to water sanitation and hygiene (WASH) interventions, further worsened the spread of the disease and its severity among the vulnerable. From the November 2015 harvest season assessment, the number of nutritional hot-spot *woredas* increased to 429, involving a total population of nearly 49 million. That same month, the public health emergency management task force received a report that the number of severely affected *woredas* in Amhara, Tigray, and Oromia had reached 32, and despite the limited surveillance program for scabies, the estimated total number of cases reached more than 250,000 with prevalence of at least 15% in some districts [6].

In October 2015, following the national government elections, prominent officials at all levels of the administration attended an official meeting. The researchers used this as an opportunity to present the preliminary data of the burden of scabies and the recommended action to be taken by the relevant officials (zonal and *woreda* administrators, zonal and *woreda* health office officers, heads of the Regional Health Bureau, and other officials) and to advocate for region wide evidence generation in preparation for the intervention.

A systematic review of scabies prevalence studies published between 1985 and 2015, included only five African countries, highlighting the paucity of prevalence data in Africa [11]. This house-to-house census and validation study of scabies provides a unique opportunity to ascertain community prevalence. Such data is more reliable than health facility-based data which generally underestimates prevalence, as individuals within communities may not present with scabies (perhaps because it is 'normalized') or because there is under-diagnosis or lack of effective treatments at clinics [12].

2. Methods

The outbreak assessment developed in two stages.

2.1. Phase 1

Following one-day face-to-face training on data recording, diagnosis, and management of scabies along with other relevant conditions for district health officials and the subsequent cascading of training to the front line care workers or health extension workers, a house-to-house census was undertaken in all the 68 hotspot *woredas* (districts) in the Amhara region (Figure 1).

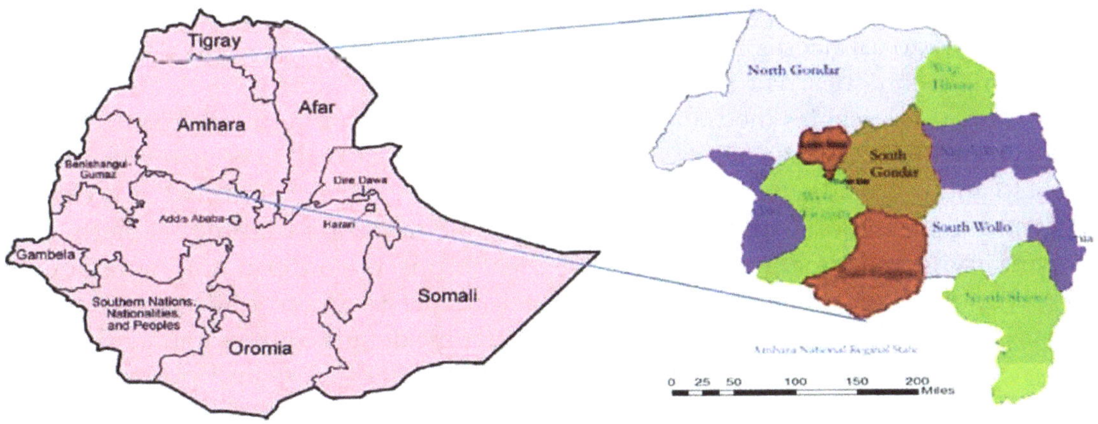

Figure 1. Amhara regional State, Ethiopia (2015/2016).

A cross-sectional house-to-house census was performed, identifying scabies cases and contacts based on regional scabies identification and management guidelines in the Amhara region as preparation for the developing a scabies outbreak control program [7]. The census was performed in all households of the previously identified 68 hot-spot districts. The sites were selected by the Regional Health Bureau and PHEM team from the routine weekly report (districts in the region that have reported scabies). In each household, all family members were screened. The study period was from October to November 2015.

The census was conducted as part of the Regional Health Bureau screening in preparation for a community-based scabies control program. The local HEW, supervised by health officers/BSc nurses from nearby health centers, registered each resident by name, age, and sex and each resident was screened for scabies. Age groups were defined as follows: <2 years, 2 to 18 years, >18 years.

Each participant was examined by a HEW trained in scabies diagnosis and treatment. The diagnosis of scabies was based on the clinical case definition (Table 1). In addition to scabies screening, the census was used for the integrated assessment of pre-determined drought-related health problems (malnutrition, measles, diarrheal diseases, meningitis, malaria, and scabies). The screening of drought related pre-determined diseases by the health extension workers in relation to scabies had, up to this point, used only a limited set of information variables to identify cases of scabies and their contacts in each district.

Table 1. Clinical case definition of scabies and contact [7].

Scabies	Presence of itching with typical lesions on hands, inter-digital, and/or genitalia and/or itching and close contact with an individual who has itching or typical lesions in a typical distribution.
Contact	A contact is a person who does not fulfill the clinical criteria for infestation with scabies (above) or a person without signs and symptoms consistent with scabies, who has had direct contact (particularly prolonged, direct, skin-to-skin contact) with a suspected or confirmed case in the two months preceding the onset of scabies signs and symptoms in the index case

The data were analyzed and results are presented using descriptive statistics. Scabies prevalence in the different age group and districts was calculated. In addition, statistical analysis was performed with SPSS 10.0 for Windows (SPSS Inc., Chicago, IL, USA). The median, interquartile range (IQR) and odds ratio (OR) were calculated and the p-value derived.

2.2. Phase 2

This study, performed between 16 October and 2 December 2015, was undertaken primarily to validate the data collected by the HEW and secondly to obtain an understanding of associated factors of the scabies epidemic. The study population was residents identified as cases in the house-to-house census. From the two zones, six districts with an estimated population of 600,000 were selected using clustered sampling techniques. The sample size was determined using a single proportion formula with consideration of the scabies median prevalence from the house-to-house census (33.5%) with a confidence level of 97% in the two zones. The reporting forms of the HEWs were used to select 474 cases. The inclusion criteria included those patients who have been identified as a case of scabies by the HEWs and the selection was performed with simple random sampling using the registration form. The team invited each patient to the village health post for a dermatology review including history, full body physical examination, and a standardized questionnaire which was completed by the dermatologist. The questionnaire included socio-demographic details of cases and additional variables such as presence of itching, severity of infestation, duration of illness and presence of secondary bacterial infection. The diagnosis of scabies was made clinically using the standardized case definition for the study (Table 1).

For clinical purposes, the severity of scabies was defined by the number of skin lesions and the presence or absence of crust. Mild: when the number of scabies associated skin lesions (papules, excoriation, and pustule) was less than or equal to ten. Moderate: The number of scabies associated skin lesions were between 10 and 50 lesions. Severe: when the number of scabies associated skin lesions were equal to or greater than 50 or the presence of scabies-associated crust. Secondary infection was defined by the presence of pustules and/or yellowish crusts.

The study received ethical approval on 14 September 2015 from the Regional Health Bureau as part of its operational research (reference number R.T.T/1/63107). A written support letter was received from the Regional Health Bureau to enlist the cooperation of the Zonal Health offices. Permission was subsequently also secured from the zonal and district health offices. The data collectors obtained verbal consent from each participant or his/her guardians. Written consent was obtained from patients who had images recorded.

The data was analyzed and results presented using descriptive statistics.

3. Results

3.1. Phase 1

The field based house-to-house survey using HEWs in the Amhara Region screened 1,125,770 individuals from October to November 2015 in 68 districts (Figure 2). A total of 379,000 confirmed cases were found. Overall, 195,665 (51.6%) of the patients were female and (60%) of confirmed cases were below 18 years of age. Children and young adults under 18 years old were 2.5 times more at risk in developing scabies (Table 2).

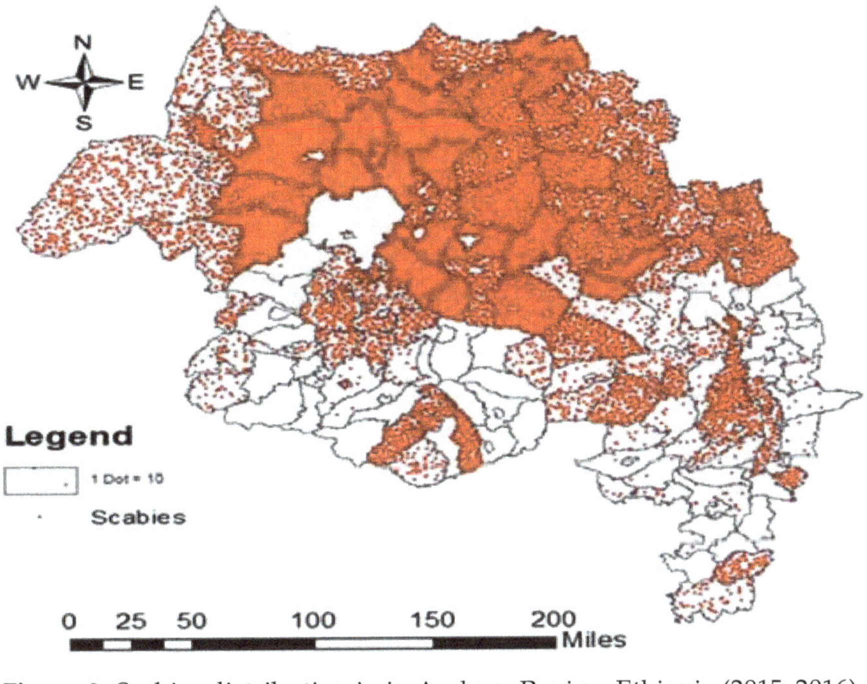

Figure 2. Scabies distribution in in Amhara Region, Ethiopia (2015–2016).

Table 2. Prevalence of scabies and bivariate analysis of demographic factors based on a house-to-house census in Amhara Region, Ethiopia (October 2015).

Variable	Total (*N*)	Affected (*n*)	Prevalence	OR *	*p* Value
Sex					
Female	585,400	195,665	33.4	Ref	Ref
Male	540,370	183,335	33.9	1.05	0.8
Total	1,125,770	379,000	33.7		
Age group (years) **					
<2	60,792	27,909	45.9	2.5	0.01
2 to 18	518,980	249,535	48.1	2.4	0.01
>18	545,998	101,556	18.6		

* Odds Ratio. ** Age groups were defined as follows: <2 years, 2 to 18 years, >18 years.

The scabies prevalence in the 68 districts ranged from 2% to 67% with a median prevalence of 33.5 (IQR 19–48%).

3.2. Phase 2

Of the 474 subjects enrolled in the 'detailed' study, 466 (98.3%) were confirmed to have scabies by a dermatologist (expert control group), which meant that the clinical diagnosis of the HEWs achieved a level of agreement with this control group of 98.3% (Figure 3). The index cases of the epidemic have been traced in both areas to the students in traditional church schools suggesting that these groups are important as sources of the infestation and in continued community transmission.

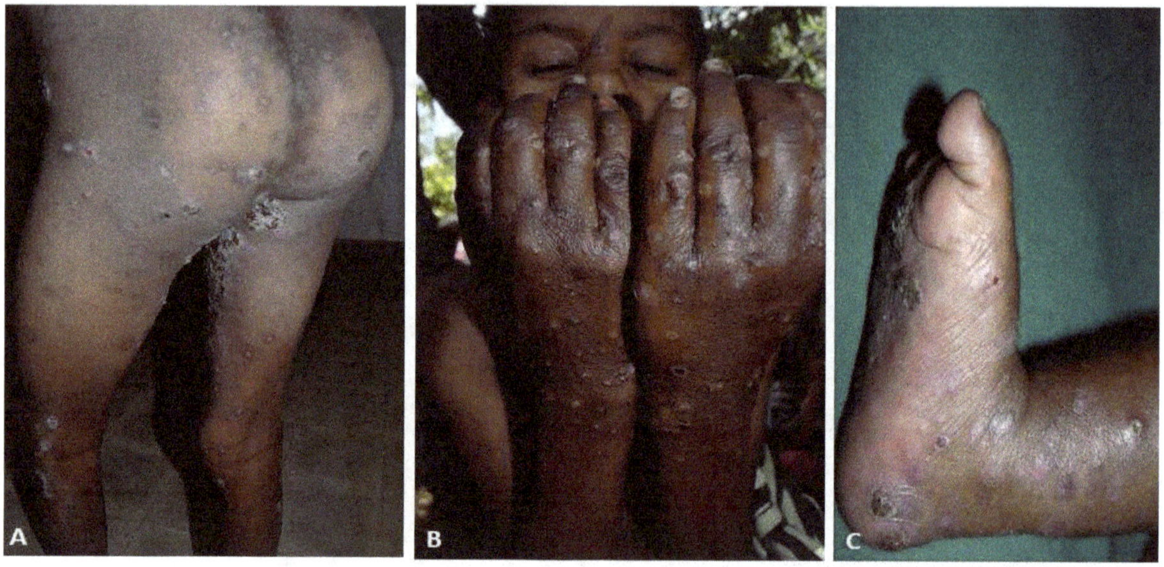

Figure 3. (**A**) Extensive crusting papules, excoriation with post-inflammatory hyperpigmentation in a 34-year-old female. (**B**) Pustules, crusts, and erosion in 12-year-old boy. (**C**) Pustules, crusts, and erosions in a 2-year-old female.

The majority (66.9%) of the scabies cases in this part of the study were in males, although the gender ratio varied with age. The proportion of males was by far the highest (113 or 87%) in those aged 18 years and above.

The median age of those affected was 10 years. The highest proportion of cases was found in those between 2 and 18 years old. 182 (39%) of the total number of cases were of school age and, of these, 63% were currently attending school, 15% never attended school, 11% had discontinued schooling prior to the drought and scabies outbreak and another 11% had discontinued their education as a result of scabies and the drought.

In the same validation study, all cases (466) had scabies skin lesions and all cases reported itching (itching and classic skin lesion are two case definitions used for scabies). The median number of lesions was found to be 10 to 49 (moderate). Approximately a quarter (116) of the cases had a history of a skin sore, of whom 94 (81%) had encrusted sores (Figure 3A). There were 14 (3%) cases with crusted scabies (Table 3).

The median duration of illness was 5 months, ranging from 0.5 to 12 months. Approximately one quarter (116) developed a secondary bacterial infection; the secondary bacterial infection rate was highest among those aged between 2 and 18 years (Table 4). On the other hand there was no significant difference in gender-specific bacterial infection rates (25% and 26% for females and males respectively). The bacterial infection rate among the school age group was 40% (Figure 3B). The rate was significantly higher 85% (95% CI of 79–91 and $p < 0.001$) among those who had dropped-out of school.

Table 3. Clinical signs and symptoms of scabies cases in the Amhara region, Ethiopia (2015).

Variables	*N* (%)
Sign and symptom	
Itching	466 (100%)
Classic scabies lesion	466 (100%)
Bacterial infection	116 (25%)
Crusted scabies	14 (3%)
Severity of the skin lesion	
Mild	13 (28%)
Moderate	191 (41%)
Severe	144 (31%)

Table 4. Scabies secondary bacterial infection rate by age, Amhara region, Ethiopia (2015).

Variable	Scabies Cases (*N*)	Infection (*N*)	Infection % (95% CI)	Odds Ratio	*p* Value
<2 years	46	7	15.2 (11.8–18.2)	1.8	0.012
2–18 years	288	101	35.1 (29.3–40.9)	4.2	<0.001
>18 years	132	11	8.3 (6.9–9.7)	Ref.	
Total	466	119	25.5 (21.3–29.7)		

4. Discussion

This regional census documenting cases of scabies and the cross-sectional validation study for the intervention campaign, documents the burden of community-based scabies in Ethiopia. This survey was noteworthy in screening the highest number of cases ever reported in the literature and, at the same time, in documenting the largest number of scabies cases. Other cross-sectional community-based studies in relatively large populations have been reported: (1) in Malawi in a village with a population of 61,735 where the prevalence was 0.7%; and (2) in Cambodia in 13 villages with a population of 14,843 where the prevalence was 4.3% [13–17]. As a community-based study the median prevalence in our survey was much larger and the range much wider (2% to 67%). This is supported by previous reports that the prevalence of scabies in community-based surveys is frequently higher than the burden reported in the Global Burden of Disease study (GBD) or reports from routine clinic data [12,18].

Even though there is no evidence on a cause and effect association, the scabies outbreak occurred following the 2015–2016 El Nino drought. In contrast, the study by Andersen et al. reported scabies to be one of the dermatological problems with a significant decrease in incidence related to El Nino [10].

Hay et al., in their review of scabies in the developing world, noted that 'the attack rate is probably equal between the sexes, and the differences in prevalence reported in some studies are probably attributable to confounding factors', which was also confirmed in this large population census [19]. Seventy-three percent of infestations were registered in those under the age 18, which correlates with the impression that in developing countries, scabies is much more common among preschool children than adolescents and rates significantly decreased in mid-adulthood [20,21].

The burden of this scabies epidemic was compounded by the high rate of secondary bacterial infection, with 30% of school-age children presenting with mild to severe secondary bacterial infection, in agreement with another population based study in the Solomon Islands [22]. This survey will strengthen the data that show that scabies infestations are an important risk factor for bacterial infection of the skin [23,24].

The key conclusions are, firstly that this community based data will serve reliable proxy indicators for the burden of the scabies epidemic in communities. Secondly this study also reaffirmed the idea that community level clinical diagnosis of scabies by community health workers using a simplified diagnostic algorithm has the potential to address the scabies burden in resource poor settings [25,26].

Finally this study will also serve as a sizeable input for the WHO's 'global strategy for scabies control' [27].

There are potential limitations in this study which are listed as follows:

1. The study used an aggregated report of the census with a limited data set (scabies case, contact, age, and sex) which could be a limitation of the study, especially for risk factor analysis.
2. In the house-to-house census of scabies cases, the examining HEWs had no other relevant experience apart from the one-day training described, which may have led to missed cases. The validation study focused only on specificity of the diagnosis.
3. Both in the census and in the validation study, the diagnosis of scabies and impetigo was made on the basis of clinical history and skin examination alone. Skin scrapings for direct microscopy or other confirmatory tests were not used.

Despite these limitations, the population survey and validation study have provided important new data about the extent of scabies in communities in northern Ethiopia and has registered the highest number of scabies cases ever reported in a single outbreak.

Author Contributions: W.E. contributed substantially to the conception and design of the house-to-house survey and validation study, the acquisition of data, the analysis and interpretation. He also drafted the article, provided final approval of the version to publish and agreed to be accountable for all aspects of the work in ensuring that questions related to the accuracy or integrity of any part of the work are appropriately investigated and resolved. A.A. contributed substantially to the design of house-to-house survey, the acquisition of data and the analysis. He also gave critical revision of the article, provided final approval of the version to publish and agreed to be accountable for all aspects of the work in ensuring that questions related to the accuracy or integrity of any part of the work are appropriately investigated and resolved.

Acknowledgments: We would like to thank Amhara Regional Health bureau for taking the leadership position and giving us all the necessary support for the implementation of the survey. Many thanks also for L. Claire Fuller and Roderick Hay from International Foundation for Dermatology for their support from encouragement for the writing and language editing of the manuscript.

References

1. Hicks, M.I.; Elston, D.M. Scabies. *Dermatol. Ther.* **2009**, *22*, 279–292. [CrossRef] [PubMed]
2. Heukelbach, J.; Feldmeier, H. Scabies. *Lancet* **2006**, *367*, 1767–1774. [CrossRef]
3. Ugbomoiko, U.; Oyedeji, S.; Babamale, O.; Heukelbach, J. Scabies in resource-poor communities in Nasarawa State, Nigeria: Epidemiology, clinical features and factors associated with infestation. *Trop. Med. Infect. Dis.* **2018**, *3*, 59. [CrossRef] [PubMed]
4. World Health Organization. *Epidemiology and Management of Common Skin Diseases in Children in Developing Countries*; WHO: Geneva, Switzerland, 2005; Available online: whqlibdoc.who.int/hq/2005/WHO_FCH_CAH_05.12_eng.pdf (accessed on 23 July 2018).
5. WHO. *El Nino and Health*; WHO Report 2016; WHO: Geneva, Switzerland, 2016; Available online: who_el_nino_and_health_global_report_21jan2016.pdf (accessed on 4 June 2017).
6. *EM-DAT: The OFDA/CRED International Disaster Database*; Universite Catholique de Louvain: Brussels, Belgium. Available online: http://www.emda.be/result-disaster-profiles?disgroup=natural&period=1900%242012&dis_type=Drought&Submit=Display+Disaster+Profile (accessed on 4 June 2017).
7. UNISDR. *Global Assessment Report on Disaster Risk Reduction: Revealing Risk, Redefining Development*; United Nations International Strategy for Disaster Reduction: Geneva, Switzerland, 2011.
8. *Scabies Outbreak Preparedness and Response Plan*; FMOH: Addis Ababa, Ethiopia, 2015; Available online: www.humanitarianresponse.info (accessed on 23 July 2018).
9. *Interim-Guideline for Multi Sectorial Scabies Outbreak Emergency Response*; FMOH: Addis Ababa, Ethiopia, 2015.

10. Andersen, L.K.; Davis, M.D. The effects of the El Nino Southern Oscillation on skin and skin-related diseases: A message from the International Society of Dermatology Climate Change Task Force. *Int. J. Dermatol.* **2015**, *54*, 1343–1351. [CrossRef] [PubMed]
11. Romani, L.; Steer, A.C.; Whitfeld, M.J.; Kaldor, J.M. Prevalence of scabies and impetigo worldwide: A systematic review. *Lancet Infect. Dis.* **2015**, *15*, 960–967. [CrossRef]
12. Engelman, D.; Andrew, I.D.; Steer, C. Control strategies for scabies. *Trop. Med. Infect. Dis.* **2018**, *3*, 98. [CrossRef] [PubMed]
13. Accorsi, S.; Barnabas, G.A.; Farese, P.; Padovese, V.; Terranova, M.; Racalbuto, V.; Morrone, A. Skin disorders and disease profile of poverty: Analysis of medical records in Tigray, northern Ethiopia, 2005-2007. *Trans. R. Soc. Trop. Med. Hyg.* **2009**, *103*, 469–475. [CrossRef] [PubMed]
14. Landwehr, D.; Keita, S.M.; Pönnighaus, J.M.; Tounkara, C. Epidemiologic aspects of scabies in Mali, Malawi, and Cambodia. *Int. J. Dermatol.* **1998**, *37*, 588–590. [CrossRef] [PubMed]
15. Carapetis, J.R.; Connors, C.; Yarmirr, D.; Krause, V.; Currie, B.J. Success of a scabies control program in an Australian aboriginal community. *Pediatr. Infect. Dis. J.* **1997**, *16*, 494–499. [CrossRef] [PubMed]
16. Nair, B.K.; Joseph, A.; Kandamuthan, M. Epidemic scabies. *Indian J. Med. Res.* **1977**, *65*, 513–518. [PubMed]
17. Dos Santos, M.M.; Amaral, S.; Harmen, S.P.; Joseph, H.M.; Fernandes, J.L.; Counahan, M.L. The prevalence of common skin infections in four districts in Timor-Leste: A cross-sectional survey. *BMC Infect. Dis.* **2010**, *10*, 61–66. [CrossRef] [PubMed]
18. Karimkhani, C.; Colombara, D.V.; Drucker, A.M.; Norton, S.A.; Hay, R.; Engelman, D.; Steer, A.; Whitfeld, M.; Naghavi, M.; Dellavalle, R.P. The global burden of scabies: A cross-sectional analysis from the Global Burden of Disease Study 2015. *Lancet Infect. Dis.* **2017**, *17*, 1247–1254. [CrossRef]
19. Hay, R.J.; Steer, A.C.; Engelman, D.; Walton, S. Scabies in the developing world—Its prevalence, complications, and management. *Clin. Microbiol. Infect.* **2012**, *18*, 313–323. [CrossRef] [PubMed]
20. Burkhart, C.G.; Burkhart, C.N.; Burkhart, K.M. An epidemiologic and therapeutic reassessment of scabies. *Cutis* **2000**, *65*, 233–240. [PubMed]
21. Kouotou, E.A.; Nansseu, J.R.N.; Sieleunou, I.; Defo, D.; Bissek, A.C.Z.K.; Ndam, E.C.N. Features of human scabies in resource-limited settings: The Cameroon case. *BMC Dermatol.* **2015**, *15*, 12. [CrossRef] [PubMed]
22. Mason, D.S.; Marks, M.; Sokana, O.; Solomon, A.W.; Mabey, D.C.; Romani, L.; Engelman, D. The prevalence of scabies and impetigo in the Solomon Islands: A population-based survey. *PLoS Negl. Trop. Dis.* **2016**, *10*, e0004803. [CrossRef] [PubMed]
23. Swe, P.M.; Zakrzewski, M.; Kelly, A.; Krause, L.; Fischer, K. Scabies mites alter the skin microbiome and promote growth of opportunistic pathogens in a porcine model. *PLoS Negl. Trop. Dis.* **2014**, *8*, e2897. [CrossRef] [PubMed]
24. Romani, L. The AIM study: A field trial of co-administration of azithromycin and ivermectin mass drug administration (MDA), CRF skin examination clinical record form, version 1, 2015. Available online: https://kirby.unsw.edu.au/project/aim-study (accessed on 23 July 2018).
25. Mahé, A.; Faye, O.; N'Diaye, H.T.; Ly, F.; Konare, H.; Keita, S.; Hay, R. Definition of an algorithm for the management of common skin diseases at primary health care level in sub-Saharan Africa. *Trans. R. Soc. Trop. Med. Hyg.* **2005**, *99*, 39–47. [CrossRef] [PubMed]
26. Steer, A.C.; Tikoduadua, L.V.; Manalac, E.M.; Colquhoun, S.; Carapetis, J.R.; Maclennan, C. Validation of an integrated management of childhood illness algorithm for managing common skin conditions in Fiji. *Bull WHO* **2009**, *87*, 173–179. [CrossRef] [PubMed]
27. World Health Organization. 9th NTD-STAG Global Working Group Meeting on Monitoring and Evaluation of Neglected Tropical Diseases. 2018. Available online: http://www.who.int/neglected_diseases/events/STAG_Working_Group_on_Monitoring_Evaluation/en/ (accessed on 12 August 2018).

3

Epidemiology and Characteristics of *Rickettsia australis* (Queensland Tick Typhus) Infection in Hospitalized Patients in North Brisbane, Australia

Adam Stewart [1,*], Mark Armstrong [1], Stephen Graves [2] and Krispin Hajkowicz [1,3]

1 Department of Infectious Diseases, Royal Brisbane and Women's Hospital, Butterfield St & Bowen Bridge Rd, Herston, Queensland 4029, Australia; mark.armstrong@health.qld.gov.au (M.A.); krispin.hajkowicz@health.qld.gov.au (K.H.)

2 Australian Rickettsial Reference Laboratory, Barwon Health, Geelong Hospital, Bellerine Street, PO BOX 281, Geelong, Victoria 3220, Australia; graves.rickettsia@gmail.com

3 School of Medicine, University of Queensland, St Lucia, Queensland 4072, Australia

* Correspondence: adm_stewart@hotmail.com;

Academic Editors: Patricia Graves, Thewarach Laha, Peter A. Leggat and Khin Saw Aye

Abstract: Queensland tick typhus (QTT; *Rickettsia australis*) is a spotted fever group (SFG) rickettsial infection endemic to Australia. It is an underreported and often unrecognized illness with poorly-defined epidemiology. This article describes epidemiological features and the geographical distribution of QTT in hospitalized patients. Cases of QTT were identified retrospectively from 2000–2015 at five sites in Northern Brisbane through a pathology database. Included cases had a four-fold rise in SFG-specific titre, a single SFG-specific titre ≥256 or an SFG-specific titre ≥128 with a clinically consistent illness. Of the fifty cases identified by serology, 36 were included. Age ranged from 3–72 years (with a mean of 39.5 years) with a male-to-female ratio of 1:1.1. Fifteen of 36 (42%) study participants had hobbies and/or occupations linked with the acquisition of the disease. Seventeen of 36 (47%) identified a tick bite in the days preceding presentation to hospital, and reported exposure to a known animal host was minimal (25%). QTT infection occurred throughout the year, with half of the cases reported between April and July. Recent ecological and sociocultural changes have redefined the epidemiology of this zoonotic illness, with areas of higher infection risk identified. Heightened public health awareness is required to monitor QTT disease activity.

Keywords: tick-borne diseases; *Rickettsia* infections; epidemiology; Queensland; Australia

---

1. Introduction

Queensland tick typhus (QTT) is an important cause of febrile illness; particularly among those exposed to the eastern coastal bushlands in Australia [1]. Currently, a diagnosis of any rickettsial infection does not require compulsory reporting in Australia, making disease surveillance incredibly difficult and inaccurate [2,3]. Although its true epidemiological impact is unknown, recently identified socio-ecological drivers of rickettsial disease could re-define QTT as a public health threat [1]. In addition, recent serological surveys point to a disease burden along the eastern coast that is greater than previously realized [1,4]. The geographical distribution and boundaries of QTT infection continue to be pushed further along the coastline, as well as inland [5]. As our understanding of host-vector interactions and ecological factors that drive disease emergence improves, informed public health interventions will become pivotal.

2. Materials and Methods

Study patients were both adults and children identified retrospectively during the period of January 2000 to January 2015 at any of the five sites in Metropolitan North Hospital and Health Service (MNHSS) in Queensland, Australia via the local pathology database. Medical records were reviewed for each identified case. Epidemiological and clinical data were recorded onto a standardized electronic case report form. Clinical features were considered present only if their presence was documented in the medical record. Confirmed or probable cases of QTT included those with a greater or equal to a four-fold rise in spotted fever group (SFG)-specific serology; a single SFG-specific titre $\geq$256; or an SFG-specific titre $\geq$128 with a clinically consistent illness [5]. A clinically consistent illness was defined as a presentation typical for QTT, without a more likely diagnosis being apparent, as well as a good clinical response to doxycycline or another appropriate antibiotic. Cases were further excluded if serology results represented an old infection, an acute illness thought to be acquired overseas, or a known cause of antibody cross-reactivity to *Rickettsia*-specific antigens (e.g. autoimmune conditions). The indirect microimmunofluorescence assay (IFA) utilizing an SFG-specific *Rickettsia rickettsii* antigen was used in serological testing.

The study was conducted in accordance with the Declaration of Helsinki, and the protocol was approved by the Royal Brisbane & Women's Hospital Ethics Committee (HREC/14/QRBW/432).

3. Results

Of the 50 cases identified by serological criteria alone through the pathology database, 36 were included after the exclusion criteria were applied. Two patient's medical records were destroyed and thus inaccessible.

3.1. Demographics

Of the studied patients, age ranged from 3–72 years (with a mean of 39.5 years) and sex distribution was approximately equal between males and females with a male-to-female ratio of 1:1.1. Fifteen of 36 (42%) study participants had hobbies and/or occupations that were linked with the acquisition of the disease, including gardening, bushwalking/orienteering, camping, and working as a botanist, wildlife ranger, groundsman, or farm worker/grazier. Eleven of 36 (31%) patients acquired their infection in association with travel away from their primary residence. Four of 36 (11%) were noted to live on a property with dense surrounding bushland. Moreover, 17 out of 36 (47%) reported a tick bite in the days preceding presentation to hospital, and 3 out of 36 (8%) reported multiple tick bites in the past, usually associated with their occupation or place of residence. Reported exposure to vertebrate animals on history was only 9 out of 36 (25%), which included exposure to cattle, dogs and horses (Table 1). Of note, eight patients reported no known risk factors for acute rickettsial infection.

3.2. Distribution of Disease

Eighteen of 36 (50%) cases occurred between April and July; 10/36 (28%) occurred from September to December; and 8/36 (22%) occurred between January and March (Figure 1). To determine the distribution of disease, the postcode of the patient's primary residence was recorded, unless there was a clear history of preceding travel to another place where the tick bite had occurred; in this case, the postcode from the site where the infection was acquired was entered into the database. A high density of infection occurred in the Samford Valley, Woodford and Mount Nebo areas (Figure 2). Eleven of 36 (31%) infections were acquired in this area alone. Six of 36 (8%) were located in the Narangba and Morayfield areas, 5–10 kilometers from the coastal area of Samford. Other infections were sporadically distributed along the eastern coast of Queensland and northern New South Wales. Interestingly, of those requiring intensive care unit (ICU) admission (4/36), 75% lived or acquired their infection within a five-kilometer radius of each other, and presented during the March/April period.

Table 1. Demographic and historical features of 36 patients with Queensland tick typhus (QTT).

Characteristic	Value
Age	3–72 years (Mean 39.5, Median 36.1)
Sex	Male-to-female ratio 1:1.1
- Male	17/36 (47%)
- Female	19/36 (53%)
Occupation	
- Groundsman/ranger	3/36 (8%)
- Farming	3/36 (8%)
Hobby/activity	
- Camping	3/36 (8%)
- Gardening	3/36 (8%)
- Bushwalking	2/36 (6%)
- Other	1/36 (3%)
Residence on acreage/property	4/36 (11%)
Recent travel (e.g., holiday)	11/36 (31%)
Tick bite	17/36 (47%)
- Single	14/36 (39%)
- Multiple	3/36 (8%)
Frequency of known risk factors	
- 0	8/36 (22%)
- 1	13/36 (36%)
- 2	13/36 (36%)
- 3	3/36 (8%)

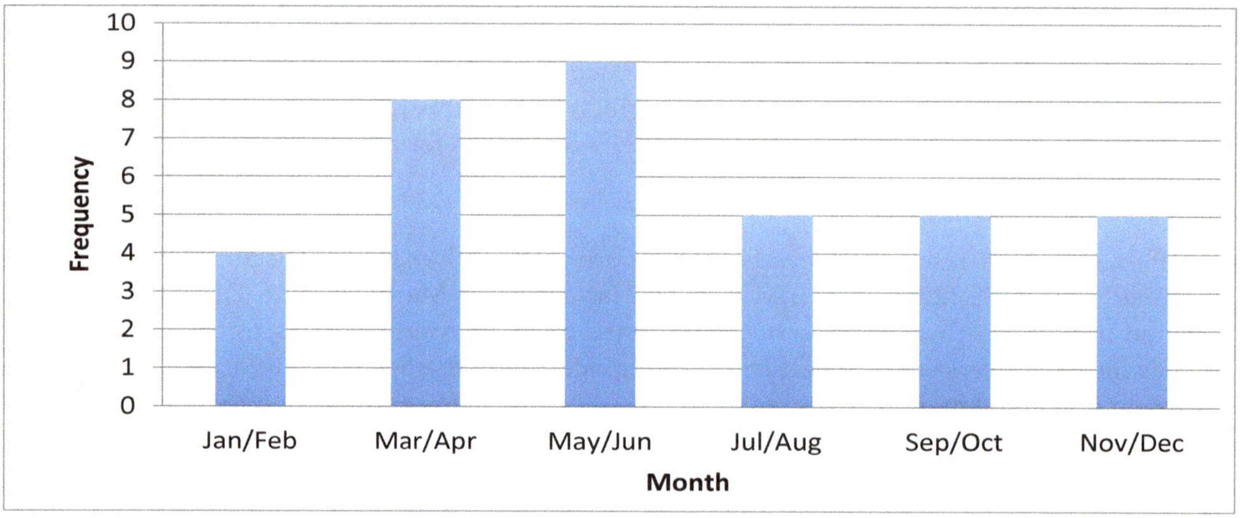

Figure 1. Seasonal variation in QTT infection in 36 hospitalized patients with Queensland tick typhus (QTT).

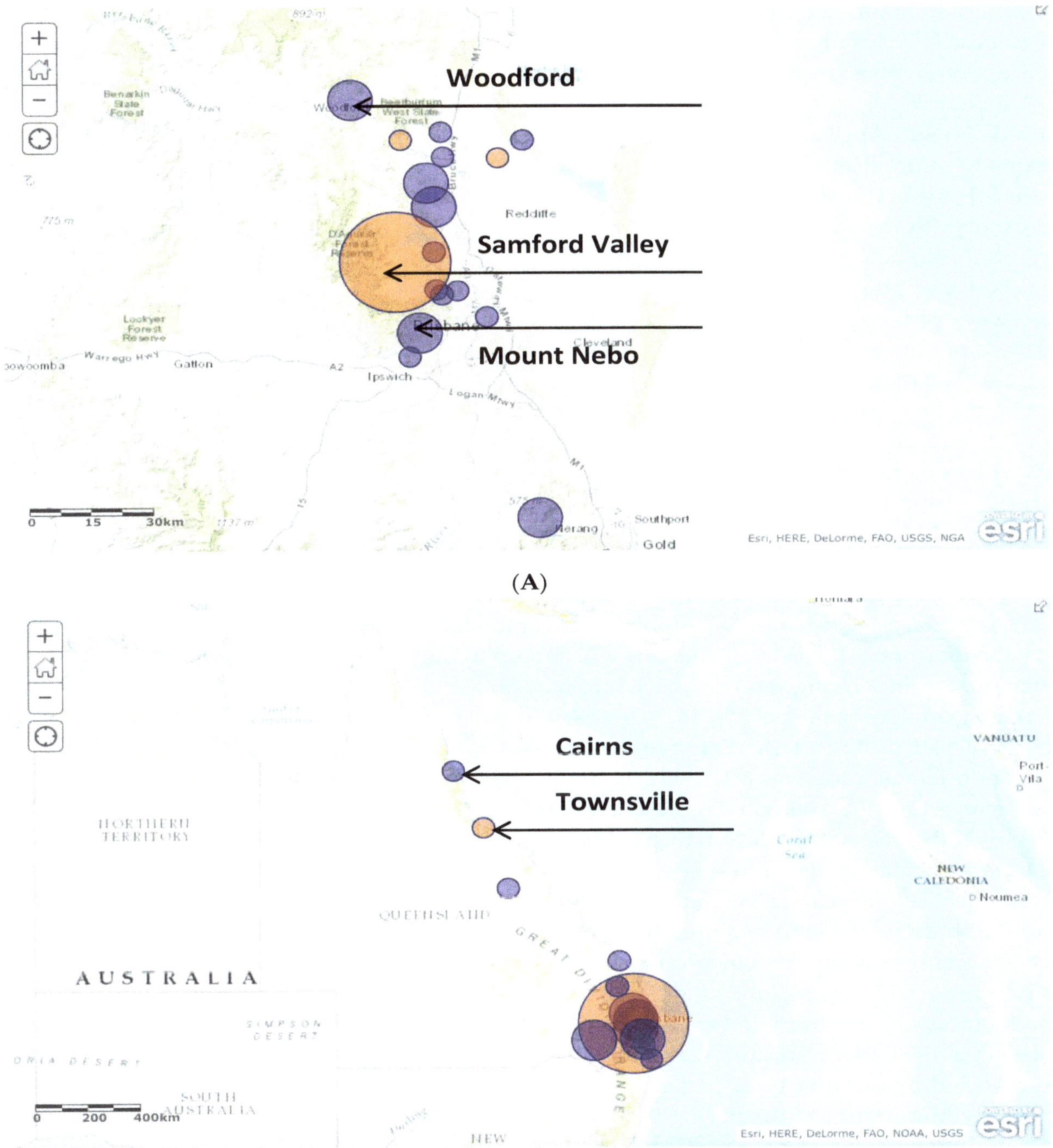

(A)

(B)

Figure 2. Location of the 36 patients who presented to the five study sites with acute *Rickettsia australis* infection within southeast (**A**) and greater Queensland (**B**) Note: Size of circle indicates relative frequency of infection; orange circles indicate where cases of severe infection occurred.

4. Discussion

Defining the distribution of each SFG rickettsial disease in Australia has been a difficult task [1]. This is largely due to inadequate reporting of infection, as well as low recognition and testing in the community and hospital settings [3,6]. In addition, there may be a larger pool of subclinical infection [1]. We relied on sporadic independent serological surveys to guide our current understanding; these are few and far between [3]. Even these can be unreliable due to assay cross-reactivity with other pathogenic and non-pathogenic rickettsia, as well as with bacteria (e.g., *Proteus species*) [7]. This report is among the few current studies documenting the features of *R. australis* infection; however, it carries significant limitations due to its retrospective nature.

Although *R. australis* infection can occur throughout the year, in this study half of the cases of QTT occurred between April and July, during the seasons of autumn and winter in Australia. This finding appeared to contradict previous reports of increasing incidence of QTT during the summer and spring months [8]. Adult female *Ixodes* spp. ticks (vector for *R. australis*) are most abundant in Queensland from October to December [9]. The reasons for this are unclear, although factors influencing vector distribution and behavior such as rainfall and climate change may play a role.

When mapping out the geographical distribution of QTT among the 36 identified cases, the postcode of the site where the infection or tick bite was thought to have occurred was recorded. If this was not immediately apparent on chart review, the patient's place of residence was used as a surrogate. The major limitation to this approach was that the tick bite was often not acquired from home, and often results from occupational or recreational exposures were not always elicited on history. Nonetheless, infection occurred along eastern coastal Queensland and northern New South Wales with none reported more than 20 kilometers inland—a finding that is consistent with previous reports [2]. A focal hyperendemic area of QTT infection was identified spanning the Samford Valley, Woodford and Mount Nebo regions, accounting for 31% of cases. A further 8% of cases were located within a 5–10 kilometer distance from this area. This identifies an area where ecological conditions for *Ixodes holocyclus* and mammalian hosts are optimal, causing increased infection among susceptible humans [1]. Increasing urbanization of this area over the last few decades has been a major contributor to this phenomenon [1]. It is likely that this will be seen in multiple locations along coastal Australia as population densities change and encroach into new areas.

The mean age of infection was 39.5 years (median 36.1 years), although there was a wide range observed (3–72 years). Extremes of age did not appear to increase the risk of infection. The male-to-female ratio was 1:1.1, which are in contrast to previous reports that revealed a male predominance (2:1) [8]. This could represent a change in occupation and recreational activities among women over the past half century, which is known to highly influence the risk of infection. Given the large number of mammalian host species for *Ixodes* spp. ticks and its predilection for wet forested areas in certain times of the year, certain human activities are high risk for acquiring infection [8,10]. Nearly half of the study participants acquired their infection through occupational or recreational activities, which was consistent with previous studies [8]. No new high-risk human behaviors were identified.

Tick bite is still a useful guide for identifying those with possible QTT, with nearly half reporting this in their history. Exposure to vertebrate animal hosts may be of less utility in diagnosis; although, this aspect of the patient's history was frequently missed or poorly documented. Multiple tick bites were reported by a minority of patients, especially those living in tick-dense areas, and may be particularly important for identifying those at risk of severe disease and sepsis [1]. Many patients discharged from hospital were given advice to avoid ticks, although none had documented lifestyle changes on follow-up; moreover, no reinfections occurred. It is difficult to conclude any benefit from this advice.

5. Conclusions

Rickettsia australis and QTT is an evolving disease with a growing public health importance [1]. A lack of current epidemiological data on its incidence and distribution limits our understanding of the disease and options for beneficial public health interventions. This study has demonstrated the current epidemiology of this infection and has identified a new area of intense QTT endemicity in eastern coastal Queensland. SFG rickettsial infections should be notifiable diseases in Australia. Furthermore, prospective studies refining our understanding of the risk of infection and hospitalization of QTT need to be carried out. In addition, serological surveys of both animal hosts and humans would identify potential hot-spot areas of QTT to limit future disease.

Author Contributions: A.S. provided data, drafted and revised the manuscript. M.A. revised the manuscript and provided intellectual content. S.G. and K.H. provided clinical expertise and intellectual content. All authors have sighted and approved the final manuscript.

References

1. Derne, B.; Weinstein, P.; Musso, D.; Lau, C. Distribution of rickettsioses in Oceania: past patterns and implications for the future. *Acta Trop.* **2015**, *143*, 121–133. [CrossRef] [PubMed]
2. Australian Rickettsial Reference Laboratory. Disease Description and/or Epidemiology. 2015. Available online: http://www.rickettsialab.org.au/-!about (accessed on 22 July 2015).
3. NNDSS. Australia's Notifiable Disease Status: Annual Report of the National Notifiable Diseases Surveillance System. Department of Health and Ageing, 2013. Available online: http://www.commcarelink.health.gov.au/internet/main/publishing.nsf/Content/cda-pubs-annlrpt-nndssar.htm (accessed on 22 July 2015).
4. Faa, A.G.; Graves, S.R.; Stenos, J. A serological survey of rickettsial infections in the Gazelle Peninsula, East New Britain and a review of the literature. *PNG Med. J.* **2006**, *49*, 1–2.
5. Graves, S.; Stenos, J. Rickettsioses in Australia. In *Rickettsiology and Rickettsial Diseases*; Hechemy, K.E., Brouqui, P., Samuel, J.E., Raoult, D.A., Eds.; Wiley-Blackwell: Hoboken, NJ, USA, 2009; Volume 1166, pp. 151–155. [CrossRef] [PubMed]
6. Graves, S. Management of rickettsial diseases and Q Fever. *Med. Today* **2013**, *14*, 65–69.
7. Sexton, D.J.; Banks, J.; Graves, S.; Hughes, K.; Dwyer, B. Prevalence of antibodies to spotted fever group rickettsiae in dogs from south-eastern Australia. *Am. J. Trop. Reed. Hyg.* **1991**, *45*, 243–248.
8. Sexton, D.J.; Dwyer, B.; Kemp, R.; Graves, S. Spotted fever group rickettsial infections in Australia. *Rev. Infect. Dis.* **1991**, *13*, 876–886. [CrossRef] [PubMed]
9. Barker, S.C.; Walker, A.R. Ticks of Australia. The species that infect domestic animals and humans. *Zootaxa* **2014**, *3816*, 1–144. [CrossRef] [PubMed]
10. Derrick, E.H. The challenge of north Queensland fevers. *Australas. Ann. Med.* **1957**, *6*, 173 188. [PubMed]

4

The Development of a Mobile Application to Support Peripheral Health Workers to Diagnose and Treat People with Skin Diseases in Resource-Poor Settings

Liesbeth F. Mieras [1,*], Anna T. Taal [1], Erik B. Post [2], Alcino G. Z. Ndeve [3] and Colette L. M. van Hees [4]

1 Technical Department, Netherlands Leprosy Relief, 1090 HA Amsterdam, The Netherlands; A.Taal@Leprastichting.nl
2 Challenge TB, KNCV Tuberculosis Foundation, Jakarta 12870, Indonesia; Erik.Post@KNCVtbc.org
3 Technical Department, Netherlands Leprosy Relief, Maputo, Mozambique; AlcinoNdeve@nlrmoz.org
4 Department of Dermatology, Erasmus Medical Centre, 3000 CA Rotterdam, The Netherlands; C.vanHees@ErasmusMC.nl
* Correspondence: L.Mieras@Leprastichting.nl;

Abstract: The high prevalence of skin diseases in resource-poor settings, where health workers with sufficient knowledge of skin diseases are scarce, calls for innovative measures. Timely diagnosis and treatment of skin diseases, especially neglected tropical diseases (NTDs) that manifest with skin lesions, such as leprosy, is crucial to prevent disabilities as well as psychological and socioeconomic problems. Innovative technological methods like telemedicine and mobile health (mHealth) can help to bridge the gap between the burden of skin diseases and the lack of capable staff in resource-poor settings by bringing essential health services from central level closer to peripheral levels. Netherlands Leprosy Relief (NLR) has developed a mobile phone application called the 'SkinApp', which aims to support peripheral health workers to recognize the early signs and symptoms of skin diseases, including skin NTDs, and to start treatment promptly or refer for more advanced diagnostic testing or disease management when needed. Further research is needed to determine how greatly mHealth in general and the SkinApp in particular can contribute to improved health outcomes, efficiency, and cost-effectiveness.

Keywords: skin diseases; mobile phone application; NTDs; dermatology; mHealth; leprosy

---

1. Introduction

1.1. Short Communication

This article is written as a short communication, describing the ongoing development process of a mobile phone application that supports peripheral health workers in diagnosing and treating skin diseases in resource-poor settings.

1.2. Epidemiology of Skin Diseases in Low- and Middle-Income Countries

It is known that skin diseases are highly prevalent, particularly in resource-poor areas, where children are disproportionally affected—though there is a lack of systematically-collected data supporting this [1,2]. The epidemiology of skin diseases varies per country and within countries, but available data show that in rural areas, usually more than 50% and sometimes as much as 80% of the population has a skin condition; especially in areas endemic for conditions like scabies, onchocerciasis or tinea capitis [1]. The Global Burden of Disease (GBD) Study 2013 indicated that skin conditions were the fourth leading cause of disability worldwide [3].

Neglected topical diseases (NTDs) that manifest in skin lesions like leprosy and lymphatic filariasis (see Table 1) are among the skin diseases that often cause disabilities such as permanent wounds, contractures, and advanced lymphedema. Timely diagnosis and treatment can prevent permanent disabilities, but skin NTDs are usually not the most prevalent skin diseases, and are therefore more likely to be missed by health workers with limited or no dermatology training.

Skin conditions are usually not fatal, but it is important to recognize those that may be, such as blistering diseases. They can also be a sign of an underlying medical condition that might be life-threatening, such as HIV/AIDS. In view of the HIV/AIDS epidemic, the importance of dermatology cannot be underestimated, as 90% of HIV/AIDS patients develop a skin problem (see Table 1) during the course of their illness, and often initially present with a skin condition [4].

Table 1. Skin Diseases in The SkinApp. NTD: neglected tropical disease.

Common Skin Diseases	NTDs Manifesting in Skin Lesions	HIV-Related Skin Diseases	Others
Acne [1]	Buruli ulcer [1]	Angular cheilitis [1]	Albinism
Atopic eczema [1]	Cutaneous leishmaniasis [1]	Herpes simplex [1]	Blistering diseases
Contact eczema [1]	Leprosy [1]	Herpes zoster [1]	Creeping eruption
Impetigo [1]	Lymphatic filiariasis [1]	Kaposi sarcoma [1]	Vitiligo
Pityriasis versicolor [1]	Mycetoma	Molluscum contagiosum [1]	
Psoriasis	Onchocerciasis [1]	Oral candidiasis [1]	
Seborrhoeic eczema [1] (*)	Podoconiosis	Pruritic papular eruption [1]	
Tinea capitis [1]	Scabies [1]		
Tinea corporis [1] (*)	Yaws		

[1] Diseases included since the first version of the SkinApp. (*) also HIV-related.

1.3. *Psycological and Socioeconomic Burden*

Physical problems caused by skin conditions can lead to deterioration of the quality of life. Additionally, skin diseases often cause psychological problems such as anxiety, depression, and exclusion. A study in Colombia to determine the impact of skin diseases on the quality of life found that even the most localized or asymptomatic skin lesion leads to a disruption at some level of patient wellness [5]. The high visibility of skin diseases contributes to the likelihood of stigmatization, and may even result in unemployment [6]. Skin diseases can negatively impact productivity at school and work, while a considerable amount of household money has to be spent on treatment that is often ineffective due to insufficient availability of health workers with basic dermatology training at the peripheral level [7]. The economic impact of accessing care and rehabilitation services can be substantial, especially when the condition is chronic or leads to disabilities [8].

1.4. *Capacity Gap*

Studies have shown that a minimum of 10% of the consultations at peripheral healthcare level relates to common skin diseases [9,10]. Unfortunately, healthcare workers often lack the knowledge and skill to diagnose and treat skin diseases due to lack of training [7,9]. There is a need to bridge the gap between the prevalence of skin conditions at community level and the availability of capable staff in peripheral health facilities. An increased capacity to diagnose and treat skin diseases will contribute to the timely diagnosis and treatment of skin diseases in general, and skin NTDs in particular, and thus to the prevention of chronic conditions and disabilities.It will also contribute to timely and appropriate referral. Seth et al. call for increased efforts to address this problem, especially in low-resource settings, using recent innovations to help provide dermatological care to underserved regions in a cost-effective manner [11].

2. Mobile Health (mHealth)

2.1. Technologies to Support Dermatology Services

There are various innovative ways to enhance the quality of peripheral dermatology care. These include, but are not limited to, technological methods such as telemedicine, artificial intelligence, and mobile health (mHealth). In teledermatology, telecommunication technologies are used to exchange information regarding skin conditions over distances that a patient would otherwise have to travel [12]. The two main methods are: 'real-time' (synchronous) videoconferencing teledermatology, when the patient and dermatologist meet simultaneously in different locations; and 'store-and-forward' (asynchronous) teledermatology, in which images are transmitted electronically to a consulting dermatologist [13]. A significant limitation regarding teledermatology is the need for a dermatologist that can be consulted when required. Additional limitations for real-time teledermatology are the need for a stable internet connection and the costs for the necessary infrastructure.

Artificial intelligence can be used to make a computer-based algorithm that is able to make diagnostic decisions regarding skin conditions to a good degree of accuracy [12]. However, these techniques are still in development and only available for a limited number of skin diseases [14].

2.2. mHealth to Improve Peripheral Services forSkin Diseases

mHealth refers to the use of mobile communication devices to support health system needs. It can be made available by and for resource managers and health workers, as well as community members, patients, and their caregivers. It can also be used for management purposes, data collection and reporting, decision support, training, emergency referrals, alerts, and supervision [15,16]. In Labrique's paper on mHealth innovations as health system strengthening tools, the focus is on mHealth applications as point of care decision support for health workers to enhance their capability in diagnosing, treating, and referring people with skin diseases [16]. A systematic review on the feasibility and effective use of mHealth strategies by frontline health workers in developing countries concluded that these tools are potentially an effective means to promote the shifting of essential health services to lower cadres of health workers, but that a balance between the technical requirements and the cost of a system is a vital factor in the scalability of such solutions [17].

There are many mobile phone applications concerning skin diseases. As of August 2017, more than 520 dermatology-related mobile phone applications are available in the Google Play Store and the Apple App Store [18]. The majority of these applications are developed for clinical use such as teledermatology consultation, as self-surveillance and self-diagnosis aids, or as general dermatology references [18,19]. General dermatology reference applications range from an information source for patients to a comprehensive guide for health professionals [19]. Teledermatology is an effective method, as it provides consultations for health professionals in remote and resource-poor areas [20,21]. Some teledermatology applications cover a broad range of diseases, such as 'Dermassistance', which combines a mobile phone application with the use of teledermatology (https://www.dermassistance.es/). There is also a variety of disease-specific applications available. In the field of leprosy, for example, there is an initiative aimed at the early recognition of leprosy using image recognition through neural network technology by the Vellore Institute of Technology (http://preleprosy.com/), but this is still in development.

2.3. Development of NLR SkinApp

To increase the capability of peripheral health workers in resource-poor settings to diagnose and treat skin diseases and thus strengthen the health system, the Netherlands Leprosy Relief (NLR) developed an application suitable for Android and Apple devices. To our knowledge, no other similar mobile phone application is available. The aim was not only to support health workers to better serve a large proportion of their patients with common skin diseases, but also to enhance the detection and treatment of less common skin diseases, such as leprosy. Knowing that correct diagnosis and timely treatment help to prevent disabilities, the use of the SkinApp can contribute to reduced suffering caused by dermatological conditions.

The SkinApp uses an algorithm to support the process of diagnosis. It was inspired by the algorithm developed by Mahé for the management of common skin diseases at the primary healthcare level [22,23]. It contains descriptions of skin diseases, supporting photos, as well as treatment and referral advice. The selected skin diseases are a combination of commonly occurring skin diseases, skin diseases that may lead to mortality, HIV/AIDS related skin diseases [24,25], and NTDs manifesting in skin lesions prevalent in sub-Saharan African countries [8,26].

The development of the NLR SkinApp went through three stages: (1) a pilot project using a paper-based algorithm in Nigeria [23]; (2) a pilot of the first version of the mobile phone application in 2015 in Zambezia Province, Mozambique; and (3) an implementation project in Nampula Province, Mozambique, 2017–2018. During all three stages, several dermatology experts with experience in resource-poor areas generously contributed to the content, narrative, and imagery, and provided feedback.

The study in Nigeria was a prospective pilot study to assess the performance of first-line healthcare providers using a paper-based algorithm to support their diagnosis and treatment of seven skin diseases. In this study, 19 patent medicine vendors and 12 traditional healers assessed a total of 4147 patients with skin lesions, and their diagnoses and treatment choices were validated by two independent dermatologists. Overall, the first-line healthcare providers using the algorithm correctly diagnosed and treated or referred 82% of patients presenting with skin lesions. Adding pictorial images of signs and symptoms was believed to further improve the algorithm [23]. On the basis of these findings, it was decided to start the development of a mobile phone application.

In the first version of the SkinApp, which was tested in Zambezia Province, in Mozambique, 21 diseases were included in the algorithm: eight common skin diseases, six NTDs that manifest in skin lesions, and seven HIV/AIDS-related skin diseases (see Table 1). The pilot project was set up to determine the user-friendliness of the application and to identify points for improvement This was done by observing and interviewing SkinApp users through semi-structured interview guides and focus group discussions. The health workers—consisting of one physician, four medical technicians and five nurses—said that they used the application in cases where the diagnosis was clear but the treatment was unknown; whenever they were in doubt; to read through signs and symptoms from diseases in their differential diagnosis; and, when necessary, to go through the algorithm step by step to see if they could come to a diagnosis. They also used the app as a training tool, going through it in their free time. The main findings were that (1) smartphone ownership is very common among health workers in Zambezia; (2) the SkinApp was easy to use after a short introduction about its functionalities; (3) not all skin diseases in the application were relevant in the context of Zambezia Province (e.g., Buruli ulcer); (4) the treatment advice was clear, but not all treatment options were available at the peripheral level in Zambezia Province; (5) a teledermatology function would enhance the usefulness of the application.

Based on the results of the pilot and advancing insight, a second version of the SkinApp was developed. While the first version presented possible diagnoses with a description of signs, symptoms, and treatment advice, the second version aligned much better with the clinical validation of a patient with a skin disease. This was achieved by integrating an improved algorithm that starts with signs and symptoms and their location on a body map, and leads to the most likely diagnosis and treatment advice. In the second version, a number of diseases and supporting photos were added. A feedback button was inserted, which could be developed into a teledermatology function if required. The second version of the SkinApp was implemented in Nampula Province in 2017–2018. A WhatsApp group was formed for SkinApp users to meet the need for a teledermatology option. This enabled them to consult with an experienced Mozambican dermatologist, if needed, though an internet connection is required. Findings from the implementation project confirmed that the SkinApp is more easily accessible than literature and books, and that it is easy to operate. The narrative and illustrative content were considered clear. However, a glossary explaining dermatological terminology would help to improve intelligibility. Adding a reporting option was also mentioned as a possible improvement. These findings helped to further improve the user-friendliness of the SkinApp, but these pilots did not address the performance of the SkinApp as a diagnostic tool.

On the basis of the experiences with the SkinApp in Mozambique and the feedback received from involved dermatologists, a third version has since been developed. Its performance is currently being validated. The third version contains a total number of 29 skin diseases (see Table 1), an improved algorithm, a glossary with frequently-used terminology, and a section on treatment options for frequently-seen skin conditions (broken skin and dry skin).

The second version of the NLR SkinApp is currently available in English and Portuguese for mobile devices with Android as well as iOS operating systems through the Google Play Store (SkinApp) and the Apple App Store (as Skin_App) respectively, free of charge. Once downloaded, the SkinApp can be used offline.

The third version will be released once the current validation study is completed. The validation study is done in clinical settings under appropriate ethical and statistical guidelines. It encompasses concordance testing of the photos used in the application. The accuracy of the SkinApp will be assessed by comparing the diagnosis made by peripheral health workers using the SkinApp, to the diagnosis made by experienced dermatologists. Further evaluation of the use of the third version is planned for in several African countries. The capacity of the health workers to diagnose and treat skin diseases at baseline will be compared to their capacity two years after the introduction of the use of the SkinApp. Furthermore, a comparison will be made between the detection and treatment of skin diseases—specifically neglected tropical diseases—before and after the introduction of the SkinApp.

Once validated, the NLR SkinApp will be made available for use in other countries, where it can be modified to the context by changing the language, adapting the included skin diseases to those prevalent in the area, and using country-specific photos and treatment advices.

3. Discussion and Conclusions

Agarwal et al. conducted a systematic review entitled 'Evidence on feasibility and effective use of mHealth strategies by frontline health workers in developing countries' [17]. They found that mHealth strategies for peripheral health workers in low-resource countries are potentially an effective means to promote the shifting of essential health services to peripheral levels. What is not known about mHealth strategies is whether they contribute to improved health outcomes, efficiency, or cost-effectiveness. Additional research is needed to determine the added value of mHealth in general, and the SkinApp in particular.

One of the success factors for the adoption of mobile tools identified by Agarwal et al. was the involvement of the health workers throughout the development and implementation process [17]. The SkinApp has been developed in three stages, during which the input of peripheral health workers regarding the use of the SkinApp was obtained. Some of their requests have not yet been integrated into the newest version of the SkinApp, such as the desire for data collection and a teledermatology option. Once the third version of the SkinApp is validated, these functionalities could be added to the application. However, in order to maximize user-friendliness, the aim is to limit the size of the application in megabytes. Furthermore, options to send and receive information not only require an internet connection, but will also need a network of professionals to process the information received and prepare information to be sent. This will increase the cost of the necessary technical support as well as human resources, while a balance between technical requirements and the cost of the system is a vital factor in the scalability of such solutions [17]. The success of an mHealth intervention also depends on the existence of an mHealth platform to facilitate not only the adoption of the tool, but also to guarantee a sustained effective use.

There is a clear need to address the mismatch between the burden of skin diseases at the community level in resource-poor areas and the capability of peripheral health workers to diagnose, treat, and refer people with skin diseases, including skin NTDs. mHealth in general and the NLR SkinApp in particular can help to bridge this gap. The technical requirements and costs to ensure the sustainability of these innovative approaches are likely to increase, especially upon usage in different countries, which requires context-specific adaptation such as the use of the local language and alignment with the epidemiological situation. Therefore, more research is needed to gather evidence on the health outcomes and (cost-) effectiveness of mHealth for skin diseases, including skin NTDs, to ensure a wider use in support of peripheral health workers.

Author Contributions: Conceptualization: E.B.P., C.L.M.v.H, A.T.T., L.F.M.; investigation: A.G.Z.N.; project administration: E.B.P., A.G.Z.N., A.T.T, L.F.M.; writing—original draft: L.F.M.; writing—review and editing: E.B.P., C.L.M.v.H., A.T.T., L.F.M.

Acknowledgments: We are grateful for the valuable comments and suggestions from experienced dermatologists in various stages of development of the SkinApp: Ben Naafs, Koos Sanders, Claire Fuller, Tahir Dahiru and others, and we would like to thank the teams in Nigeria and Mozambique and Marloes Frijters for the fieldwork related to the development of the SkinApp.

References

1. Hay, R.; Fuller, L. The assessment of dermatological needs in resource-poor regions. *Int. J. Dermatol.* **2011**, *50*, 552–557. [CrossRef] [PubMed]
2. Vos, T.; Allen, C.; Arora, M.; Barber, R.; Bhutta, Z.; Brown, A.; Carter, A.; Casey, D.; Charlson, F.; Murray, C.; et al. Global, regional, and national incidence, prevalence, and years lived with disability for 310 diseases and injuries, 1990–2015: A systematic analysis for the Global Burden of Disease Study 2015. *Lancet* **2016**, *388*, 1545–1602. [CrossRef]
3. Hay, R.; Johns, N.; Williams, H.; Bolliger, I.; Dellavalle, R.; Margolis, D.; Marks, R.; Naldi, L.; Weinstock, M.; Wulf, S.; et al. The global burden of skin disease in 2010: An analysis of the prevalence and impact of skin conditions. *J. Investig. Dermatol.* **2014**, *134*, 1527–1534. [CrossRef] [PubMed]
4. Hu, J.; McKoy, K.; Papier, A.; Klaus, S.; Ryan, T.; Grossman, H.; Masenga, E.J.; Sethi, A.; Craft, N. Dermatology and HIV/AIDS in Africa. *J. Glob. Infect. Dis.* **2011**, *3*, 275–280. [PubMed]
5. Sanclemente, G.; Burgos, C.; Nova, J.; Hernández, F.; González, C.; Reyes, M.; Córdoba, N.; Arévalo, Á.; Meléndez, E.; Colmenares, J.; et al. The impact of skin diseases on quality of life: A multicenter study. *Actas Dermosifiliogr.* **2017**, *108*, 244–252. [CrossRef] [PubMed]
6. Barankin, B.; DeKoven, J. Psychosocial effect of common skin diseases. *Can. Fam. Physician* **2002**, *48*, 712–716. [PubMed]
7. Figueroa, J.; Fuller, L.; Abraha, A.; Hay, R. Dermatology in southwestern Ethiopia: Rationale for a community approach. *Int. J. Dermatol.* **1998**, *37*, 752–758. [CrossRef] [PubMed]
8. Mitjà, O.; Marks, M.; Bertran, L.; Kollie, K.; Argaw, D.; Fahal, A.; Fitzpatrick, C.; Fuller, L.; Garcia Izquierdo, B.; Hay, R.; et al. Integrated control and management of neglected tropical skin diseases. *PLoS Negl. Trop. Dis.* **2017**, *11*, e0005136. [CrossRef] [PubMed]
9. Mahe, A.; N'Diaye, H.; Bobin, P. The proportion of medical consultations motivated by skin diseases in the health centers of Bamako (Republic of Mali). *Int. J. Dermatol.* **1997**, *36*, 185–186. [CrossRef] [PubMed]
10. Odueko, O.M.; Onayemi, O.; Oyedeji, G.A. A prevalence survey of skin diseases in Nigerian children. *Niger. J. Med.* **2001**, *10*, 64–67. [PubMed]
11. Seth, D.; Cheldize, K.; Brown, D.; Freeman, E. Global burden of skin disease: Inequities and innovations. *Curr. Dermatol. Rep.* **2017**, *6*, 204–210. [CrossRef] [PubMed]

12. Surovi, N.A.; Kiber, A.; Kashem, A.; Babi, K.N. Study and Development of Algorithm of Different Skin Diseases Analysis Using Image Processing Method. Available online: http://www.alliedacademies.org/articles/study-and-development-of-algorithm-of-different-skin-diseases-analysis-using-image-processing-method.html (accessed on 26 June 2018).
13. Desai, B.; McKoy, K.; Kovarik, C. Overview of international teledermatology. *Pan Afr. Med. J.* **2010**, *6*, 3. [CrossRef] [PubMed]
14. Yadav, N.; Narang, V.; Shrivastava, U. Skin diseases detection models using image processing: A survey Utpal Shrivastava. *Int. J. Comput. Appl.* **2016**, *137*, 34–39.
15. WHO. Classification of Digital Health Interventions v1.0. World Health Organization. Available online: http://www.who.int/reproductivehealth/publications/mhealth/classification-digital-health-interventions/en/ (accessed on 26 June 2018).
16. Labrique, A.; Vasudevan, L.; Kochi, E.; Fabricant, R.; Mehl, G. mHealth innovations as health system strengthening tools: 12 common applications and a visual framework. *Glob. Health Sci. Pract.* **2013**, *1*, 160–171. [CrossRef] [PubMed]
17. Agarwal, S.; Perry, H.; Long, L.; Labrique, A. Evidence on feasibility and effective use of mHealth strategies by frontline health workers in developing countries: Systematic review. *Trop. Med. Int. Health* **2015**, *20*, 1003–1014. [CrossRef] [PubMed]
18. Flaten, H.K.; Claire, C.S.; Schlager, E.; Dunnick, C.A.; Dellavalle, R.P. Growth of mobile applications in dermatology 2017 update. *Dermatol. Online J.* **2018**, *24*, 13.
19. Brewer, A.C.; Endly, D.C.; Henley, J.; Amir, M.; Sampson, B.P.; Moreau, J.F.; Dellavalle, R.P. Mobile applications in dermatology. *JAMA Dermatol.* **2013**, *149*, 1300–1304. [CrossRef] [PubMed]
20. Lipoff, J.B.; Cobos, G.; Kaddu, S.; Kovarik, C.L. The Africa Teledermatology Project: A retrospective case review of 1229 consultations from sub-Saharan Africa. *J. Am. Acad. Dermatol.* **2015**, *72*, 1084–1085. [CrossRef] [PubMed]
21. Nguyen, A.; Tran, D.; Uemura, M.; Bardin, R.L.; Shitabata, P.K. Practical and sustainable teledermatology and teledermatopathology: Specialty care in Cameroon Africa. *J. Clin. Aesthet. Dermatol.* **2017**, *10*, 47–56. [PubMed]
22. Mahe, A.; Faye, O.; N'Diaye, H.T.; Ly, F.; Konare, H.; Keita, S.; Traore, A.K.; Hay, R. Definition of an algorithm for the management of common skin diseases at primary health care level in sub-Saharan Africa. *Trans. Soc. Trop. Med. Hyg.* **2005**, *99*, 39–47. [CrossRef] [PubMed]
23. Taal, A.; Hussaini, T.; Gayus, B.; Dahiru, T.; Post, E. First-line health care provider performance in the management of common skin diseases using an algorithmic approach as a diagnostic tool in Kano State, Nigeria. *Res. Rep. Trop. Med.* **2015**, *6*, 85–94. [CrossRef]
24. Van Hees, C.; Naafs, B. *Common Skin Diseases in Africa, an Illustrated Guide*, 3rd ed.; Stichting Troderma: Voorburg, The Netherlands, 2014.
25. Kousa, M.; Sanders, C. HIV Related Skin Diseases and Sexually Transmitted Infections. Available online: https://www.ntvg.nl/artikelen/hiv-related-skin-diseases-and-sexually-transmitted-infections-africa/volledig (accessed on 29 June 2018).
26. WHO. Neglected Tropical Diseases. Available online: http://www.who.int/neglected_diseases/en/ (accessed on 16 July 2018).

5

Evaluation of Rapid Extraction Methods Coupled with a Recombinase Polymerase Amplification Assay for Point-of-Need Diagnosis of Post-Kala-Azar Dermal Leishmaniasis

Rajashree Chowdhury [1,†], Prakash Ghosh [1,*,†], Md. Anik Ashfaq Khan [1], Faria Hossain [1], Khaledul Faisal [1], Rupen Nath [1], James Baker [1], Ahmed Abd El Wahed [2], Shomik Maruf [1,3], Proggananda Nath [4], Debashis Ghosh [1], Md. Masud-Ur-Rashid [5], Md. Utba Bin Rashid [1], Malcolm S. Duthie [6] and Dinesh Mondal [1]

1 Nutrition and Clinical Service Division (NCSD), International Centre for Diarrhoeal Disease Research, Bangladesh, (icddr,b), Dhaka 1212, Bangladesh; r.chowdhury@icddrb.org (R.C.); anik.khan@icddrb.org (M.A.A.K.); faria.hossain@icddrb.org (F.H.); khaledul.faisal@icddrb.org (K.F.); rupen.nath@icddrb.org (R.N.); james.baker@icddrb.org (J.B.); shomik.maruf@icddrb.org (S.M.); debashis@icddrb.org (D.G.); utbabinrashid@icddrb.org (M.U.B.R.); din63d@icddrb.org (D.M.)

2 Institute of Animal Hygiene and Veterinary Public Health, University of Leipzig, D-04103 Leipzig, Germany; abdelwahed@gwdg.de

3 London School of Hygiene and Tropical Medicine, University of London, London WC1E 7HT, UK

4 Infection and Tropical Medicine, Mymensingh Medical College and Hospital (MMCH), Mymensingh 2200, Bangladesh; progganath@yahoo.com

5 Department of Cardiovascular and Thoracic Surgery, National Heart Foundation Hospital and Research Institute, Dhaka 1216, Bangladesh; mrashid1580@gmail.com

6 Host Directed Therapeutics (HDT) Bio Corp, Seattle, WA 98102, USA; malcolm.duthie@hdtbiocorp.com

* Correspondence: prakash.ghosh@icddrb.org;

† These authors contributed equally to this work.

Abstract: To detect Post-kala-azar leishmaniasis (PKDL) cases, several molecular methods with promising diagnostic efficacy have been developed that involve complicated and expensive DNA extraction methods, thus limiting their application in resource-poor settings. As an alternative, we evaluated two rapid DNA extraction methods and determined their impact on the detection of the parasite DNA using our newly developed recombinase polymerase amplification (RPA) assay. Skin samples were collected from suspected PKDL cases following their diagnosis through national guidelines. The extracted DNA from three skin biopsy samples using three different extraction methods was subjected to RPA and qPCR. The qPCR and RPA assays exhibited highest sensitivities when reference DNA extraction method using Qiagen (Q) kit was followed. In contrast, the sensitivity of the RPA assay dropped to 76.7% and 63.3%, respectively, when the boil & spin (B&S) and SpeedXtract (SE) rapid extraction methods were performed. Despite this compromised sensitivity, the B&S-RPA technique yielded an excellent agreement with both Q-qPCR (k = 0.828) and Q-RPA (k = 0.831) techniques. As expected, the reference DNA extraction method was found to be superior in terms of diagnostic efficacy. Finally, to apply the rapid DNA extraction methods in resource-constrained settings, further methodological refinement is warranted to improve DNA yield and purity through rigorous experiments.

Keywords: post-kala-azar dermal leishmaniasis (PKDL); point-of-need diagnosis; DNA extraction; recombinase polymerase amplification (RPA); real-time PCR

1. Introduction

Post kala-azar dermal leishmaniasis (PKDL) is a sequelae of *Leishmania donovani* infection that mostly affects individuals after successful treatment for visceral leishmaniasis (VL) [1]. PKDL usually manifests as macules (hypopigmented patches), papules, and nodules, or a combination of the three, known as polymorphic skin lesions, mainly on the face, trunk, legs, arms, and genitals [2,3]. For unknown reasons, the incidence of PKDL cases with different types of lesions varies across *L. donovani* endemic regions [2]. In Sudan, 50–60% of treated VL patients develop PKDL within six months, whereas in the Indian subcontinent, PKDL is reported to develop in 5–10% of VL patients within two to four years after treatment [3–5]. Surprisingly, the incidence rate of PKDL increases two fold within five years of completion of VL treatment [6]. In addition, 15–20% of PKDL cases present without a documented history of VL, suggesting that these individuals may have had a prior subclinical *L. donovani* infection that was not detected [4]. PKDL, unlike VL, is not life threatening if it remains untreated, but PKDL patients often unfortunately experience stigma within their society [7,8]. Of further concern, the Leishmania parasites harbored within skin lesions of PKDL patients serve as the known reservoir of VL, and this plays a pivotal role in their interepidemic transmission through sandfly bites, particularly in the Indian subcontinent [9–11]. This vector-borne parasitic disease is anthroponotic in the Indian subcontinent, whereas animal reservoirs are responsible for disease transmission in particular endemic regions [12,13].

Kala-azar elimination programme (KEP) activities in the Indian subcontinent (ISC) have contributed to a remarkable decline in the incidence of kala-azar in recent years, and the KEP is now considered to be in the consolidation phase. However, PKDL is identified as a potential threat to the sustained success of the programme and its ultimate goal of kala azar elimination. Proper diagnosis and management of PKDL has consequently been set as an essential component of the KEP [14,15]. The control programme is facing challenges regarding early diagnosis and treatment of PKDL, however, because of its symptomatic resemblance to other skin diseases such as leprosy, vitiligo, secondary syphilis, and sarcoidosis, and the lack of sensitive field-friendly diagnostic methods [16,17]. The lack of awareness and poor treatment-seeking behavior of PKDL patients further complicate control activities [18,19].

Currently, diagnosis of PKDL relies on clinical assessments with support from parasitological approaches [2]. Direct demonstration of *Leishmania* amastigotes in either slit skin or skin biopsy smear provides 60–100% sensitivity in nodular lesions, but has poor sensitivity in macular lesions (7–50%) [20–22]. Furthermore, several antibody-based serological methods such as direct agglutination test, enzyme linked immunosorbent assay, and rK39-based rapid diagnostic tests (RDT) have been considered as ancillary diagnostic tests for PKDL diagnosis, because all of the treated VL patients give a positive result for antibody-based methods, even after being cured [16,23]. In contrast, molecular methods can detect *L. donovani* DNA, and several conventional as well as real time PCR assays have been developed with high sensitivities and specificities for laboratory diagnosis of both VL and PKDL [20,24]. These methods can help confirm the diagnosis of PKDL in 40–94% of clinically suspected individuals [4,25], and we previously developed a promising real time PCR assay for the diagnosis of PKDL that provided excellent sensitivity (91.2%) for macular PKDL cases in endemic regions of Bangladesh [20]. The application of qPCR in resource-limited settings, including primary and secondary health-care facilities, is challenging because it requires a well-equipped laboratory, trained personnel, and reliable storage conditions for the reagents. Therefore, the need for a user-friendly, design-locked, and field-feasible diagnostic method for PKDL detection remains. In this regard, the recombinase polymerase amplification (RPA) assay has recently emerged as a novel alternative isothermal amplification technology for the detection of nucleic acid [26,27] with the potential to overcome the limitations of poor-resourced settings. RPA provides results faster than conventional and even real time-PCR, despite amplifying nucleic acid at a constant temperature (42 °C), and requiring less expensive and simpler equipment [26]. Due to the many advantages of the RPA assay, we developed an RPA assay for detection of *Leishmania donovani* (LD) parasites that showed absolute sensitivity and specificity in correspondence with real-time PCR [28]. Furthermore, our newly devised RPA assay can detect both *L. donovani* and *L. infantum*. Eventually, this assay might have broader implications in endemic regions where the disease is both zoonotic and anthroponotic.

In addition to the detection method, an important parameter for the optimum sensitivity of molecular diagnostic approaches is the extraction of high-quality genomic DNA extraction from clinical specimens. Generally, the spin-column-based extraction method produces pure DNA, but requires use of high-speed multiple centrifugation with enhanced washing steps, which is costly and usually not feasible in field settings. On the other hand, the SpeedXtract (SE) method that has been incorporated with the RPA assay in several studies involves a magnetic bead-based lysis protocol to avoid the creation of aerosols and the use of a high-speed centrifuge. The SE method has not, however, been evaluated using skin samples. Alternatively, we found a relatively simple DNA extraction method based on an in-house lysis buffer to be suitable for loop-mediated isothermal assays [29,30]. This rapid boil & spin (B&S) DNA extraction method does not require multiple washing steps with commercial buffers; however, an end-stage centrifugation step is needed to separate DNA containing aqueous layer from the pellet with cellular debris. In an effort to develop a field-friendly diagnostic algorithm for detecting *L. donovani* DNA in skin samples from PKDL patients, we therefore assessed various nucleic acid extraction techniques in combination with an RPA assay.

2. Materials and Methods

2.1. Study Sites and Participants

The study entailed both field and laboratory activities. Field activities were performed at Surja Kanta Kala-azar Research Centre (SKKRC), Mymensingh, Bangladesh, a region highly endemic for VL, and laboratory activities at Emerging Infections and Parasitology, icddr,b, Dhaka, following the approval of the International Centre for Diarrhoeal Disease Research, Bangladesh (icddr,b) Institutional Review Board (IRB) (PR-17041). In total, thirty treatment-seeking, suspected PKDL cases residing in the endemic zone were enrolled at the Surya kanta kala-azar research centre (SKKRC), the only specialized hospital for treatment of VL, PKDL, and their associated complications. The majority of the recruited PKDL patient had a history of VL and all exhibited characteristic skin rashes. All PKDL patients were positive in rk39 RDT and were diagnosed based on clinical characteristics by the hospital physician. Following initial examination, each patient was invited to participate in the study, and written informed consent was obtained from either the participant or the legal guardian of children participants before samples were collected. Following standard procedures, the study physician collected three 3 mm skin biopsy samples from each participant. Each biopsy was preserved in NET buffer for subsequent DNA extraction. All PKDL patients were referred for treatment following national guidelines, and each was found to be responsive to treatment. To determine the specificity of our investigative assays, thirty DNA samples were extracted from buffy coat of cured VL patients and were also subjected to laboratory analyses.

2.2. DNA Extraction from Clinical Specimen

DNA was isolated following three DNA extraction methods:

Spin column-based method: This reference method was involved DNA extraction using a QIAamp DNA tissue & blood mini kit (Cat no #69506, Qiagen, Hilden, Germany) according to the manufacturer's protocol with a minor modification: skin biopsy materials were kept at 37 °C overnight after addition of ATL buffer and protease K. The following day, the material was homogenized then incubated at 56 °C for two hours before purification.

SpeedXtract Extraction (SE) method: A simple and rapid blood lysis protocol (SpeedXtract, Qiagen, Hilden, Germany) was modified to suit DNA extraction from skin as follows: 100 µL of Buffer SL and 30 µL of Suspension A (Cat no # 703060, SpeedXtract, Qiagen, Lake Constance, Germany) was added with 3 mm skin punch biopsy in a 2 mL tube and was mixed thoroughly by vortexing for

10 s. Thereafter, the mix was incubated at 95 °C for 10 min and after incubation, the skin biopsy was pressed with grinding pestle and mixed by vortexing. The mix was incubated at 95 °C for another 10 min, then the tube was transferred to a magnetic stand and incubated at room temperature for 1 min. Finally, the supernatant was carefully transferred to a new tube.

Boil & spin (B&S) method: Skin biopsy materials were kept in 37 °C overnight after addition of an in-house-prepared simple lysis buffer (400 mM NaCl, 40 mM Tris pH 6.5, 0.4% SDS) [28] following addition of protease K (Qiagen, Hilden, Germany). The following day, the skin materials were homogenized, then incubated at 70 °C for 15 min. After incubation, the mixture was vortexed, spun, and incubated for 5 min at 95 °C before centrifugation for 3 min at 10,000× *g*. After centrifugation, 30 µL of clear supernatant was transferred to a dilution tube containing 345 µL of PCR-grade water.

2.3. DNA Purity and Concentration

To assess the purity of each extracted DNA sample, OD values at 260 nm and 280 nm were measured by a Thermo Scientific Nanodrop™ 2000 Spectrophotometer (Thermo Scientific, Hilden, Germany) and the ratio calculated (the standard ratio for purified DNA ranges between 1.8 and 2.0). Subsequently, DNA concentration/quantity was determined from the OD value at 260 nm following the standard method [31].

2.4. Molecular Detection of LD-DNA

Recombinase polymerase amplification (RPA) assay: The RPA assay was performed with the extracted DNA samples following the previously published method [28]. In brief, the assay was performed in a 50 µL volume using a TwistAmp exo kit (Product code#TAEXO02KIT, TwistAmp exo kits, TwistDx, Cambridge, UK). Master mix was prepared in a tube with 420 nM of RPA primer, 120 nM of RPA Probe, and 1× rehydration buffer, and was added to the RPA lyophilized pellet. Then, 14 mM Mg acetate was pipetted into the tube lids. Subsequently, template DNA was added to the tubes, and the tube was closed and mixed well. The tubes were immediately placed into the tubescanner (Twista, TwistDx, Cambridge, UK) and incubated for 15 min at 42 °C. The emitted fluorescence signals were measured at 20 s intervals. A combined threshold and first derivative analysis were used for signal interpretation. The total reaction time for RPA was approximately 20 min.

Real time PCR: Real time PCR was performed by a previously published method [32]. Briefly, Taqman primers and probes were designed targeting conserved region of Leishmania REPL repeats (L42486.1) specific for *L. donovani* and *L. infantum* and synthesized by Applied Biosystems [32]. Briefly, a 20 µL reaction mix was prepared, containing 5 µL template, 10 µL of TaqMan® Gene Expression Master Mix (2X), 1 µL preordered primer–probe mix, and PCR grade water. Amplification was performed on a Bio-Rad CFX96 iCycler system with following reaction conditions: 10 min at 95 °C, followed by 45 cycles of 15 s at 95 °C and 1 min at 60 °C. Samples with cycle threshold (Ct) > 40 were considered negative. The total reaction time for real time PCR was approximately 120 min.

2.5. Reagent Cost and Time Analysis

The reagent costs associated with this study were assessed similarly to previous studies [33–35]. We estimated the cost of each qPCR or RPA reaction including DNA extraction for each individual sample, where only the operational costs of supplies, kit, and reagents were considered. Costs for infrastructure, labor, training, and supervision were not included in the calculation. The time required for each assay was estimated through inclusion of sample processing time prior to each respective DNA extraction method and detection time associated with either qPCR or RPA.

2.6. Statistical Analysis

Parametric and nonparametric tests were performed based on the distribution of data. Kappa and McNemar's test were performed to determine the concordance and discordance among the three extraction methods in combination with the RPA assay. Standard statistical formulas were followed to determine the sensitivity and specificity of the test with 95% CI. Furthermore, receiver operating characteristic (ROC) curve analysis was performed to determine the accuracy of each of the extraction method when coupled with RPA/qPCR assay. All statistical analyses were performed using SPSS (Version 20.0) and GraphPad Prism (Version 8.1.2). p value < 0.05 was considered as statistically significant.

2.7. Ethics

This study was approved by the International Centre for Diarrhoeal Disease Research, Bangladesh (icddr,b) Institutional Review Board (IRB) and ethical review committee (ERC), research protocol number PR-17041. Informed written consent was collected from each participant or the legal guardian in the case of children.

3. Results

3.1. Participants' Indices

Among the 30 clinically confirmed PKDL cases recruited, 60% were male, and the mean age of the participants was 26.47 ± 12.41 years. Previous history of VL was reported in 93.3% of the PKDL patients, and 23.3% were relapse cases (Table 1). The clinical examination confirmed 22 (73.3%) as macular cases, whereas the remaining cases presented with either nodular (6.7%) or mixed (20%) lesions.

Table 1. Clinical and demographic parameters of the Post-kala-azar leishmaniasis (PKDL) patients enrolled in the study (n = 30).

Variable		Value
Male, n (%)		18/30 (60%)
Age in years, mean ± SD		26.47 ± 12.41
Children (<17 years), n (%)		9/30 (30%)
Adults (>17 years), n (%)		21/30 (70%)
Past history of VL, n (%)		28/30 (93.3%)
Past history of PKDL, n (%)		7/30 (23.3%)
Type of Rash, n (%)	Macular	22/30 (73.3%)
	Nodular	2/30 (6.7%)
	Mixed	6/30 (20%)

3.2. Extraction Method-Based Performance of RPA/qPCR Assay

The qPCR assay detected 26 out of 30 clinically confirmed PKDL patients with a sensitivity of 86.67%, when DNA was extracted with the spin column (Qiagen) method. Likewise, the RPA assay showed elevated performance with a sensitivity of 93.33% when the same DNA extraction method was followed. On the other hand, when the B&S (23/30) and SE (19/30) methods were performed (Figure 1), the RPA assay showed compromised diagnostic efficacy, with a sensitivities of 76.7% and 63.3%, respectively (Table 2). As expected, Q-RPA (20/22) and Q-qPCR (18/22) exhibited a considerably higher positive rate (90.9% and 81.8%) than B&S-RPA and SE-RPA (69.6% and 59.1%) among the macular PKDL cases. In addition, all nodular and mixed cases were detected by both Q-RPA and Q-qPCR, whereas one nodular case was not detected by B&S-RPA, and two mixed cases remained undetected by the SE-RPA assay. Both qPCR and RPA assays showed absolute specificity for all of the extraction methods.

Table 2. Analysis of the performance of three DNA extraction methods with qPCR and recombinase polymerase amplification (RPA) assay.

DNA Extraction Methods	Mean DNA conc. (ng/µL) [95% CI] N = 30	Mean OD 260/280 ratio [95% CI] N = 30	Sensitivity of qPCR [95% CI] (Pos/Neg)	Sensitivity of RPA [95% CI] (Pos/Neg)	Specificity of Q-qPCR and RPA [95% CI] (Pos/Neg)	App. Time (per Sample)		App. Cost (in US$ per Sample)	
						qPCR	RPA	qPCR	RPA
Spin-column method (Qiagen)	21.6 ± 10.4 [17.71–25.49]	1.85 ± 0.09 [1.81–1.88]	86.67% [69.28–96.24%] (26/4)	93.33% [77.93–99.18%] (28/2)		17 h [30]	15 h [20] min [26]	16.5 [27]	7.5 [26,33]
Boil & Spin (B&S)	22.9 ± 9.3 [19.47–26.44]	0.91 ± 0.11 [0.87-0.95]	N/A	76.67% [57.72–90.07%] (23/7)	100.00% [88.43–100.00%] (0/30)	15 h [27,30]	13 h [27]	14.0 [31]	5.0 [31]
SpeedXtract (SE)	140.7 ± 50.5 [121.89–159.63]	0.77 ± 0.22 [0.68–0.85]	N/A	63.33% [43.86–80.07%] (19/11)		2 h 20 min [26]	40 min [26]	15.5 [33]	6.5 [26,33]

The ROC analysis showed the superior diagnostic accuracy of Q-RPA, as presented by the highest value of area under the curve (AUC) (AUC = 0.967). As the least efficacious technique, SE-RPA gave the lowest AUC value (AUC = 0.817) (Figure 2C). Notwithstanding the poor performance, B&S-RPA presented an excellent agreement with both the Q-qPCR (k = 0.828) and Q-RPA (k = 0.831) techniques, whereas SE-RPA showed good agreement with the Q-qPCR (k = 0.755), Q-RPA (k = 0.692), and B&S-RPA (k = 0.635) assay (Table 3) techniques. Furthermore, SE-RPA showed significant discordance with both Q-qPCR (p = 0.02) and Q-RPA (p = 0.004) (Table 3). Overall, among the 30 clinically diagnosed PKDL cases, 16 cases were found to be pan-positive and two cases were pan-negative.

Table 3. Agreement between different DNA extraction methods coupled with the RPA assay and spin-column-based (Qiagen) DNA extraction method together with qPCR assay.

Methods Comparison	Kappa (k)	Agreement	McNemar (p Value)
Q-RPA vs. B&S-RPA	0.831	Excellent	0.06
Q-RPA vs. SE-RPA	0.692	Good	0.004
B&S-RPA vs. SE-RPA	0.635	Good	0.34
Q-RPA vs. Q-qPCR	0.933	Excellent	0.50
B&S-RPA vs. Q-qPCR	0.828	Excellent	0.38
SE-RPA vs. Q-qPCR	0.755	Good	0.02

3.3. *Efficiency of DNA Extraction Methods*

The DNA concentration was highest for the SpeedXtract method, with an average concentration of 140.7 ± 50.5 ng/µL compared to the Qiagen (21.6 ± 10.4 ng/µL) and boil & spin (22.9 ± 9.3 ng/µL) methods (Table 2). However, the spin-column-based extraction method (Qiagen) gave the most purified DNA with a mean OD 260/280 ratio of 1.85 ± 0.09, while the SE extraction method gave the least purified DNA with a mean OD 260/280 ratio of 0.77 ± 0.22 (Table 2). To be noted, a significant difference was found between RPA positive and negative samples regarding the DNA concentration ($p < 0.001$) and purity ($p < 0.0001$) for the B&S method, which was not observed for the two other methods (Figure 2A,B).

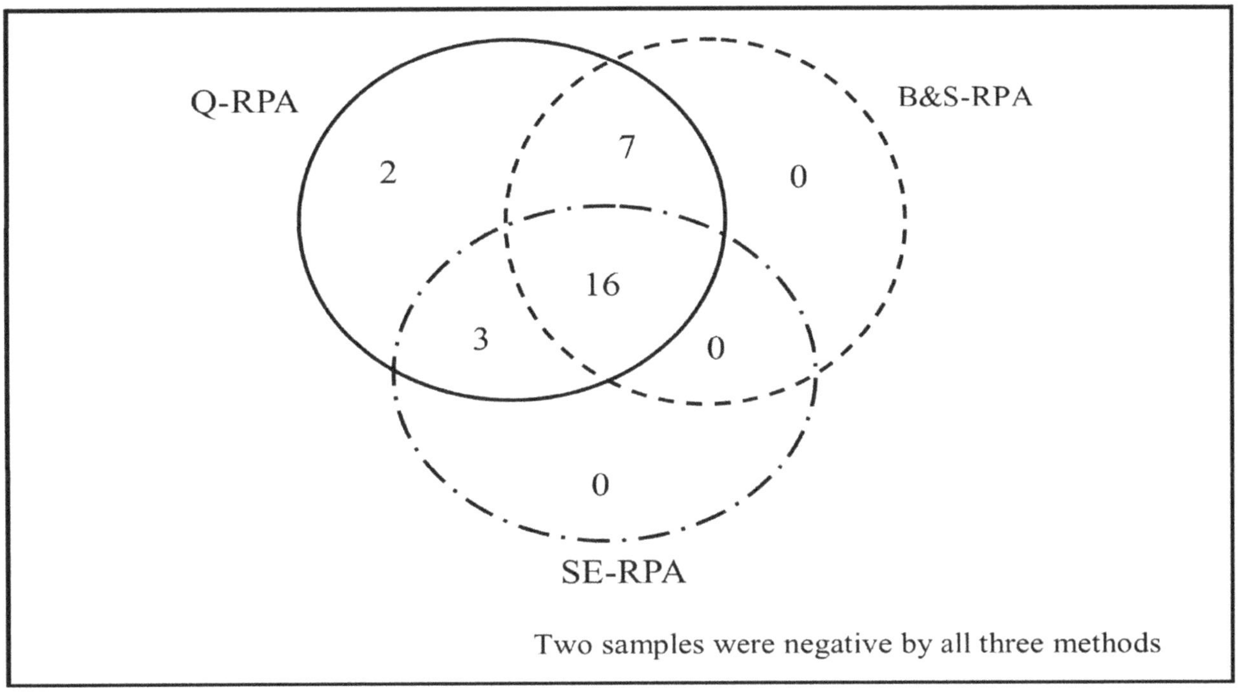

Figure 1. Venn diagram depicting the distribution of Post-kala-azar leishmaniasis detected through Q-RPA, B&S-RPA, and SE-RPA. Among 30 skin biopsy samples from PKDL patients, 28 were positive for *L. donovani* by Q-RPA, whereas 23 and 19 samples were positive by B&S-RPA and SE-RPA, respectively.

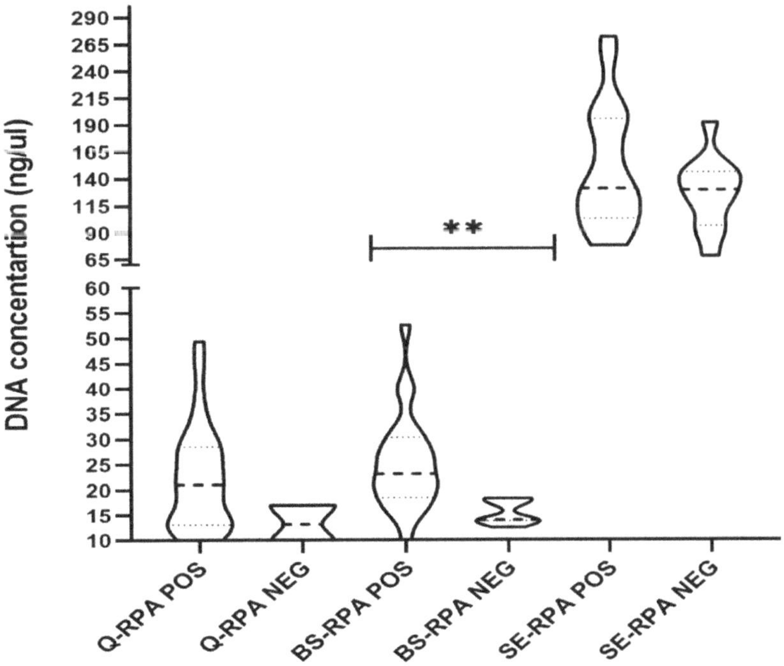

(**A**)

Figure 2. *Cont.*

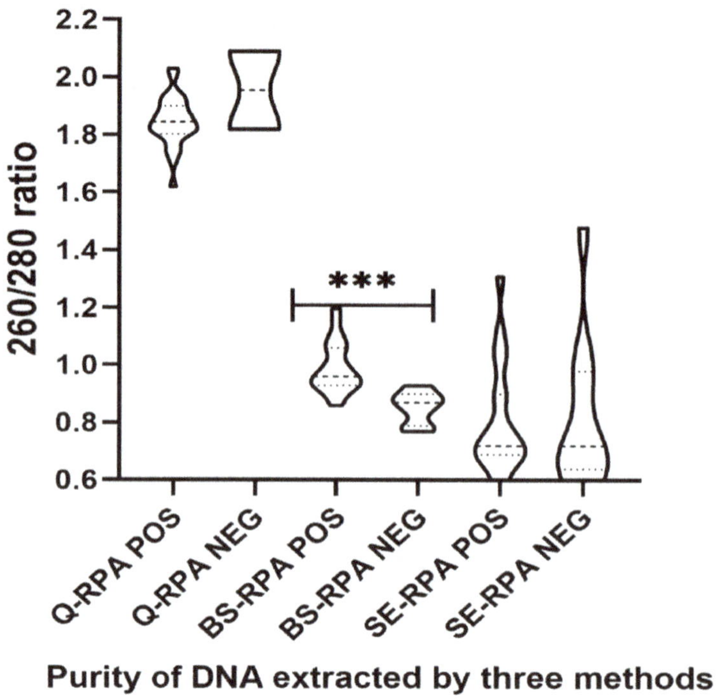

(B)

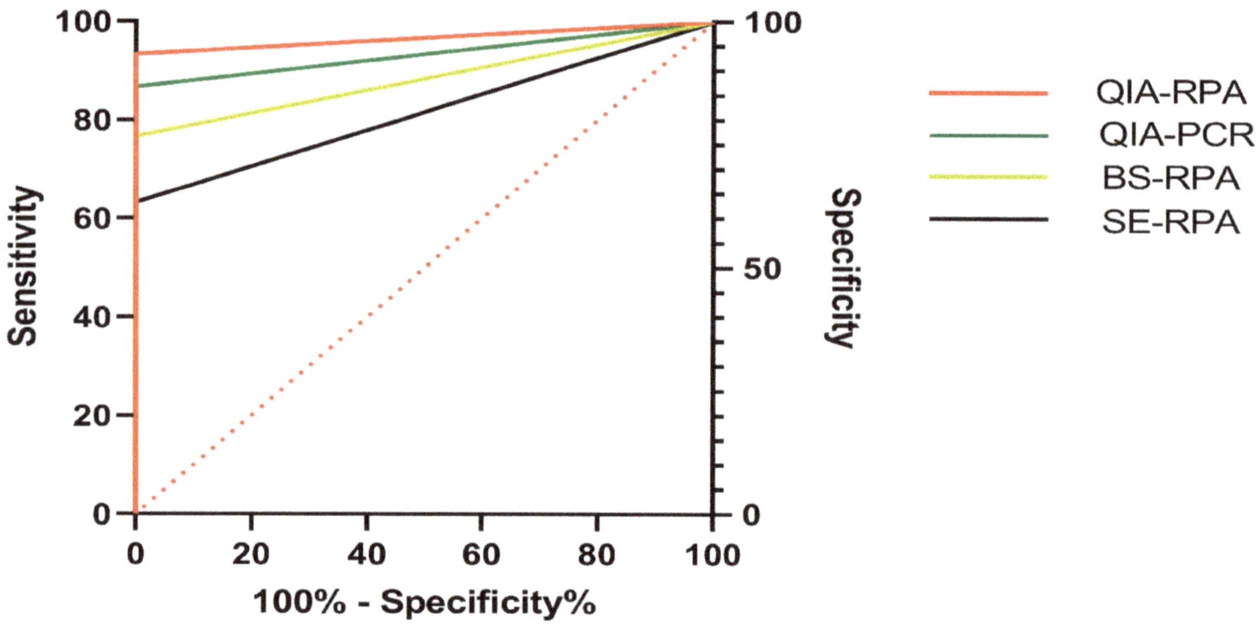

(C)

Figure 2. Illustration of the performance of three DNA extraction methods coupled with the RPA assay. In (**A**), the graph presents the concentration of DNA by the spin column (Qiagen), boil & spin, and SpeedXtract extraction methods, ** $p < 0.001$. In (**B**), the purity of DNA through the spin column (Qiagen), boil & spin, and SpeedXtract extraction methods is shown, *** $p < 0.0001$. In (**C**), the receiver operating characteristic (ROC) curve shows the diagnostic accuracy of the qPCR and RPA assays coupled with the spin-column-based (Qiagen), boil & spin, and SpeedXtract extraction methods for the detection of *Leishmania* parasites in skin biopsy samples.

3.4. Comparison of Assay Time and Cost-Effectiveness

The cost and time estimation analysis showed that the cost and time required for the spin-column-based (Qiagen) DNA extraction method coupled with the qPCR assay were approximately US$16.5 and 17 h, respectively, for each sample, whereas the RPA assay has a lower cost per sample of US$7.5 and requires less performance time (15 h 20 min). We found the B&S-RPA assay to be the least expensive (US$5) assay, and the SE-RPA assay was less time-consuming (40 min) compared to Q-RPA (15 h 20 min) and B&S-RPA (13 h).

4. Discussion

Tremendous declines in the incidence/rate of VL and its mortality due to the initiatives of KEP indicate substantial advancement towards the elimination of kala-azar from the ISC, including Bangladesh. The regional VL initiative is actively pursuing elimination targets by 2020, and Bangladesh has already succeeded in reaching the targets in over 90% of its endemic subdistricts [36–38]. Following the success of the attack phase, the KEP has moved to the consolidation phase with the aim of identifying and controlling potential sources of *L. donovani* infection in endemic areas. Our recent studies have demonstrated that, in addition to VL patients, PKDL cases can competently transmit the parasites to generate new VL cases [10]. PKDL cases are now considered as important reservoirs for parasites and are deemed to be key contributors to interepidemic disease transmission. Therefore, early diagnosis and treatment of PKDL should be prioritized as additional means to control the transmission of *Leishmania* parasites and to ensure elimination is sustained. In a recent review, Zijlstra et al. suggested that validation and implementation of diagnostic methods, including qPCR or isothermal amplification techniques, are essential for diagnosis of PKDL to sustain the success of VL elimination efforts in the ISC [11]. In addition to clinical parameters, qPCR is considered to be the most promising method for diagnosis and assessments of cure [19,23]. The RPA assay has, however, shown comparable diagnostic efficacy to qPCR, while surpassing PCR-based molecular methods with a multitude of practical and technological advantages [28]. A simple and inexpensive method of DNA extraction would make the RPA assay even more feasible and sustainable in poorly resourced settings. We therefore evaluated three DNA extraction methods together with the RPA assay and compared to the reference DNA extraction method (Qiagen) coupled with the qPCR assay to determine if we could generate a field-friendly and cost-effective diagnostic method for diagnosis of PKDL.

Our data indicate that, relative to other extraction methods, considerably higher detection rates are achieved by the RPA (93.3%) and qPCR (86.7%) assays when DNA extraction was performed with the spin-column-based method. We found similar sensitivity (83.4–96.1%) for qPCR in our previous study where only macular cases with low parasite burden were included [19]. In the current study, all nodular and mixed PKDL cases were positive in both RPA and qPCR, a result that is consistent with their higher parasite abundance [15]. These data clearly indicate the promising diagnostic efficacy of Q-RPA assay in detecting Leishmania parasites in skin biopsies from PKDL patients. However, the sensitivity of the RPA assay was compromised when rapid DNA extraction methods such as boil & spin (B&S) and SpeedXtract (SE) were used. Although several studies have reported excellent performance of isothermal amplification-based assays such as LAMP and RPA assays conducted on nucleic acid extracted from whole blood samples by boil & spin and SpeedXtract methods [28–30], our finding is similar to that of an earlier study performed in Sri Lanka on CL patients that reported 65.5% sensitivity of SE-RPA [39].

The comparatively lower sensitivity of boil & spin and SpeedXtract DNA extraction methods in the RPA assay might be attributed to the inherent limitations of these techniques. Notably, the absence of washing steps and deproteination agent, such as proteinase K (SpeedXtract), leads to poor quality DNA with impurities that may inhibit the activity of recombinase and polymerase enzymes in the RPA assay [40]. In addition, the 2.5-fold lower A260/A280 ratio in SE method provides another empirical demonstration of the underperformance of the RPA assay due to the protein impurities in the DNA. Moreover, we noted that skin samples were only partially digested at the end of the recommended ten minutes in the SE method (notably, the digestion time for two other methods was longer). Surprisingly, we found a significant difference in A260/A280 ratio ($p < 0.0001$) of DNA being extracted by the boil & spin method between RPA positive and negative samples, suggesting promise for this extraction method by increasing the DNA yield. Considering the cost and time for each of the assays, we estimated that the B&S-RPA assay is 3-fold less expensive (at ~US$5 per sample) than Q-qPCR (at ~US$16.5 per sample). On the other hand, SE-RPA assay was far less time-consuming and can produce results significantly faster (within 40 min) than the other combinations. Last but not least, the B&S-RPA assay showed excellent agreement with the Q-RPA and Q-qPCR assays, and the SE-RPA assay presented good agreement with the Q-qPCR, Q-RPA, and B&S-RPA assays (Table 3), further indicating the promise of the B&S-RPA and SE-RPA assays in detecting LD in clinical samples.

The major limitation of this study is that we performed RPA and qPCR assays with DNA extracted by three different DNA extraction methods using different skin biopsies. This might have generated some variance, and an over- or underestimation of the performance of any of the methods, as the parasites are not evenly distributed in the lesions of PKDL patients [5]. The skin biopsy procedure is invasive and requires surgical set-up, which limits the ability to collect multiple biopsies without negatively impacting patient participation and use as an active field-based case detection method. Several recent studies have indicated the satisfactory diagnostic efficacies of the less invasive slit skin, microbiopsy, and fine needle biopsy methods [21,41,42]. Further evidence is required, however, before these invasive sample collection procedures can be applied for diagnosis of PKDL. Another limitation to our study is that, due to ethical issues, we used buffy coat samples from cured VL patients instead of the skin biopsy samples to determine assay specificity. Our previous study provided a basis for the use of blood samples for evaluating the specificity of an index method in PKDL diagnostic studies [19].

Considering the diagnostic performance, operational cost, and feasibility, our data indicate that a spin-column-based (Qiagen) DNA extraction method coupled with the RPA assay can be routinely performed as an alternative to qPCR for diagnosis of PKDL cases. Moreover, this method has the potential to be used for diagnosis of canine leishmaniasis, which implicates the broader application of this rapid molecular technique. In addition, we recommend a refined B&S method as an alternative method to the reference DNA extraction method. Further modification of the SpeedXtract method to achieve better sensitivity could generate a SE-RPA assay that could be used as a point-of-contact tool for rapid diagnosis of PKDL. Further large-scale studies are both warranted and required to generate a Q-RPA assay that can be used for the molecular diagnosis of leishmaniasis involving dermatological complications.

5. Conclusions

The findings of this study demonstrate the superior diagnostic performance of reference DNA extraction method (Qiagen) over the boil & spin (B&S) and SpeedXtract (SE) methods in detecting LD DNA through RPA assay from skin biopsy of PKDL patients. We recommend a spin-column-based (Qiagen) DNA extraction method coupled with the RPA assay as a surrogate mode of diagnosis of PKDL that can be routinely performed as an alternative of qPCR. We believe our findings, and the recommendations we make from them, could help policy-makers adopt a cost-effective diagnostic method for PKDL that could be implemented in resource-limited settings to help the KEP sustain their successes. Further, considering the promises of this assay, clinical studies are imperative for the detection of visceral leishmaniasis both in human and animal reservoirs.

Author Contributions: P.G., D.M., P.N., M.S.D. and A.A.E.W. conceived and designed the study. P.G., R.C., F.H., M.A.A.K., K.F., S.M., D.G., J.B., M.M.-U.-R., M.U.B.R. and R.N. performed the experiments and maintained the data source. PG, RC and M.AA.K. performed the statistical analysis. R.C. and PG drafted the manuscript. P.G., D.M., M.S.D. and A.A.E.W. revised the manuscript. All authors have read and agreed to the published version of the manuscript.

Acknowledgments: We are grateful to all of the participants for their valuable participation in this study. The authors are grateful to core donors which provide unrestricted support to icddr,b. Current donors include the Government of the People's Republic of Bangladesh; Global Affairs Canada GAC), Canada; Swedish International Development Cooperation Agency (Sida); and the Department for International Development (UKAid). Prakash Ghosh was supported as a Clinical Research and Development Fellow (CRDF) by UNICEF/UNDP/World Bank/WHO Special Programme for Research and Training in Tropical Diseases (TDR) during the study period.

References

1. Verma, S.; Bhandari, V.; Avishek, K.; Ramesh, V.; Salotra, P. Reliable diagnosis of post-kala-azar dermal leishmaniasis (PKDL) using slit aspirate specimen to avoid invasive sampling procedures. *Trop. Med. Int. Heal.* **2012**, *18*, 268–275. [CrossRef]
2. Mondal, D.; Khan, G.M. Recent advances in post-kala-azar dermal leishmaniasis. *Curr. Opin. Infect. Dis.* **2011**, *24*, 418–422. [CrossRef]
3. Zijlstra, E.; Musa, A.; Khalil, E.; El Hassan, I.; El-Hassan, A. Post-kala-azar dermal leishmaniasis. *Lancet Infect. Dis.* **2003**, *3*, 87–98. [CrossRef]
4. Rahman, K.M.; Islam, S.; Rahman, M.W.; Kenah, E.; Galive, C.M.; Zahid, M.M.; Maguire, J.; Rahman, M.; Haque, R.; Luby, S.; et al. Increasing Incidence of Post–Kala-Azar Dermal Leishmaniasis in a Population-Based Study in Bangladesh. *Clin. Infect. Dis.* **2010**, *50*, 73–76. [CrossRef] [PubMed]
5. Ganguly, S.; Saha, P.; Chatterjee, M.; Roy, S.; Ghosh, T.K.; Guha, S.K.; Kundu, P.K.; Bera, D.K.; Basu, N.; Maji, A.K. PKDL—A Silent Parasite Pool for Transmission of Leishmaniasis in Kala-azar Endemic Areas of Malda District, West Bengal, India. *PLoS Neglected Trop. Dis.* **2015**, *9*, e0004138. [CrossRef]
6. Islam, S.; Kenah, E.; Bhuiyan, M.U.; Rahman, K.M.; Goodhew, B.; Ghalib, C.M.; Zahid, M.M.; Ozaki, M.; Rahman, M.W.; Haque, R.; et al. Clinical and Immunological Aspects of Post–Kala-Azar Dermal Leishmaniasis in Bangladesh. *Am. J. Trop. Med. Hyg.* **2013**, *89*, 345–353. [CrossRef]
7. Mondal, D.; Hasnain, M.G.; Hossain, M.S.; Ghosh, D.; Ghosh, P.; Hossain, H.; Baker, J.; Nath, R.; Haque, R.; Matlashewski, G.; et al. Study on the safety and efficacy of miltefosine for the treatment of children and adolescents with post-kala-azar dermal leishmaniasis in Bangladesh, and an association of serum vitamin E and exposure to arsenic with post-kala-azar dermal leishmaniasis: An open clinical trial and case–control study protocol. *BMJ Open* **2016**, *6*, e010050. [CrossRef]
8. Garapati, P.; Pal, B.; Siddiqui, N.A.; Bimal, S.; Das, P.; Murti, K.; Pandey, K. Knowledge, stigma, health seeking behaviour and its determinants among patients with post kalaazar dermal leishmaniasis, Bihar, India. *PLoS ONE* **2018**, *13*, e0203407. [CrossRef]
9. Molina, R.; Ghosh, D.; Carrillo, E.; Monnerat, S.; Bern, C.; Mondal, D.; Alvar, J. Infectivity of Post-Kala-azar Dermal Leishmaniasis Patients to Sand Flies: Revisiting a Proof of Concept in the Context of the Kala-azar Elimination Program in the Indian Subcontinent. *Clin. Infect. Dis.* **2017**, *65*, 150–153. [CrossRef]
10. Mondal, D.; Bern, C.; Ghosh, D.; Rashid, M.; Molina, R.; Chowdhury, R.; Nath, R.; Ghosh, P.; Chapman, L.A.C.; Alim, A.; et al. Quantifying the Infectiousness of Post-Kala-Azar Dermal Leishmaniasis Toward Sand Flies. *Clin. Infect. Dis.* **2019**, *69*, 251–258. [CrossRef]
11. Zijlstra, E.E.; Alves, F.; Rijal, S.; Arana, B.; Alvar, J. Post-kala-azar dermal leishmaniasis in the Indian subcontinent: A threat to the South-East Asia Region Kala-azar Elimination Programme. *PLoS Neglected Trop. Dis.* **2017**, *11*, e0005877. [CrossRef]
12. Hirve, S.; Boelaert, M.; Matlashewski, G.; Mondal, D.; Arana, B.; Kroeger, A.; Olliaro, P. Transmission Dynamics of Visceral Leishmaniasis in the Indian Subcontinent—A Systematic Literature Review. *PLoS Neglected Trop. Dis.* **2016**, *10*, e0004896. [CrossRef]
13. Alemayehu, B. Leishmaniasis: A Review on Parasite, Vector and Reservoir Host. *Heal. Sci. J.* **2017**, *11*, 1. [CrossRef]
14. WHO. *Regional Strategic Framework for Elimination of Kala-Azar from the South-East Asia Region (2011–2015)*; WHO Regional Office for South-East Asia: New Delhi, India, 2012; p. 24.
15. Moulik, S.; Chaudhuri, S.J.; Sardar, B.; Ghosh, M.; Saha, B.; Das, N.K.; Chatterjee, M. Monitoring of Parasite Kinetics in Indian Post–Kala-azar Dermal Leishmaniasis. *Clin. Infect. Dis.* **2017**, *66*, 404–410. [CrossRef]

16. Salotra, P.; Kaushal, H.; Ramesh, V. *Containing Post Kala-Azar Dermal Leishmaniasis (PKDL): Pre-requisite for Sustainable Elimination of Visceral Leishmaniasis (VL) from South Asia. Kala Azar in South Asia*; Springer: Cham, Switzerland, 2016; pp. 7–22.
17. Adams, E.R.; Versteeg, I.; Leeflang, M. Systematic Review into Diagnostics for Post-Kala-Azar Dermal Leishmaniasis (PKDL). *J. Trop. Med.* **2013**, *2013*, 1–8. [CrossRef]
18. Huda, M.M.; Hirve, S.; Siddiqui, N.A.; Malaviya, P.; Banjara, M.R.; Das, P.; Kansal, S.; Gurung, C.K.; Naznin, E.; Rijal, S.; et al. Active case detection in national visceral leishmaniasis elimination programs in Bangladesh, India, and Nepal: Feasibility, performance and costs. *BMC Public Heal.* **2012**, *12*, 1001. [CrossRef]
19. Basher, A.; Nath, P.; Nabi, S.G.; Selim, S.; Rahman, F.; Sutradhar, S.R.; Faiz, A.; Bhuiyan, M.R.; Ahmed, B.-N.; Rahman, R. A Study on Health Seeking Behaviors of Patients of Post-Kala-Azar Dermal Leishmaniasis. *BioMed Res. Int.* **2015**, *2015*, 1–8. [CrossRef]
20. Ghosh, P.; Hasnain, G.; Hossain, F.; Khan, A.A.; Chowdhury, R.; Faisal, K.; Mural, M.A.; Baker, J.; Nath, R.; Ghosh, D.; et al. Evaluation of Real-time PCR for Diagnosis of Post-Kala-azar Dermal Leishmaniasis in Endemic Foci of Bangladesh. *Open Forum Infect. Dis.* **2018**, *5*, ofy234. [CrossRef]
21. Salotra, P.; Singh, R. Challenges in the diagnosis of post kala-azar dermal leishmaniasis. *Indian J. Med Res.* **2006**, *123*, 295.
22. Verma, N.; Singh, D.; Pandey, K.; Das, V.N.R.; Lal, C.S.; Verma, R.B.; Sinha, P.K.; Das, P. Comparative Evaluation of PCR and Imprint Smear Microscopy Analyses of Skin Biopsy Specimens in Diagnosis of Macular, Papular, and Mixed Papulo-Nodular Lesions of Post-Kala-Azar Dermal Leishmaniasis. *J. Clin. Microbiol.* **2013**, *51*, 4217–4219. [CrossRef]
23. Chappuis, F.; Rijal, S.; Soto, A.; Menten, J.; Boelaert, M. A meta-analysis of the diagnostic performance of the direct agglutination test and rK39 dipstick for visceral leishmaniasis. *BMJ* **2006**, *333*, 723. [CrossRef]
24. Hossain, F.; Ghosh, P.; Khan, A.A.; Duthie, M.S.; Vallur, A.C.; Picone, A.; Howard, R.F.; Reed, S.G.; Mondal, D. Real-time PCR in detection and quantitation of Leishmania donovani for the diagnosis of Visceral Leishmaniasis patients and the monitoring of their response to treatment. *PLoS ONE* **2017**, *12*, e0185606. [CrossRef]
25. Srivastava, P.; Mehrotra, S.; Tiwary, P.; Chakravarty, J.; Sundar, S. Diagnosis of Indian Visceral Leishmaniasis by Nucleic Acid Detection Using PCR. *PLoS ONE* **2011**, *6*, e19304. [CrossRef] [PubMed]
26. Faye, O.; Faye, O.; Soropogui, B.; Patel, P.; El Wahed, A.A.; Loucoubar, C.; Fall, G.; Kiory, D.; Magassouba, N.; Keita, S.; et al. Development and deployment of a rapid recombinase polymerase amplification Ebola virus detection assay in Guinea in 2015. *Eurosurveillance* **2015**, *20*, 30053. [CrossRef] [PubMed]
27. Piepenburg, O.; Williams, C.H.; Stemple, D.L.; Armes, N.A. DNA Detection Using Recombination Proteins. *PLoS Boil.* **2006**, *4*, e204. [CrossRef] [PubMed]
28. Mondal, D.; Ghosh, P.; Khan, A.A.; Hossain, F.; Böhlken-Fascher, S.; Matlashewski, G.; Kroeger, A.; Olliaro, P.; El Wahed, A.A. Mobile suitcase laboratory for rapid detection of Leishmania donovani using recombinase polymerase amplification assay. *Parasites Vectors* **2016**, *9*, 281. [CrossRef]
29. Mukhtar, M.; Ali, S.S.; Boshara, S.A.; Albertini, A.; Monnerat, S.; Bessell, P.; Mori, Y.; Kubota, Y.; Ndung'U, J.M.; Cruz, I. Sensitive and less invasive confirmatory diagnosis of visceral leishmaniasis in Sudan using loop-mediated isothermal amplification (LAMP). *PLoS Neglected Trop. Dis.* **2018**, *12*, e0006264. [CrossRef]
30. Hopkins, H.; González, I.J.; Polley, S.D.; Angutoko, P.; Ategeka, J.; Asiimwe, C.; Agaba, B.; Kyabayinze, D.J.; Sutherland, C.J.; Perkins, M.D.; et al. Highly sensitive detection of malaria parasitemia in a malaria-endemic setting: Performance of a new loop-mediated isothermal amplification kit in a remote clinic in Uganda. *J. Infect. Dis.* **2013**, *208*, 645–652. [CrossRef]
31. Desjardins, P.; Conklin, D. NanoDrop Microvolume Quantitation of Nucleic Acids. *J. Vis. Exp.* **2010**, *45*, 2565. [CrossRef]
32. Vallur, A.C.; Duthie, M.S.; Reinhart, C.; Tutterrow, Y.; Hamano, S.; Bhaskar, K.; Coler, R.N.; Mondal, D.; Reed, S.G. Biomarkers for intracellular pathogens: Establishing tools as vaccine and therapeutic endpoints for visceral leishmaniasis. *Clin. Microbiol. Infect.* **2013**, *20*, O374–O383. [CrossRef]
33. Burke, R.; McKenna, J.; Cox, C.; Coyle, P.V.; Shields, M.D.; Fairley, D. A comparison of different pre-lysis methods and extraction kits for recovery of Streptococcus agalacticae (Lancefield group B Streptococcus) DNA from whole blood. *J. Microbiol. Methods* **2016**, *129*, 103–108. [CrossRef]
34. De Assis, T.S.M.; Azeredo-Da-Silva, A.L.F.; Werneck, G.L.; Rabello, A. Cost-effectiveness analysis of diagnostic tests for human visceral leishmaniasis in Brazil. *Trans. R. Soc. Trop. Med. Hyg.* **2016**, *110*, 464–471. [CrossRef]

35. Xing, W.; Yu, X.; Feng, J.; Sun, K.; Fu, W.; Wang, Y.; Zou, M.; Xia, W.; Luo, Z.; He, H.; et al. Field evaluation of a recombinase polymerase amplification assay for the diagnosis of Schistosoma japonicum infection in Hunan province of China. *BMC Infect. Dis.* **2017**, *17*, 164. [CrossRef]
36. Sundar, S.; Singh, O.P.; Chakravarty, J. Visceral leishmaniasis elimination targets in India, strategies for preventing resurgence. *Expert Rev. Anti-infective Ther.* **2018**, *16*, 805–812. [CrossRef] [PubMed]
37. Singh, O.P.; Hasker, E.; Boelaert, M.; Sundar, S. Elimination of visceral leishmaniasis on the Indian subcontinent. *Lancet Infect. Dis.* **2016**, *16*, e304–e309. [CrossRef]
38. Hirve, S.; Kroeger, A.; Matlashewski, G.; Mondal, D.; Banjara, M.R.; Das, P.; Be-Nazir, A.; Arana, B.; Olliaro, P. Towards elimination of visceral leishmaniasis in the Indian subcontinent—Translating research to practice to public health. *PLoS Neglected Trop. Dis.* **2017**, *11*, e0005889. [CrossRef] [PubMed]
39. Gunaratna, G.; Manamperi, A.; Böhlken-Fascher, S.; Wickremasinghe, R.; Gunawardena, K.; Yapa, B.; Pathirana, N.; Pathirana, H.; De Silva, N.R.; Sooriyaarachchi, M.; et al. Evaluation of rapid extraction and isothermal amplification techniques for the detection of Leishmania donovani DNA from skin lesions of suspected cases at the point of need in Sri Lanka. *Parasites Vectors* **2018**, *11*, 665. [CrossRef]
40. Daher, R.K.; Stewart, G.; Boissinot, M.; Bergeron, M.G. Recombinase Polymerase Amplification for Diagnostic Applications. *Clin. Chem.* **2016**, *62*, 947–958. [CrossRef] [PubMed]
41. Kirstein, O.D.; Abbasi, I.; Horwitz, B.Z.; Skrip, L.; Hailu, A.; Jaffe, C.; Lin, L.L.; Prow, T.W.; Warburg, A. Minimally invasive microbiopsies: A novel sampling method for identifying asymptomatic, potentially infectious carriers of Leishmania donovani. *Int. J. Parasitol.* **2017**, *47*, 609–616. [CrossRef]
42. Bandyopadhyay, A.; Majumdar, K.; Gangopadhyay, M.; Koley, S. Fine-needle sampling provides appreciable diagnostic yield in lesions of post kala azar dermal leishmaniasis: Analysis of four cases from North Eastern India. *Diagn. Cytopathol.* **2013**, *42*, 525–529. [CrossRef]

6

A Teledermatology Pilot Programme for the Management of Skin Diseases in Primary Health Care Centres: Experiences from a Resource-Limited Country

Ousmane Faye [1,*], Cheick Oumar Bagayoko [2], Adama Dicko [1], Lamissa Cissé [1], Siritio Berthé [1], Bekaye Traoré [1], Youssouf Fofana [1], Mahamoudan Niang [2], Seydou Tidiane Traoré [2], Yamoussa Karabinta [1], Mamadou Gassama [1], Binta Guindo [1], Alimata Keita [1], Koreissi Tall [1], Somita Keita [1], Antoine Geissbuhler [4], Antoine Mahé [3] and Teledermali Team [†]

1 Department of Dermatology, Faculty of Medicine and Odontostomatology, Bamako, Mali; adadicko@yahoo.fr (A.D.); lamissa05@gmail.com (L.C.); siritio_b@yahoo.fr (S.B.); b_traore@ymail.com (B.T.); youssouffofana346@yahoo.fr (Y.F.); ykarabinta@yahoo.com (Y.K.); gasdiaby@yahoo.fr (M.G.); binta.guindo@yahoo.fr (B.G.); alimatakeita@yahoo.fr (A.K.); koreissit@yahoo.fr (K.T.); somitak@yahoo.fr (S.K.)

2 CERTES, Bamako, Mali; cob281@yahoo.fr (C.O.B.); mniang@certesmali.org (M.N.); trawore@keneya.net (S.T.T.)

3 Service de Dermatologie, Hôpital Pasteur, Colmar 68000, France; antoine.mahe@ch-colmar.fr

4 Département de Radiologie et Informatique médicale, Université de Genève, Genaven 1211, Switzerland; antoine.Geissbuhler@hcuge.ch

* Correspondence: faye_o@yahoo.fr;

† Teledermali Team: Samba Ba, Dokala Diarra, Aoua Togora, Issa Koné, Modibo Traoré, Aissata Diallo, Chaka Koné, Drissa Traoré, Diakalia Berthé, Ousmane Cissé, Boubacar Sidiki Nanacassé, Abdoul Karim Doumbia, Sidi Niaré, Mamady Yattara, Bakary Traoré, Moussa Traoré.

Abstract: In sub-Saharan Africa, in particular in rural areas, patients have limited access to doctors with specialist skills in skin diseases. To address this issue, a teledermatology pilot programme focused on primary health centres was set up in Mali. This study was aimed at investigating the feasibility of this programme and its impact on the management of skin diseases. The programme was based on the store-and-forward model. Health care providers from 10 primary centres were trained to manage common skin diseases, to capture images of skin lesions, and to use an e-platform to post all cases beyond their expertise for dermatologists in order to obtain diagnosis and treatment recommendations. After training, the cases of 180 patients were posted by trained health workers on the platform. Ninety-six per cent of these patients were properly managed via the responses given by dermatologists. The mean time to receive the expert's response was 32 h (range: 13 min to 20 days). Analysis of all diseases diagnosed via the platform revealed a wide range of skin disorders. Our initiative hugely improved the management of all skin diseases in the targeted health centres. In developing countries, Internet accessibility and connection quality represent the main challenges when conducting teledermatology programmes.

Keywords: teledermatology; Africa; primary health care; skin diseases; tele-expertise

---

1. Introduction

To date, there is a general agreement that skin diseases (SDs) should be considered a public issue, in particular in developing countries [1] where their management is subject to several challenges.

Prevalence studies from different continents have pointed to a high prevalence of SDs, especially in children, at an average of 30% (range 6 to 87%) [2–10]. While SDs are the fourth leading cause of consultations in health centres [11,12], patients have limited access to skin doctors with specialist skills in skin disease; these generally prefer to settle in big cities. In Africa, the situation is critical; the ratio of dermatologists to the population is extremely low, and ranges from 1 for every 500,000 to 1 million inhabitants. Mali, a country of 17 million inhabitants, had only 10 dermatologists in 2015; all were posted in the capital city. The pressure for skin care is mainly borne by front-line health facilities, and most of those personnel are swamped with other health priority programmes (immunization, malaria, tuberculosis, HIV, etc.). The capacity of such agents to manage common SDs and leprosy has been questioned [13]. The overall context of care provision in developing countries represents an additional challenge. Warm climate and overcrowded settings are likely to foster the skin infections that represent almost 70% of the skin disorders that motivate consultations [14]. Hitherto, there are no international guidelines or treatment recommendations, with the exception of leprosy, a disease that has been eliminated in most endemic countries. A previous study [15] identified the effectiveness of one-day training to improve the management of common SDs in primary health care centres. The issue remains as to how the remaining cases that need the expertise of a specialist dermatologist can be managed. The recent boom of information and communication technologies (ICTs) and their use in medicine, particularly dermatology (teledermatology), have transformed the way in which skin disorders can be properly managed in remote areas. By the year 2013, more than 560 papers were published on this subject [16] and 2000 patients were evaluated, with good kappa concordance test values ranging from 0.63 to 0.95 [17–21]. This growing awareness for teledermatology prompted us to take advantage of this technology to improve skin care in Mali through a pilot programme.

The aim of this study was to test the feasibility and the impact of a teledermatology programme on the management of skin diseases, at primary health care level.

2. Methods

2.1. Ethical Statements

The study protocol was approved by the Institutional Review Board of the National Ethical Committee for Health and Life Sciences of Mali (*Comité National d'éthique pour la santé et les sciences de la vie, CNESS*). Prior to the study, informed consent was obtained from adult participants andfrom the parents or legal guardians of minors after detailed explanation of the study protocol. In accordance with the ethical review committee requirements, patient information was made confidential. Our intervention was only focused on the health system and the management of patient care so that this could be improved in Mali. There was no new drug tested nor blood test performed in the study.

2.2. Health Care System in Mali

In Mali, as in many African countries, the health care system in the public sector comprises three levels of care. The first level, also called primary health care level, comprises community health centres (*centre de santé communautaire*) and district referral health care centres (*centre de santé de référence*) where the first-level administration (district) is sited. Regional hospitals and regional health administrations represent the second health care level (region). The capital city hosts the third health care level, represented by teaching hospitals and the national health administration, where the national health policy is elaborated. In 2015, the country had 5 teaching hospitals, 8 regional hospitals covering 10 health regions, 63 district referral centres, and 1215 community health centres. The present study was focused on this last group, the primary health care centres that represent the entry point to the health system where health care is delivered by general physicians, nurses, and in a few cases, minimally trained health care workers (HCWs).

2.3. Study Design, Sites, and Duration

From July 2015 to February 2017, we carried out a pilot teledermatology programme based on the store-and-forward (SAF) model, focused on front-line health care delivery services. Of the 10 health regions in Mali, we selected three regions for the purpose (Koulikoro, Sikasso, and Mopti); the rest were excluded for either security reasons or the close presence of a dermatologist. In each health region, selected three health districts were also selected: the administrative centre of the health region plus two or three more health districts randomly selected thereafter, depending on the size of the region (Figure 1). Overall, 9 health districts were involved in the study planned to last for 18 months: 6 months for pre and post programme evaluation and training, and 12 months for utilization of the system.

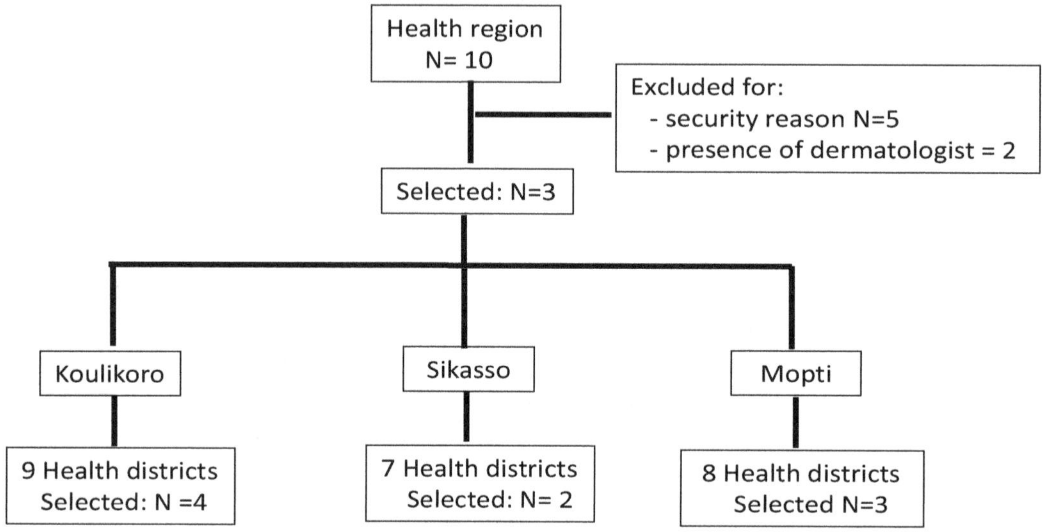

Figure 1. Flow chart of the selection of study sites: health region and districts.

2.4. Intervention—Equipment and Participants

The first step of our intervention was training. In each health centre, two health care workers were invited to participate in the training session which was held in the main dermatological ward, at the Marchoux Institute in the capital city Bamako where expert dermatologists were posted. During three consecutive days, the selected HCWs were respectively given information on the algorithmic approach for the management of common skin diseases identified in the pilot project [15], the use of a digital camera, and computer skills including type writing, the use of Internet (email), and the tele-expertise platform named '*Bogou*' [22] (that means mutual assistance or help in all situations in the Djerma and Songhoï languages spoken in Mali, Niger, and Cameroon). This e-platform is a web-based application with secured access through a personal login and password [23]. It was developed with Java to run on several operating systems and work reliably with unstable and low-bandwidth connections. All data in *Bogou* are encrypted using a public and private key system [23]. Dermatological training was focused on common SDs, i.e pyoderma, superficial mycoses including tinea capitis, scabies, and conditions with pale patches inclusive of leprosy; attendees were encouraged to refer via the platform all skin disorders assessed as being beyond their competency and any case that did not fit with the algorithm. Theoretical training was also completed with clinical case studies and practical exercises. At the end of the training session, participants were issued with a booklet addressing the management of common SDs as cited above, a digital camera, and a kit for Internet connection including a 3G key USB.

2.5. Teledermatology Operating Procedures

In practice, when encountering a case that needed a consultation with a dermatologist, the health agent captures one or more pictures with a digital camera, logs on to a computer, uploads the images from the camera, connects to the platform, and uploads the pictures with a short medical history of the patient. The dermatologist (expert) immediately receives an email alert indicating an assignment for a case for diagnosis that has been sent. The expert also will log onto the platform, analyse the images, and send back concise details on the disorders and treatment recommendations. At any time, all participating HCWs could access pictures and responses. Importantly, the workload involved in responding to the HCWs relied mainly on one individual (OF) backed by a second in case the first one was not available; only one response to each request was given. The validity of all diagnoses and management strategies given was checked by another dermatologist based in France, who had expertise in tropical dermatology (AM). Clinical supervision was performed quarterly by a team (dermatologist and computer scientists) to confirm difficult diagnoses through skin biopsy and to solve technical issues.

2.6. Evaluation

We planned to evaluate the feasibility of the study and its impact on the management of common SD. While implementing and performing the programme, all relevant issues and challenges were recorded. The following indicators were also evaluated: total number of store-and-forward teledermatology consults via the *Bogou* platform, the number of cases that received a clear diagnosis and treatment, the turnaround time to receive the response from experts, the pattern of SDs referred to experts, the diagnosis concordance between experts, and the proportion and pattern of SDs as seen by HCWs before and after intervention. All SDs diagnosed via teledermatology were also compared to those seen in a dermatological setting where experts were working over the same period of time. Patient and care provider feedback was also assessed to measure the level of satisfaction and acceptance of the system.

2.7. Data Collection and Statistical Analysis

A standardized questionnaire was used to collect the data from patients who visited the targeted health centres for skin diseases and patients managed via the system. The opinions of both HCWs and the patients were also collected and then sorted by level of satisfaction. The software SPSS.16.0 (IBM Company, Chicago, IL, USA) was used for data capture and analysis. The chi-squared test was used to compare two proportions.

3. Results

3.1. Characteristics of the Study Sites and Trainees:

Overall, 20 HCW from 9 health centres were involved in the study: 9 nurses and 11 general physicians. Before the study, 6 out of 20 HCW had never touched a computer and had no email address (nurses only). Of the 9 health centres, only 4 had an Internet connection (Table 1). Not a single centre had a digital camera.

3.2. Skin Diseases Diagnosed by HCWs

Before the intervention, the proportion of dermatological consultation varied from 8% (Ngolobougou, 51/612) to 65% (Sikasso, 692/1067) with a mean of 20%. After the training session, these proportions were respectively 9% and 63% (Table 1). There was a slight increase in the dermatological activity of all centres, but the difference was not significant.

The pre-programme evaluation revealed that the five top diagnoses of SDs retrieved in the health centre logbook were: wounds (10.8%), allergies (8.8%), mycosis (5%), genital infection (7.3%), and pruritus (4.7%) (Table 2). At the post-programme evaluation, pyoderma (28.4%), eczema (13.5%), dermatophytosis (6.9%), tinea capitis (5.3%), and prurigo (4.4%) were the most common SDs. There was a huge decrease in the proportion of patients with unclear diagnosis, which decreased from 53.7%

(322/599) to 12.4% (84/679) before and after training, respectively ($p < 10^{-6}$). Clearer diagnoses were also observed during the post-programme period.

Table 1. Evaluation of health centres: proportion of skin diseases before and after training and distribution of trainees and cases posted via the platform.

Health Centre	Number of Trainees	Number of Cases Posted via the Platform	Before Training		After Training	
			Number of Skin Diseases (%)	Number of Consults	Number of Skin Diseases (%)	Number of Consults
Koulikoro [a]	2	9	82	900	76	756
Banamba [a]	3	32	185	1512	185	1426
Nara	2	3	95	542	85	501
Sikasso [a]	2	16	692 (65)	1067	706 (63)	1121
Ngolobougou	1	36	51 (8)	612	65 (9)	723
Kadiolo	2	6	60	415	79	608
Mopti [a]	4	35 [b]	108	902	166	1091
Douentza	2	17 [b]	45	480	60	461
Bankass	2	26	78	678	106	816
TOTAL	20	180	1396	7108	1528	7503

[a] Centres where the Internet connection was available before teledermatology intervention; [b] centre exclusively run by a nurse.

Table 2. Pattern of skin diseases observed in health centres before and after intervention: report on the six-month period.

Skin Diseases	Before Intervention	After Intervention
Dermatosis	322	84
Eczema	6	92
Dermatophytosis	-	47
Mycoses	30	7
Tinea capitis	3	36
Pyoderma	16	193
Wounds	65	-
Urticaria	-	11
Allergy	53	14
Follicular infection	8	-
Pruritus	28	-
Scabies	3	15
Onychodystrophy	-	13
Candidiasis	-	20
Measles	-	12
Herpes zoster	-	3
Herpes labialis	-	5
Genital infection	44	8
Prurigo		30
Erysipelas	7	11
Rash	4	8
Molluscum contagiosum	-	3
Aphthous ulcers	-	3
Patches	6	-
Intertrigo	-	6
Chickenpox	-	20
Vitiligo	-	4
Lipoma	-	1
Miliaria	-	22
Burn	4	-
Keloid	-	4
Ulceration	-	7
Total	**599**	**679**

3.3. *Management of Skin Diseases via Teledermatology*

This started immediately after training and continued over one year, from October 2015 to October 2016. Overall, 180 patients who consulted at the targeted health facilities were diagnosed and treated via our platform. The mean number of patients managed per month was 15, with a range of 5 (January) to 24 (August). Regarding the centre activity, the number of patients seen ranged from 3 patients (Nara) to 36 patients (Banamba) (Table 1). The number of images sent per patient varied from 0 to 13, with an average of 3.6. All patients except one accepted being photographed. The average turnaround time to receive the expert's response was 32 h (range from 13 min to 20 days). Except in two cases referred to the dermatological ward in the capital city (one case of bullous pemphigoid and one case of psoriasis) all patients were managed locally. Analysis of diseases diagnosed via the platform illustrated a wide range of conditions (Table 2) (Figures 2–5). The five top diagnoses were: eczema (25/180), dermatophytosis (22/180), pyoderma (10/180), prurigo (11/180), and psoriasis (7/180). However, other conditions such as keratoderma plantaris, vitiligo, small pox, pemghigus, drug-related eruption, and psoriasis were also seen. Miscellaneous diseases included lupus erythematosus (2 cases), leprosy (1 case), transient pustular melanosis (1 case), haemangioma (1 case), epidermal cyst (1 case), syringoma (1 case), and alopecia areata (1 case) (Table 3). The overall diagnosis concordance between dermatologists involved in the programme was 95% amongst the 40 cases randomly selected. Experts had divergent diagnoses in two cases in which the quality of the images was judged unsuitable for correct diagnosis. Importantly, clinical supervision of the health centres enabled the diagnosis of five patients through skin biopsy: two cases of psoriasis and one case each of pemphigus, lichen planus, and epidermal cyst, respectively. The quality of information and photographs given to experts was considered not good enough for diagnosis in six patients (3%). In addition, we failed to diagnose five more cases. Overall, 11 patients had no diagnosis.

Table 3. Miscellaneous skin conditions diagnosed via the platform in 22 cases out of 180 cases posted from health centres.

Skin Disorders	Frequency
Sun burn	2
Eczematised miliaria	2
Hemangioma	1
Alopecia areata	2
Epidermal cyst	1
Vulvovaginitis	1
Leprosy	1
Viral exanthema	1
Multiple keloid	2
Transient pustular melanosis	1
Onychodystrophy	1
Eruptive hidradenoma	1
Lichen simplex	1
Plantar ulcer	1
Congenital keratoderma	2
Varicose veins	2
Total	**22**

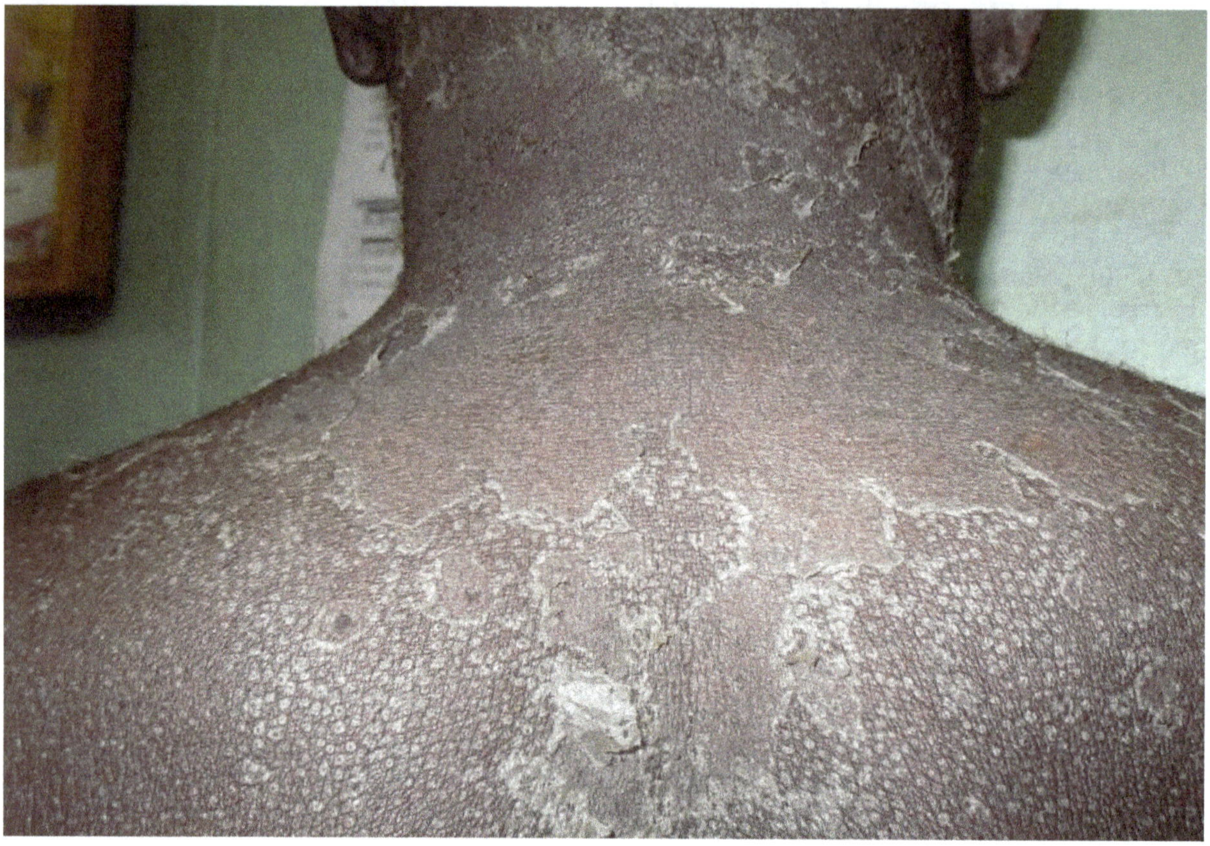

Figure 2. Drug eruption caused by amoxicillin intake following dental extraction.

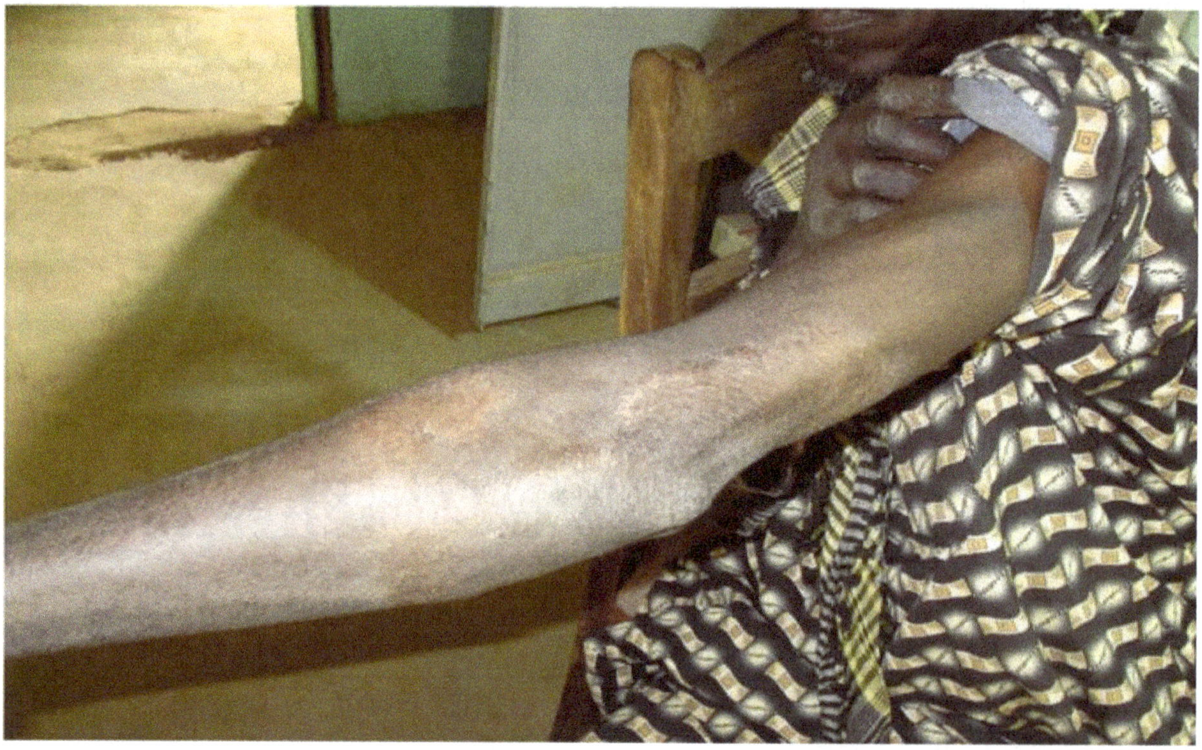

Figure 3. Paucibacillary leprosy: note the large hypochromic patch of the arm.

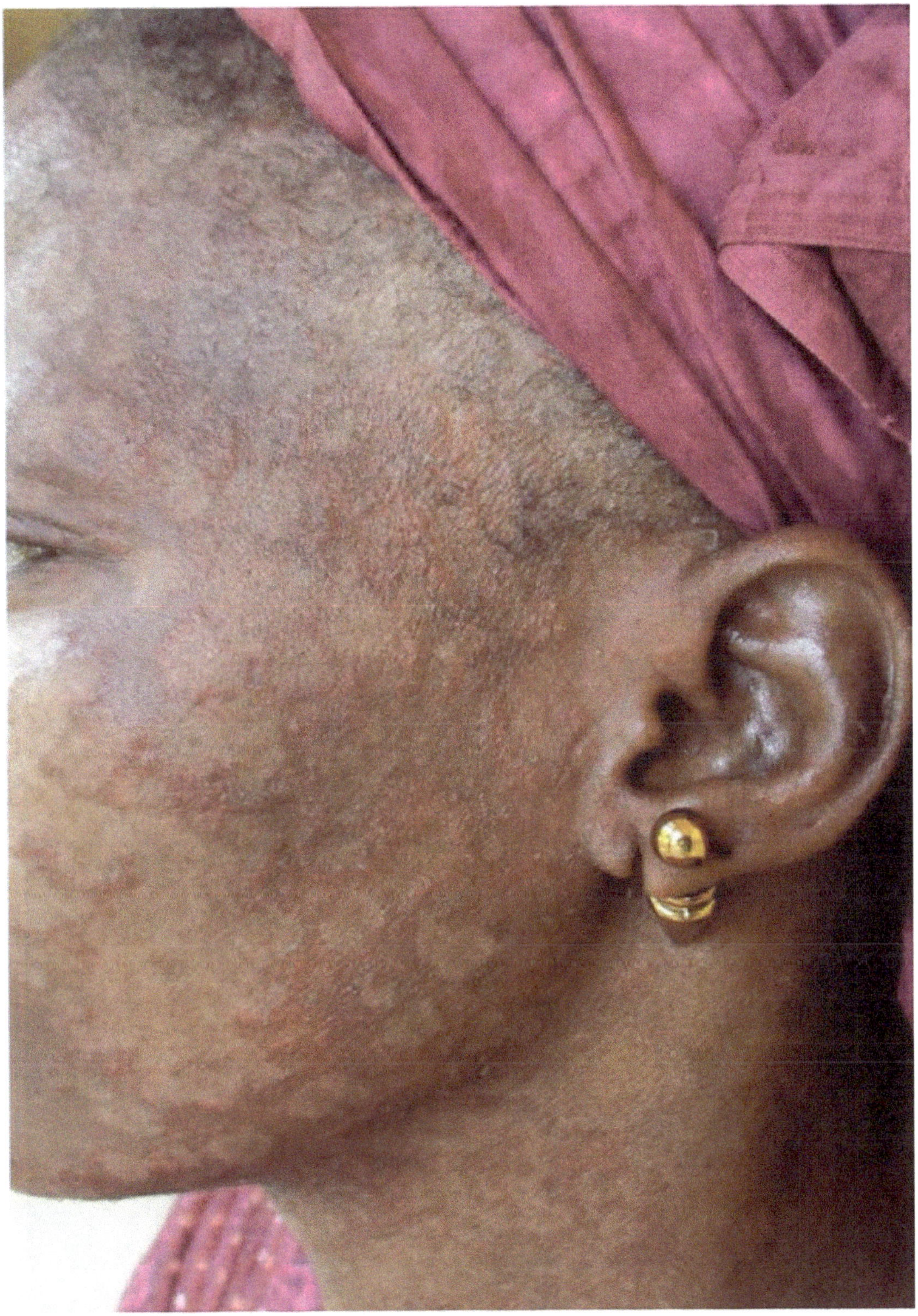

Figure 4. Tinea facei in women using skin bleaching creams (clobetasol and hydroquinone).

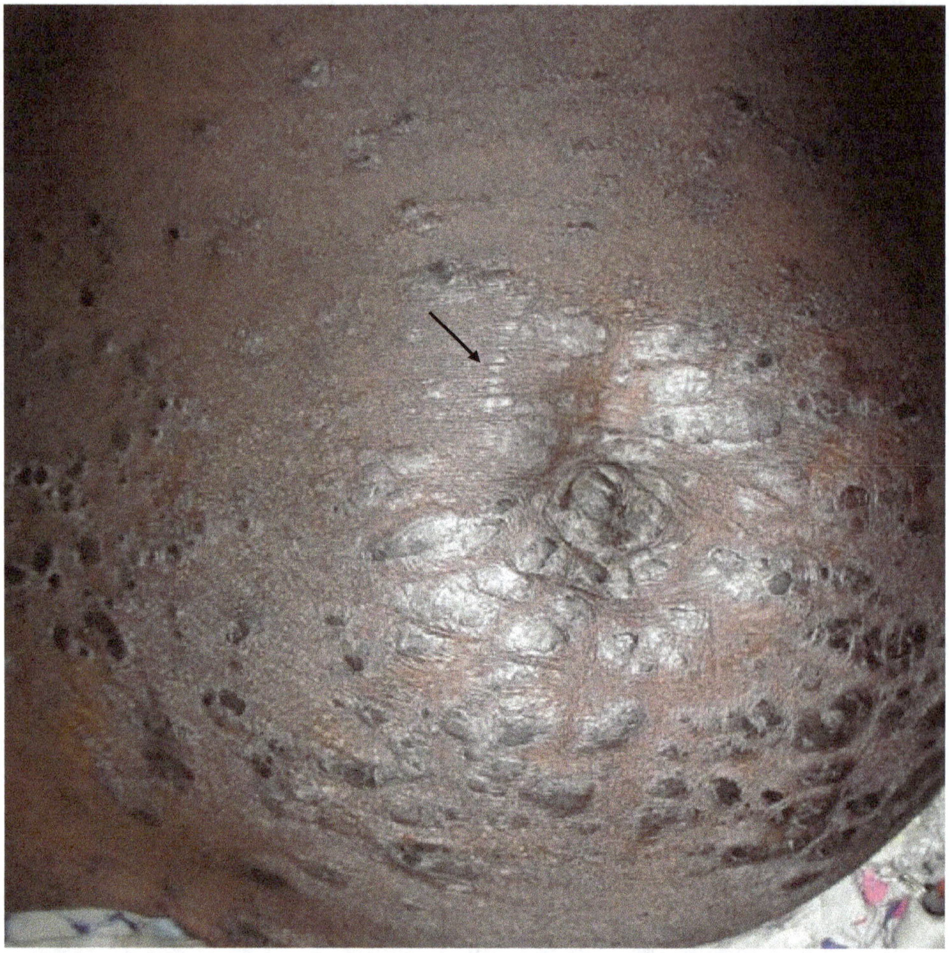

(**A**)

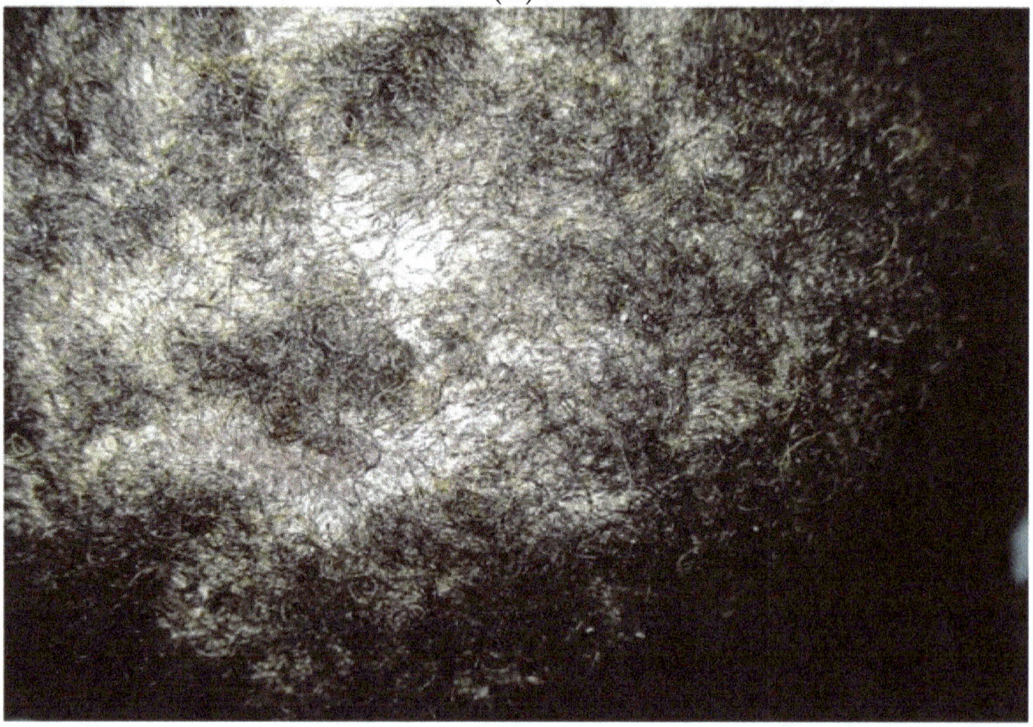

(**B**)

Figure 5. (**A**) Psoriasis in a 35-year-old woman: erythematous papules and plaque over the abdomen. Note the Köbner phenomenon; (**B**) Scalp involvement of the patient.

In the dermatology clinic of the capital city, 24,520 patients were consulted during the study period. The five top diagnoses observed in these patients were: eczema, dermatophytosis, bacterial infection and prurigo, or pruritus and plantar keratoderma. This pattern was similar to that of cases managed via teledermatology during the same period (Figures 6 and 7).

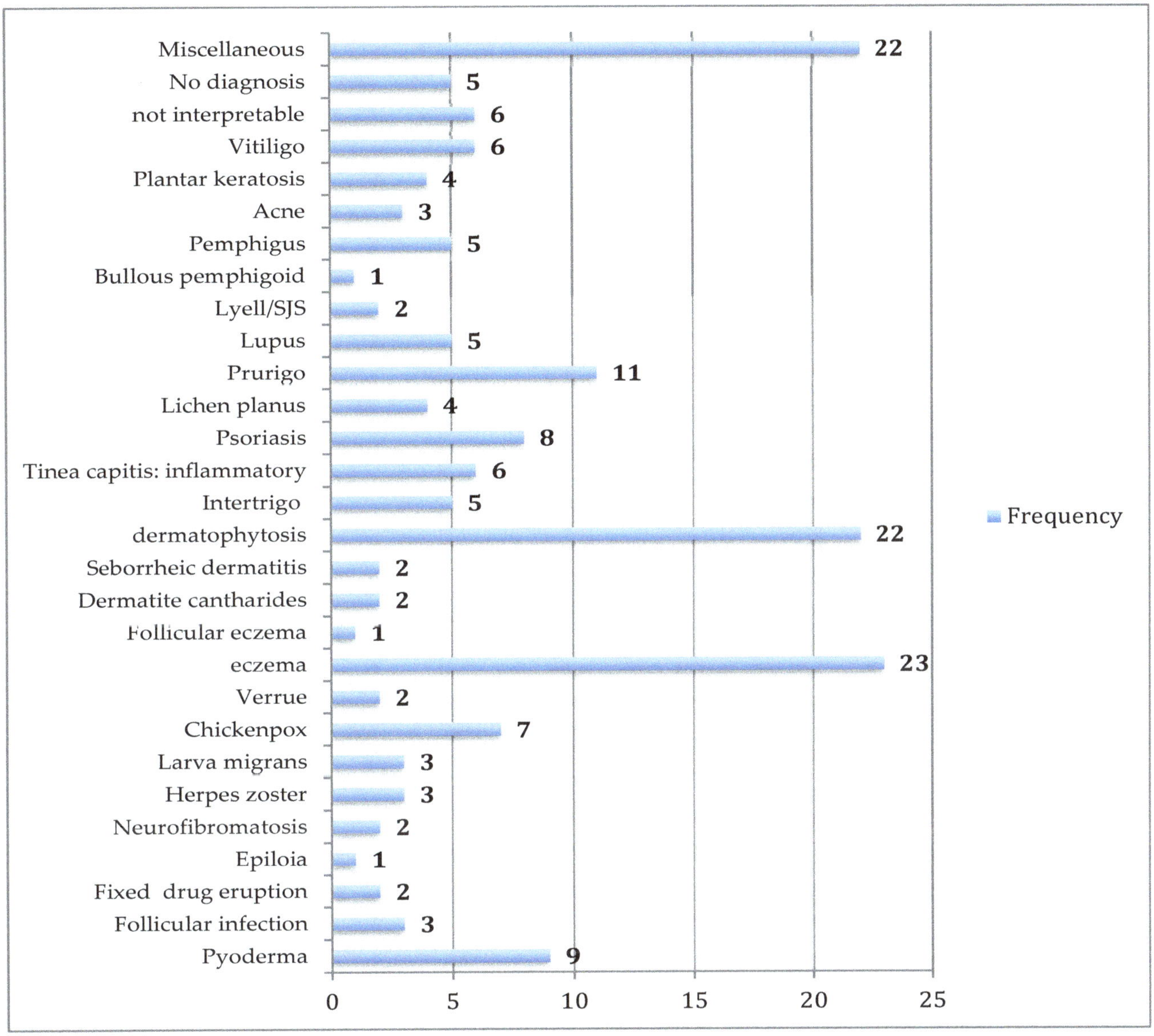

Figure 6. Pattern of skin diseases diagnosed via the platform in 180 cases posted by primary health care workers.

3.4. Satisfaction of HWCs and Patients

Interviews regarding the level of satisfaction involved 10 health providers and 37 patients managed via the system. Eight out of 10 HCWs declared that they were satisfied by the management of patients via the platform, this included four who were strongly satisfied. The time to receive the response from the expert was considered to be reasonable for seven out of 10 HCWs and response times for two were 'moderately' acceptable. According to some health care providers, our intervention enhanced both health centres and general health care practices. They stated: "I felt more confident when facing a patient with SD"; or: "presently, people look at me differently (with more attention) when compared to the time before the programme started". They also though that some programme aspects could be improved: the time to receive the response from the expert, and the platform. The concept of an android version for mobile phones and improved quality of the Internet connection in each region were considered relevant.

All the 37 patients interviewed stated that they were strongly satisfied and would recommend teledermatology to other patients. The fact that they were locally managed was very much appreciated. They also expressed the need to sustain this initiative.

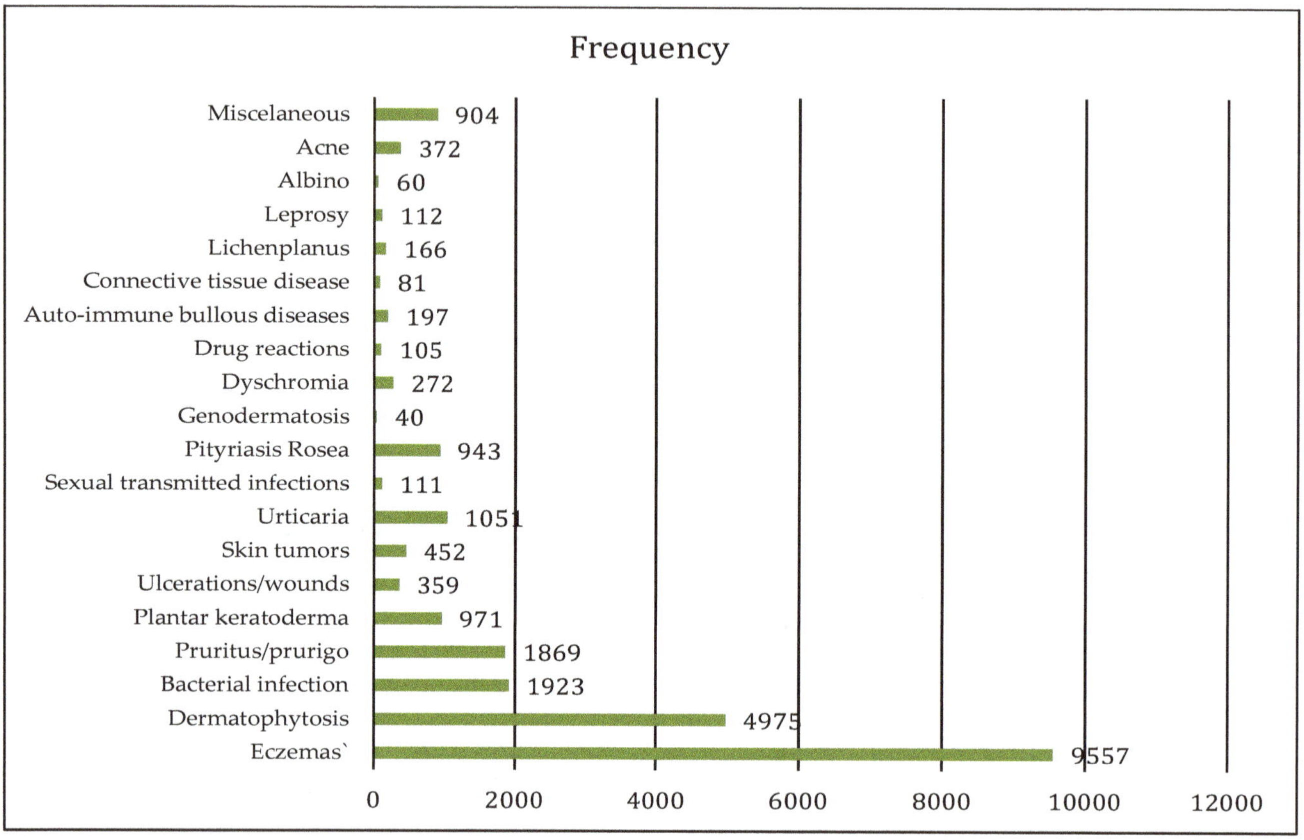

Figure 7. Pattern of skin diseases seen in the Referral centre of Dermatology at the Marchoux Institute in 2015: 24,520 cases.

4. Discussion

This study was a teledermatology pilot programme based on a store-and-forward model and designed to work at a primary health care level in a developing country. Its implementation and evaluation definitely validated the feasibility of a teledermatology programme in a resource-limited area. The usefulness and challenges of such a programme has also been highlighted. There was a huge improvement in the management of all skin diseases in the targeted primary centres, for both common skin diseases and those beyond the expertise of the HCWs. A large number skin diseases were identified and managed locally by health care workers whose knowledge was also improved as long as the intervention continued. The equipment used for connection in this study was very simple, low-cost, and suitable when compared to a live interactive model that requires more equipment and greater technological expertise.

However, several limitations should be addressed. These include the selection of only three health regions, the small number of randomly selected health centres as compared to the total number of health centres in Mali, and the small number of teledermatology requests from one centre (Banamba) due to either the quality of the Internet connection or the lack of HCW commitment to ask for help.

Several papers have addressed the usefulness and effectiveness of teledermatology programmes [16,24]. The greatest number of published studies were performed in the United States, followed by the United Kingdom, Spain, the Netherlands, Italy, and Austria [25] Very few studies were conducted in Africa [26] or in sites such as prisons with greater health care needs [27]. As used in our study, store-and-forward continued to be the most common delivery modality [28]. The present study helps to bridge the gap of health care quality between front line health facilities and dermatologic wards. In rural areas where is a high prevalence of SDs and lack of specialists the needs of care for many people are also met.

The post-programme evaluation of health centres revealed that the management of common SDs was improved as shown by the decrease in the proportion of patients with either unclear diagnosis or 'dermatoses' (allergy, mycosis), and an increase in the number of clear diagnoses, i.e. pyoderma, dermatophytosis, scabies, and eczema. In the pre-programme evaluation, not a single case of very common disorders such as prurigo, urticaria, chickenpox, and miliaria was recorded in the centre logbook. After training, there was a huge improvement in the management of these disorders due to the dermatologic training. Along with this management shift, the skills of HCWs regarding computer science were also improved. One of our HCWs, who had never touched a computer, sent 17 requests for tele-expertise. In addition, two health centres were completely run by nurses, who were beginners in terms of computer science and the Internet. While no case of prurigo was mentioned in the pre-programme evaluation, many cases were noticed after intervention. This improvement could be in part related to the training module of common SDs to which participants have been exposed. It also confirmed the effectiveness of one-day training of primary HCWs in the management of common SDs with an algorithmic approach [15] that was likely to have helped to control the number of requests for teledermatology and avoided experts being swamped by HCW requests. We assume that the trained health staff managed many skin disorders themselves and e-referred only those for which dermatological expertise was required; this indicates that the programme expectations were met. The improvement in the diagnosis of SD in the targeted health centres as shown in the post-intervention evaluation might also have been a result of the continuing medical education created by the regularly-sent responses of experts via the e-platform that all HCW had the possibility to see and learn from. The clinical supervision by dermatologist confirmed cases in which the diagnosis was uncertain. The similarity of leading causes for visits in both primary and specialized health centres, as shown in this study, indicates that the pattern of SDs is not related to the level of health care facilities, but to the epidemiology of SDs. It also points out the necessity to set up and to sustain such initiatives, particularly in areas with poor geographic accessibility and weak coverage by dermatologists.

Despite the profound penetration of information and communication technology in Africa, the actual functioning of such tools has been repeatedly questioned given the frequent shortages of electric power, maintenance issues, and the low quality of connectivity. This prompted us to choose low-level technology with an adapted tool that comprised a 3G key connection and digital camera, as computers were available in all centres. This equipment worked well, and more than 90% of patients were properly managed. It should be underlined that the estimated cost of the teledermatology kit tool can be can easily covered by the cost of referral of one patient from Mopti to Bamako, the capital city. The mobile version of *Bogou*, which has been recently put into production, will lead in the future to a considerable drop in equipment costs. Indeed, almost every HWC has a smartphone in Mali.

Some issues not addressed in this study should be addressed further, in particular in developing countries when setting up a teledermatology programme. These include privacy issues as well as ethical and medicolegal responsibility in cases of injury and unsolved cases.

5. Conclusions

The implementation of a teledermatology programme based on a store-and-forward process in primary health care services is feasible and can positively impact the management of skin disorders. Development and testing of specific and secure applications for the e-management of skin disorders should be promoted. The expansion of such programmes is appealing in resource-limited countries where there are financial constraints and dermatologists are lacking.

Author Contributions: Conceptualization, O.F., C.O.B.; Methodology, O.F., C.O.B., S.K.; Software, C.O.B., M.N., A.G.; Training, Y.F., Y.K., M.G., B.G., A.K., K.T.; Validation, A.M.; Formal Analysis, O.F., L.C., B.T.; Investigation, A.D., L.C., S.B., B.T., B.K.; Resources, S.T.T.; Data Curation, S.T.T.; Writing—Original Draft Preparation, O.F., C.O.B., A.G.; Writing—Review and Editing, O.F., A.M.; Supervision, S.K.; Project Administration, O.F.; Funding Acquisition, O.F.

Acknowledgments: We are grateful to Prof. Roderick J Hay (London) for advice concerning the manuscript and Dr. Florence Poli for her constant support to Malian dermatologists.

References

1. Anonymous. Skin disease and public health medicine. *Lancet* **1991**, *337*, 1008–1009. [CrossRef]
2. Figueroa, J.I.; Fuller, L.C.; Abraha, A.; Hay, R.J. Dermatology in southwestern Ethiopia: Rationale for a community approach. *Int. J. Dermatol.* **1998**, *37*, 752–758. [CrossRef] [PubMed]
3. Mahé, A.; Prual, A.; Konaté, M.; Bobin, P. Skin diseases of children in Mali: A public health problem. *Trans. R. Soc. Trop. Med. Hyg.* **1995**, *89*, 467–470. [CrossRef]
4. Walker, S.L.; Shah, M.; Hubbard, V.G.; Pradhan, H.M.; Ghimire, M. Skin disease is common in rural Nepal: Results of a point prevalence study. *Br. J. Dermatol.* **2008**, *158*, 334–338. [CrossRef] [PubMed]
5. Saw, S.M.; Koh, D.; Adjani, M.R.; Wong, M.L.; Hong, C.Y.; Lee, J.; Chia, S.E.; Munoz, C.P.; Ong, C.N. A population-based prevalence survey of skin diseases in adolescents and adults in rural Sumatra, Indonesia, 1999. *Trans. R. Soc. Trop. Med. Hyg.* **2001**, *95*, 384–388. [CrossRef]
6. Abdel-Hafez, K.; Abdel-Aty, M.A.; Hofny, E.R. Prevalence of skin diseases in rural areas of Assiut Governorate, Upper Egypt. *Int. J. Dermatol.* **2003**, *42*, 887–892. [CrossRef] [PubMed]
7. Leekassa, R.; Bizuneh, E.; Alem, A.; Fekadu, A.; Shibre, T. Community diagnosis of common skin diseases in the Zay community of the Zeway Islands, Ethiopia. *Ethiop. Med. J.* **2005**, *43*, 189–195. [PubMed]
8. Dogra, S.; Kumar, B. Epidemiology of skin diseases in school children: A study from northern India. *Pediatr. Dermatol.* **2003**, *20*, 470–473. [CrossRef] [PubMed]
9. Bechelli, L.M.; Haddad, N.; Pimenta, W.P.; Pagnano, P.M.; Melchior, J.E.; Fregnan, R.C.; Zanin, L.C.; Arenas, A. Epidemiological survey of skin diseases in schoolchildren living in the Purus Valley (Acre State, Amazonia, Brazil). *Dermatologica* **1981**, *163*, 78–93. [CrossRef] [PubMed]
10. Gibbs, S.A.M. Skin disease and socioeconomic conditions in rural Africa: Tanzania. *Int. J. Dermatol.* **1996**, *35*, 633–639. [CrossRef] [PubMed]
11. National Health Administration of the Minister of Health. *Direction Nationale de la Santé. Données du Système d'Information Sanitaire National: Annuaire Statistique 2007*; Ministère de la Santé: Bamako, Mali, 2007; p. 145. (In French).
12. Karimkhani, C.; Dellavalle, R.P.; Coffeng, L.E.; Flohr, C.; Hay, R.J.; Langan, S.M.; Nsoesie, E.O.; Ferrari, A.J.; Erskine, H.E.; Silverberg, J.I.; et al. Global skin disease morbidity and mortality: an update from the global burden of disease study 2013. *JAMA Dermatol.* **2017**, *153*, 406–412. [CrossRef] [PubMed]
13. Faye, O.; Keita, S.; N'diaye, H.; Konare, H.; Coulibaly, I. Evaluation du niveau de connaissance des agents de santé sur le diagnostic de la lèpre à Bamako (MALI): Proposition pour l'avenir de la lutte anti-lépreuse. *Mali. Méd.* **2003**, *18*, 32–34. (In French)
14. Mahé, A.; Cissé, I.A.; Faye, O.; N′ Diaye, H.T.; Niamba, P. Skin diseases in Bamako (Mali). *Int. J. Dermatol.* **1998**, *37*, 673–676. [CrossRef] [PubMed]
15. Mahé, A.; Faye, O.; N'Diaye, H.T.; Konaré, H.D.; Coulibaly, I.; Kéita, S.; Traoré, A.K.; Hay, R.J. Integration of basic dermatological care into primary health care services in Mali. *Bull World Health Organ.* **2005**, *83*, 935–943. [PubMed]
16. Warshaw, E.M.; Hillman, Y.J.; Greer, N.L.; Hagel, E.M.; MacDonald, R.; Rutks, I.R.; Wilt, T.J. Teledermatology for diagnosis and management of skin conditions: A systematic review. *J. Am. Acad. Dermatol.* **2011**, *64*, 759–772. [CrossRef] [PubMed]

17. Heffner, V.A.; Lyon, V.B.; Brousseau, D.C.; Holland, K.E.; Yen, K. Store-and-forward teledermatology versus in-person visits: A comparison in pediatric teledermatology clinic. *J. Am. Acad. Dermatol.* **2009**, *60*, 956–961. [CrossRef] [PubMed]
18. Edison, K.E.; Ward, D.S.; Dyer, J.A.; Lane, W.; Chance, L.; Hicks, L.L. Diagnosis, diagnostic confidence, and management concordance in live-interactive and store-and-forward teledermatology compared to in-person examination. *Telemed. E-Health,* **2008**, *14*, 889–895. [CrossRef] [PubMed]
19. Moreno-Ramirez, D.; Ferrandiz, L.; Nieto-Garcia, A.; Carrasco, R.; Moreno-Alvarez, P.; Galdeano, R.; Bidegain, E.; Rios-Martin, J.J.; Camacho, F.M. Store-and-forward teledermatology in skin cancer triage: Experience and evaluation of 2009 teleconsultations. *Arch. Dermatol.* **2007**, *143*, 479–483. [CrossRef] [PubMed]
20. Moreno-Ramirez, D.; Ferrandiz, L.; Bernal, A.P.; Duran, R.C.; Martin, J.J.; Camacho, F. Teledermatology as a filtering system in pigmented lesion clinics. *J. Telemed. Telecare* **2005**, *11*, 298–303. [CrossRef] [PubMed]
21. Oliveira, M.R.; Wen, C.L.; Neto, C.F.; Silveira, P.S.; Rivitti, E.A.; Böhm, G.M. Web site for training nonmedical health-care workers to identify potentially malignant skin lesions and for teledermatology. *Telemed. J. E-Health* **2002**, *8*, 323–332. [CrossRef] [PubMed]
22. Bogou. Available online: http://raft.unige.ch/bogou/ (accessed on 18 July 2018).
23. Bediang, G.; Perrin, C.; Ruiz de Castañeda, R.; Kamga, Y.; Sawadogo, A.; Bagayoko, C.O.; Geissbuhler, A. The RAFT telemedicine network: Lessons learnt and perspectives from a decade of educational and clinical services in low-and middle-incomes countries. *Front. Public Health* **2014**, *2*, 180. [CrossRef] [PubMed]
24. Tran, K.; Ayad, M.; Weinberg, J.; Cherng, A.; Chowdhury, M.; Monir, S.; Hariri, M.; Kovarik, C. Mobile teledermatology in the developing world: Implications of a feasibility study on 30 Egyptian patients with common skin diseases. *J. Am. Acad. Dermatol.* **2011**, *64*, 302–309. [CrossRef] [PubMed]
25. Trettel, A.; Eissing, L.; Augustin, M. Telemedicine in dermatology: Findings and experiences worldwide—A systematic literature review. *J. Eur. Acad. Dermatol. Venereol.* **2018**, *32*, 215–224. [CrossRef] [PubMed]
26. Delaigue, S.; Bonnardot, L.; Olson, D.; Morand, J.J. Overview of teledermatology in low-resource settings. *Med. Sante Trop.* **2015**, *25*, 365–372. [PubMed]
27. Khatibi, B.; Bambe, A.; Chantalat, C.; Resche-Rigon, M.; Sanna, A.; Fac, C.; Bagot, M.; Guibal, F. Teledermatology in a prison setting: A retrospective study of 500 expert opinions. *Ann. Dermatol. Venereol.* **2016**, *143*, 418–422. [CrossRef] [PubMed]
28. Yim, K.M.; Florek, A.G.; Oh, D.H.; McKoy, K.; Armstrong, A.W. Teledermatology in the United States: An Update in a Dynamic Era. *Telemed. J. E-Health* **2018**, in press. [CrossRef] [PubMed]

7

A One Health Approach for Guinea Worm Disease Control: Scope and Opportunities

Matthew R. Boyce *, Ellen P. Carlin, Jordan Schermerhorn and Claire J. Standley

Center for Global Health Science & Security, Georgetown University, Washington, DC 20057, USA; ec1223@georgetown.edu (E.P.C.); js4904@georgetown.edu (J.S.); Claire.Standley@georgetown.edu (C.J.S.)

* Correspondence: mb2266@georgetown.edu

Abstract: Guinea worm disease (GWD) is a neglected tropical disease that was targeted for eradication several decades ago because of its limited geographical distribution, predictable seasonality, straightforward diagnosis, and exclusive infection of humans. However, a growing body of evidence challenges this last attribute and suggests that GWD can affect both humans and animal populations. The One Health approach emphasizes the relatedness of human, animal, and environmental health. We reviewed epidemiological evidence that could support the utility of a One Health approach for GWD control in the six countries that have reported human GWD cases since 2015—Angola, Cameroon, Chad, Ethiopia, Mali, and South Sudan. Human GWD cases have dramatically declined, but recent years have seen a gradual increase in human case counts, cases in new geographies, and a rapidly growing number of animal infections. Taken together, these suggest a need for an adjusted approach for eradicating GWD using a framework rooted in One Health, dedicated to improving disease surveillance and in animals; pinpointing the dominant routes of infection in animals; elucidating the disease burden in animals; determining transmission risk factors among animals and from animals to humans; and identifying practical ways to foster horizontal and multidisciplinary approaches.

Keywords: animal health; *Dracunculus medinensis*; guinea worm; human health; infectious disease; one health; zoonoses

---

1. Introduction

Guinea worm disease (GWD), also known as dracunculiasis or Medina worm disease, is a neglected tropical disease (NTD) caused by a nematode, *Dracunculus medinensis*. Humans usually become infected by ingesting water containing copepods (small aquatic crustaceans) infected with Dracunculus larvae [1]. While the copepods are killed in the stomach, the larvae mature into adult Guinea worms and copulate. Male worms die following copulation, but approximately one-year post-infection, adult female Guinea worms migrate to the skin and breach the surface through a blister. When these wounds are exposed to a water source, the female worm releases embryos (i.e., L1 larvae) and the cycle repeats.

Secondary infections are common, and complications can result in abscess formation, tetanus, septic arthritis, or systemic sepsis [1]. Though rarely fatal, GWD can cause permanent disability and impose major economic burdens [1,2]. Like many other NTDs, GWD primarily affects poor, rural communities. Neither a vaccine nor effective medical prophylaxis is currently available [3,4]. Case management is limited to carefully and safely removing the whole worm and tending the exit wound to prevent infection.

Following the success of the smallpox eradication campaign in 1979, public health experts identified GWD as a candidate for eradication [4]. GWD was considered a suitable candidate because its geographical distribution was limited to tropical or subtropical areas, it adhered to seasonal transmission patterns [5,6], the diagnosis was straightforward [7], and, critically, there were no known animal reservoirs [3,4].

Led by the Carter Center and supported by the World Health Organization, United Nations Children's Fund, and United States Centers for Disease Control and Prevention (CDC), the Global Dracunculiasis Eradication Campaign began in 1980 and has significantly reduced the global burden of the disease [8]. Since it began, when there were more than 3 million cases of GWD in 20 countries, the eradication campaign has dramatically reduced GWD prevalence and as few as 22 cases were reported in four countries in 2015 [9]. However, recent years have seen an increase in the number of reported cases, as well as human cases and animal infections reported in new countries and countries that had previously been certified free of GWD. Consequently, the eradication target has been delayed until 2030 [10].

These delays are the result of numerous factors, including conflict and social unrest, that have limited the ability of field teams to conduct active searches for cases [2,10–12]. However, an emerging body of evidence also suggests that eradication efforts have been further impeded by the presence of other non-human animal species (hereafter "animals") that act as hosts and maintain transmission. Dogs, cats, and baboons, and potentially fish and frogs, are now recognized as playing a role in the parasite's transmission to human populations [3,13–19]. Of these, widespread reservoir infections in dogs are considered the largest threat to eradication efforts [11,20]. Adult Guinea worms emerging from humans and these other animals are genetically indistinguishable, with evidence that worms emerging from animals have subsequently caused infections in humans by releasing larvae into shared water sources [13].

That multiple countries now report animal infections underscores the need for novel intervention and eradication strategies [21]. The identification of the worm in so many species complicates eradication and necessitates an interdisciplinary approach. One Health is a concept that acknowledges the relatedness of human, animal, and environmental health and the importance of interdisciplinary efforts in achieving positive health outcomes across these populations [22,23]. Although the body of work to eradicate GWD has been substantial, relatively little research has been undertaken to elucidate the role that animals may play in transmission or to isolate the impact of specific interventions on the number of animal infections. Accordingly, this paper reviews the epidemiological evidence as it relates to animal epidemiology, and in turn to potential animal-level interventions toward the goal of human eradiation, and creates a conceptual framework for how such an approach could be applied to create new GWD control paradigms that support eradication efforts.

2. Materials and Methods

We conducted a review to identify GWD surveillance data for humans and animals and to identify interventions being implemented to control the spread of disease. We performed a literature review using the PubMed and Web of Science databases. Synonyms for "Dracunculiasis", "dog", "cat", "baboon", "frog", and "fish" were combined with a list of the countries that have reported GWD cases since 2015 (i.e., Angola, Cameroon, Chad, Ethiopia, Mali, and South Sudan). A supplementary file provides the complete search syntax (Supplementary Table S1). Our last search was conducted in January 2020.

We attempted to obtain detailed monthly human and animal surveillance data, including through outreach to the Carter Center, but found no sources. To address this, we collected all Guinea Worm Wrap-Up reports—reports periodically co-published by the Carter Center and the U.S. CDC that contain human and animal surveillance data—published between January 2015 and January 2020 and reviewed their surveillance data for human cases and animal infections [24]. The monthly human surveillance data were robust, but the monthly animal surveillance data were not publicly reported. As a result, for animals, we gathered monthly surveillance data when available, but focused efforts primarily on annual data. These were supplemented with data from the World Health Organization. Gathered data were compiled in a Microsoft Excel spreadsheet (Supplementary Table S2).

We then reviewed and analyzed the identified peer-reviewed literature and surveillance data to synthesize a conceptual framework for how such an approach that emphasizes the nexus of human, animal, and environmental health could enhance efforts to eradicate GWD.

3. Results

3.1. Epidemiological Data

In 2010, a collective 1786 human GWD cases were reported in the five countries considered in this study, with a majority of these coming from South Sudan (Table 1). By 2015, total reported human cases declined to 22, from which point they gradually rose to reach 53 in 2019 (Figure 1), with a majority of these cases coming from Chad. Four countries reported human GWD cases from 2010–2015, three from 2016–2018, and four in 2019. Angola and Chad were the only two countries to report more human GWD cases in 2019 than in 2010. After no previous reports of cases (with the caveat that no GWD-specific case search programs had ever been active in the country), Angola reported one human GWD case in 2018 and another in 2019 (Table 1). Chad reported 10 human cases in 2010, and a low of 9 cases in 2015, before reported cases began to increase, reaching 47 in 2019.

A variety of mammalian species have long been established as potential reservoirs of GWD; however, there was limited evidence that these species were transmitting Guinea worm to humans [3,15]. Sporadic infections in dogs and other animals have been historically reported in Cote d'Ivoire, Ghana, India, Kazakhstan, and Pakistan, but studies to definitively assess animals as a transmission risk factor for humans are limited. In the countries listed, infections in animals are thought to have ceased after human infections were eliminated [28]. Whether these animal infections were instances of anthroponosis (i.e., the transmission of a pathogen from humans to a nonhuman species) that were then interrupted via interventions in the human host is not known as studies have not assessed this question.

Table 1. Reported Human Cases of Guinea Worm Disease in Considered Countries, 2010–2019.

Year	Country						Total
	Angola	Cameroon	Chad	Ethiopia	Mali	South Sudan	
2010	0	0	10	21	57	1698	1786
2011	0	0	10	8	12	1028	1058
2012	0	0	10	4	4	521	539 [1]
2013	0	0	14	7	11	113	145 [2]
2014	0	0	13	3	40	70	126
2015	0	0	9	3	5	5	22
2016	0	0	16	3	0	6	25
2017	0	0	15	15	0	0	30
2018	1	0	17	0	0	10	28
2019	1	1 [3]	47	0	0	4	53

[1] An additional three cases were reported in Niger in 2012, but none have been reported since. These were thought to have been imported from Mali [25]. [2] An additional three cases were reported in Sudan in 2013, but none have been reported since. While the cases were not classified as imported, they were detected in an area of southwest Sudan that borders South Sudan and the Central African Republic [26]. [3] A 2019 case in Cameroon was found close to the Chad border; the origin of infection remains unclear, though human cases and reports of animal infections from the same part of Cameroon could suggest localized transmission [27].

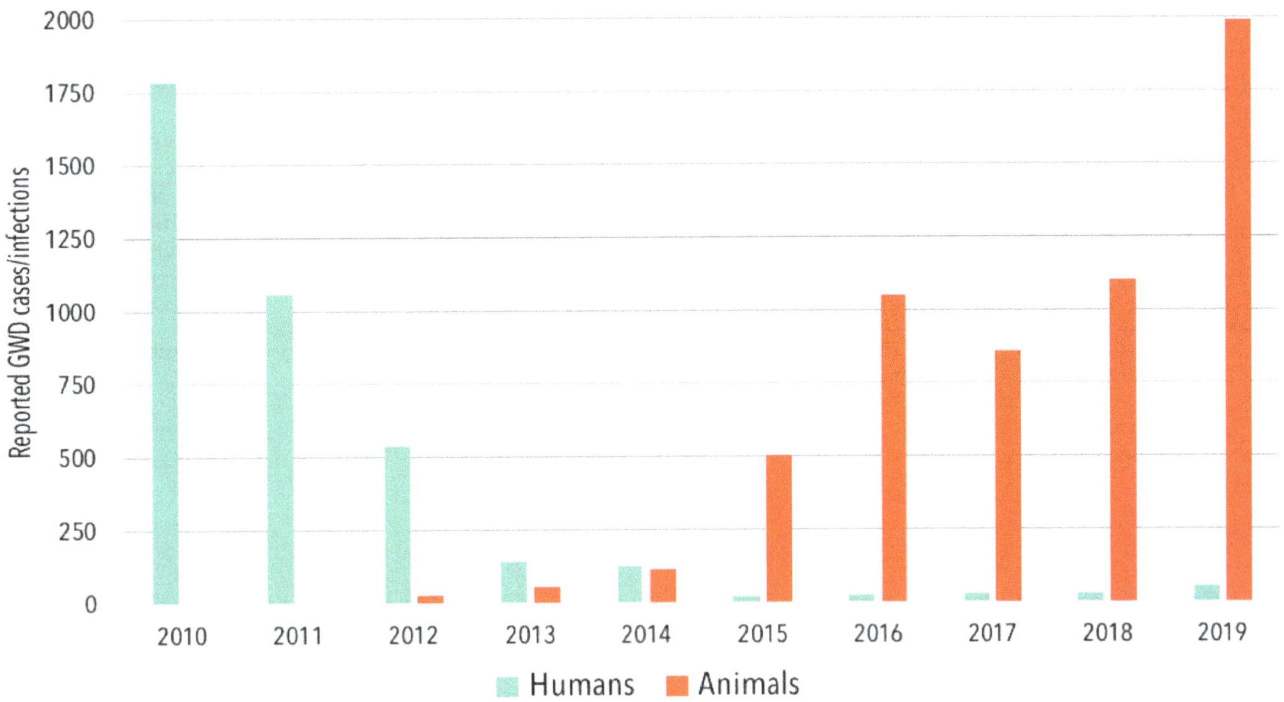

Figure 1. The total annual reported human cases and animal infections of Guinea worm disease in Angola, Cameroon, Chad, Ethiopia, Mali, and South Sudan, 2010–2019.

There has been an increase in reported animal Guinea worm infections since 2015. Most reported animal Guinea worm infections have involved dogs in Chad. The total number of reported canine infections has grown from 498 in 2015 to 1943 infections in 2019 (Table 2). The pathways by which dogs are infected remain unconfirmed, but it is hypothesized they can acquire Guinea worm infection in the same way as humans (i.e., from drinking water containing infected copepods), or possibly by consuming infected paratenic hosts [15]. The consumption of raw fish entrails, discarded by humans during food preparation, has been considered a potential source of transmission and addressed by the human behavioral intervention of promoting burial of entrails in all known-endemic villages since 2015 [21]. A study conducted in Chad found that dogs in households where water was provided for animals were less likely to have had Guinea worm and that dogs with a higher proportion of fish in their diets were more likely to have had Guinea worm [19]. However, dogs with less fish in their diets and those more likely to consume provided water may also live further from natural water sources and therefore less likely to be infected via the traditional waterborne route. A similar study conducted in Ethiopia found no evidence to support the hypothesized paratenic host transmission pathway [29]. Further, although the phenomenon of canine infections with Guinea worm was only recently realized, evidence suggests that this was the result of insufficient surveillance rather than the absence of infection [13].

Guinea worm infections have also been reported in cats, baboons, a leopard [27], and a donkey [28]. The incident involving the leopard was later removed from official counts because the worm was found while dissecting the dead animal, and had not emerged as is required for official case counts [27,30]. Excluding dogs, animal infection counts rose from 5 reported infections in 2015 to 53 in 2019 (Table 2).

Chad has reported the most animal infections, including dogs, of any country and there appears to be a temporal alignment between patterns of reported human cases and animal infections (Figure 2). After first reporting 27 infections in dogs in 2012 [32], the number has risen steadily, peaking at 1927 infections in 2019 [30]. Humans and dogs are infected by shared populations of worms in Chad and it has been hypothesized that this may be driving the increase in human GWD cases [13,15]. Chad also reported four Guinea worm infections in cats in 2015, rising to 46 infections in 2019 following intensified education and surveillance efforts targeting cats.

Table 2. Reported Animal Infections of Guinea Worm Disease in Considered Countries, 2015–2019; (Canine Infections).

Year	Country						Total
	Angola	Cameroon	Chad	Ethiopia	Mali	South Sudan	
2015	0	0	487 (483)	14 (13)	1 (1)	1 (1)	503 (498)
2016	0	0	1022 (1011)	16 (14)	11 (11)	0	1049 (1036)
2017	0	0	830 (817)	15 (11)	10 (9)	0	855 (837)
2018	0	1 (1)	1065 (1040)	17 (11)	20 (18)	0	1103 (1070)
2019	1 (1)	5 (5) [1]	1973 (1927)	8 (2)	9 (8)	0	1996 (1943)

[1] This number includes only reported infections explicitly mentioned in a Carter Center update [31], and does not include other unconfirmed rumors discovered by WHO investigators.

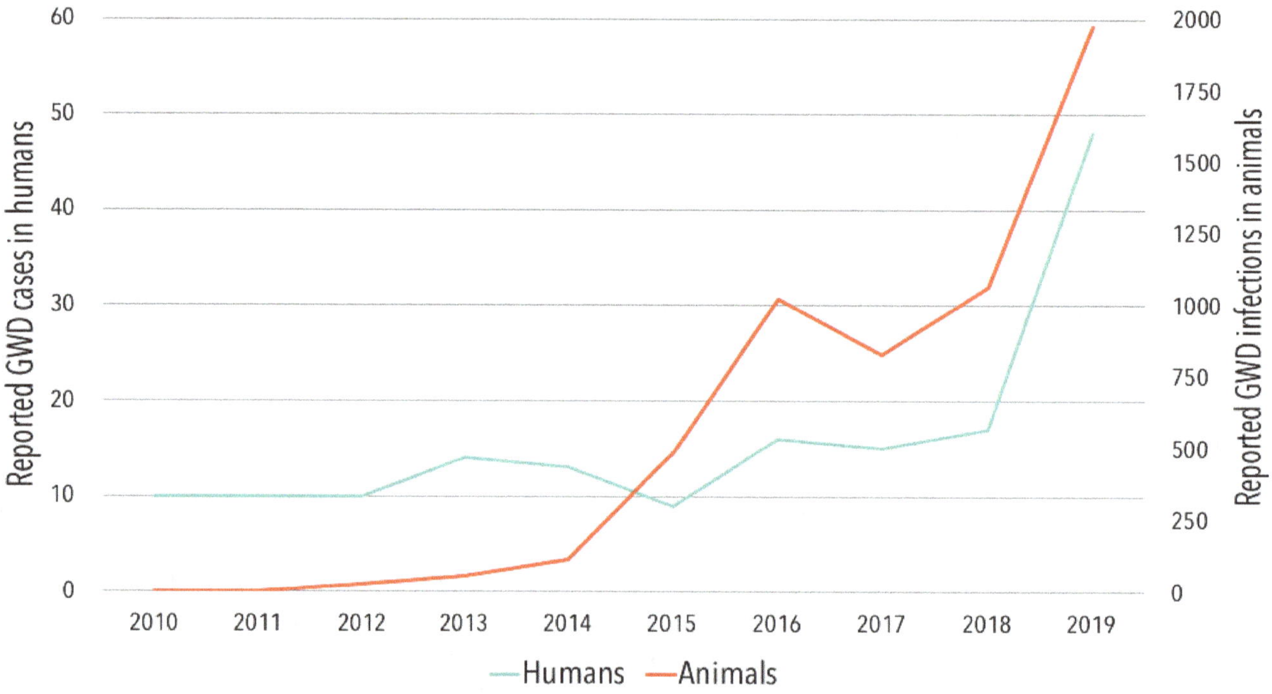

Figure 2. Reported human cases and animal infections of Guinea worm disease in Chad, 2010–2019.

Ethiopia reported one Guinea worm infection in baboons annually from 2013–2015 [28,33], two infections in 2016 [34], four infections in 2017 [35], one infection in 2018 [36], and six infections in 2019 [30]; Ethiopia also reported five infections in cats in 2018 [36]. Mali reported one infection in a cat in 2017 [35], two infections in 2018 [31], and one infection in 2019 [30]. From 2015–2019, Angola and South Sudan each reported one Guinea worm infection in dogs [30,35], and neither has reported infections in other animals.

3.2. Interventions Used to Reduce the Burden of Guinea Worm Disease in Humans and Animal Populations

GWD eradication efforts primarily rely on behavioral- and environmental-based interventions and associated health education campaigns to break the cycle of transmission between humans and the environment [37]. Countries that are endemic for GWD often endorse layered approaches that emphasize the implementation of multiple interventions with the understanding that no single intervention will be perfectly executed [38].

Many GWD eradication programs are based on the provision of improved water sources for human populations [4,18,20,39,40] (Figure 3). Specific interventions include the use of water filtration devices [4,18,20,39,40] and providing clean water from underground sources by hand-dug or bore-hole wells or other similar means [4,18,39,40]. Sand, steel mesh, and finely woven cloth water filtration devices prevent GWD in humans by removing the copepods from drinking water. Portable pipe filters—straws with a filter inside—allow people to filter their water when traveling or away from home [40]. A more communal solution involves drilling boreholes to provide clean water from underground sources, which protects against other infectious diseases in addition to GWD [40].

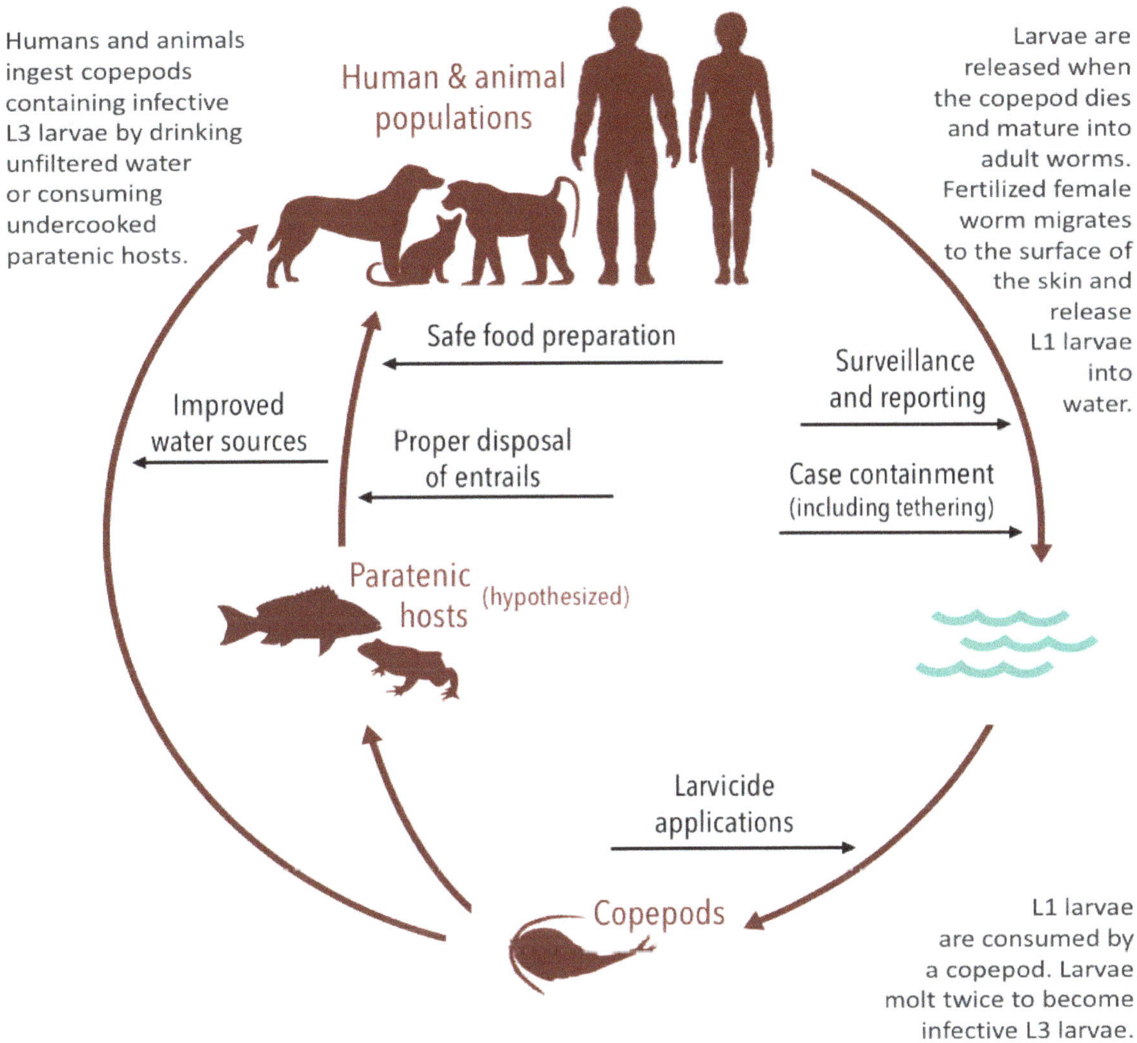

Figure 3. Transmission and life cycle of the Guinea worm with impact points of existing interventions.

To supplement interventions focused on drinking water, eradication campaigns also treat water sources with larvicides to reduce and control vector populations. Temephos is a colorless, odorless, and tasteless larvicide that is harmless to humans, fish, and plants at recommended concentrations, but lethal to the copepods that act as intermediate hosts for Guinea worm [40]. Accordingly, it is frequently used to treat contaminated or potentially contaminated sources of surface water to reduce transmission risk [2–4,12,18,20,40–42]. It may be proactively applied at monthly intervals [4], or reactively following the known contamination of a water source by an infected human or animal within 10–14 days [28].

Challenges related to treating water sources with temephos include the intensity of labor, difficulties in reaching remote areas, difficulties in identifying which surface water sources require treatment, and effectively treating larger or flowing bodies of water (which is generally less successful than treatments of smaller or stagnant bodies) [3,4,18]. Because animals may infect and utilize water sources that are not used by humans, some programs endeavor to map and apply larvicide to hidden water sources in at-risk areas; however, seasonal flooding and the drying of many water sources make this difficult to track [2,19]. Overall, there is some evidence that suggests vector control interventions are an effective method for suppressing GWD infections via the traditional water-based infection route; in theory, it should also reduce hypothesized paratenic transmission if the infected copepods are killed prior to consumption by paratenic hosts.

Other interventions focus on the containment of human and animal cases before they have an opportunity to enter and contaminate water sources [14,18,20,41,42]. Eradication programs have promoted the tethering of domestic dogs and cats with signs of infection, to prevent them from contaminating water sources once the worms fully emerge; Ethiopia and Chad have piloted preventative tethering of animals without symptoms in villages identified as high-risk [14,41,42]. Eradication programs have provided monetary incentives for complying with tethering protocols; the Ethiopia program has also imposed fines for persons found releasing animals from tethering prematurely [43]. GPS collars have also been piloted to track the movement of baboons [19,36,44], with the goal of monitoring the potential contamination of water sources even in densely forested areas [45].

To increase the sensitivity of surveillance efforts, programs have also introduced cash rewards for reporting suspected cases of GWD in animals and humans that are subsequently confirmed [2,4,18]. This form of active surveillance depends on the rapid investigation of rumors, a robust network of staff and volunteers, and a reliable reporting system [20]. Rewards are generally higher for reporting human cases of GWD and generally increase as countries report fewer human cases. Cash rewards for reporting infections in dogs are occasionally split between the person who reports the dog and the owner of the dog, in exchange for tethering the animal until the worm emerges [35,46–48].

Health education and awareness campaigns are also used to reduce transmission. Campaigns frequently focus on educating people about the transmission cycle, how the infection is acquired, and how it can be prevented [2,18,20,21,40,41]. These efforts are designed to inform people about the aforementioned interventions but have also encouraged other behavioral interventions, such as sufficiently cooking, drying or smoking hypothesized paratenic hosts before eating [2,18,21,41], and burning or burying fish entrails that may contain infected copepods to prevent animals from eating them [2,18,21,41,42]. Campaigns occur in person, through radio and television programming, via printed materials (e.g., posters), and through existing community structures like school systems and houses of religion to achieve maximum reach [48]. These efforts are of importance in endemic communities, neighboring communities, and at-risk non-endemic areas [2].

Some additional interventions have aimed at using medical treatment to prevent or cure infections in dogs. Topical and oral anthelmintics commonly used in dogs as preventives for other nematode infections, such as heartworm, have been tested with limited effects [38,48]. Trials of ivermectin and imidacloprid/moxidectin have not demonstrated effectiveness in preventing or curing infections in dogs and were discontinued [49]; an oral trial with flubendazole is ongoing [38,50]. These recent, limited efforts at incorporating veterinary treatment into human eradication goals may benefit from more laboratory research prior to field trials and, if successful in controlled environments, incorporation into a systemic, long-term interdisciplinary strategy.

4. Discussion

Pathogens with complex transmission cycles that involve multiple hosts can be exceptionally challenging to eliminate and eradicate. The massive mid-21st century campaign to eradicate smallpox was successful because of the comparatively simple, single-host epidemiology of the smallpox virus. Most pathogens of humans are characterized by more complex transmission pathways. Indeed, most infectious diseases of humans have zoonotic origins [51], meaning that, by definition, animals can serve as reservoirs, paratenic or dead-end hosts, or transmitters of the pathogen in question.

GWD, once believed to have been exclusively a disease of humans, has proven capable of infecting other animals. As the lack of zoonotic reservoirs has traditionally been considered a key factor for identifying human diseases with the potential for eradication [52]; this begs the question of whether

GWD should no longer be considered eradicable; whether GWD should be considered eradicable, but only with respect to the disease in humans, and not entirely removed from the ecosystem (i.e., alter the current definition of "eradicated"); or pursue the full eradication of Guinea worm across both humans and animals, and use it as evidence that the previous tenets of "eradicable" are flawed. We advocate for the last of these options and believe that more intensive and holistic interventions and approaches that consider environmental, human, and animal elements as part of an interacting whole are more likely to be successful.

The veterinary profession has targeted prevention and treatment of gastrointestinal worms in dogs and cats as a way not only to keep pets healthy but also to prevent transmission of worms to humans. There is some evidence for success. For instance, higher-income nations often report much lower rates of toxocariasis than lower-income nations [53]. Yet, *Toxocara* seroprevalence and other indicators remain alarmingly high, even in the industrialized world, in part because of earlier misconceptions about the parasite's lifecycle, lack of access to animal care, and practical challenges of treating street dog populations—all challenges similar to those associated with GWD.

Rabies represents another example of successful coordination between human and veterinary health specialists working in lock-step toward the common goal of eliminating rabies in human populations. Many countries have had success with a case management mechanism that spans human and animal healthcare-seeking known as integrated bite case management [54,55]. In addition, countries that have eliminated rabies in people often have dedicated and aggressive canine and feline rabies vaccination programs implemented through legal requirements on pet owners to vaccinate their animals. Indeed, the World Health Organization's strategy for eliminating human rabies in countries where it remains endemic is to eliminate it in dogs through mass vaccination campaigns [56].

While existing interventions for GWD have generally been successful in controlling the disease in human populations, they have been unsuccessful in halting transmission, as infections in animals have recently been detected in all of the remaining endemic countries. The increasing presence of animal infections suggests that improved adherence to existing interventions and/or new interventions targeting animals are necessary [2], especially given that people will likely be at risk so long as the parasite continues to infect animals. Zoonotic diseases, like GWD, may therefore benefit from strategies that explicitly integrate public health, veterinary medicine, animal management, and ecological approaches [57].

A renewed approach to eradicating GWD in affected countries can be achieved through a framework and set of targeted activities that improve disease surveillance in humans and animals; pinpoint the dominant routes of infection in animal hosts; elucidate the burden of disease in animals; determine risk factors for transmission among animals and from animals to humans; and identify practical ways to foster horizontal and multidisciplinary intervention approaches.

The eradication of GWD will require a holistic understanding of the burden of disease and the identification and containment of every case. While daunting, as mentioned earlier, this is necessary because humans and animals are infected by shared populations of Guinea worms, and as a result, humans be at risk for infections so long as the parasite continues to infect animals. This makes disease surveillance, case finding, and case containment a priority [58]. In Chad, a consistent pattern has been the discovery of dog infections with the expansion of active surveillance following identified human cases in new areas. For instance, after 13 human cases were detected in the Moyen-Chari region of Chad between 2010 and 2014, the initiation of active surveillance in 2015 uncovered hundreds of infected dogs in subsequent years; the region reported 409 dog infections in 2018 and 855 dog infections in 2019 [59,60]. A similar discovery may come to pass in Chad's Tandjile region, which only initiated active surveillance in 2019 following sporadic detection of human cases since 2011 [38]. Surveying communities about the year they first noticed worms emerging from dogs—and comparing responses to initiation of active surveillance programs—may provide further insights. Given the relative numbers, it seems more likely that transmission among dogs is driving cases in humans rather than vice-versa, and active surveillance with an equal focus on animal transmission should immediately follow the detection of human cases in new areas. Because dogs, unlike humans, are not able to report their own infections, exploratory surveillance efforts outside of areas known to be endemic should also be considered. These efforts should include periodic capture and examination of free-ranging and feral dogs in areas known to be endemic, as these animals may perpetuate transmission even when infections in domestic dogs are fully contained.

To this end, identifying practical ways to foster horizontal and multidisciplinary approaches could improve surveillance and control efforts. Coordinating interventions with other human and animal public health initiatives, and leveraging existing One Health efforts, represent opportunities to achieve this goal. For example, in Mali, NTD control efforts use predominantly vertical approaches, and while there is a One Health platform, it is not currently involved in the Guinea worm effort. Integrating surveillance activities in humans and animal populations could ensure more routine activities for both populations also help to ensure that GWD is not reintroduced to areas where it had previously been eliminated. Further, integrating NTD control programs with other health programs has proven to be a practical option for improving accountability, efficiency, and cost-effectiveness [61], and both of the human cases in Angola and Cameroon were initially recognized by healthcare workers who were involved in national immunization campaigns [27,35]. Future work should investigate the cost-effectiveness of current strategies, as well as that of new interventions to help determine which approaches for eradication are most appropriate for areas that remain at risk.

With regard to surveillance in animal populations, integrating Guinea worm and rabies could represent a feasible option, as some countries have robust rabies vaccination programs that could also be used to conduct Guinea worm infection exams. Integrating GWD control efforts with these initiatives may improve the reach, cost-effectiveness, and sustainability of surveillance for dog infections in particular, and may help flag areas endemic for animal transmission for expansion of both active surveillance and control interventions before human cases appear. Different levels of integration could include surveying rabies vaccination teams for reports of rumored dog infections; training rabies teams to identify symptoms, report infections, and inform dog owners about reward money; or, most intensively, providing rabies field staff with sample collection tubes and reward money for identifying confirmed infections in areas beyond the reach of active surveillance. Further, for countries that do not have robust rabies control programs, integrating GWD and rabies control efforts could incentivize collaboration between veterinary and human health departments and correspondingly improve rabies vaccination rates—which would benefit both GWD and rabies control efforts.

Beyond simply detecting infections, understanding relevant risk factors for transmission and how transmission is occurring among dogs, cats, and other animal species would allow for the implementation of timely and more effective control measures. It is possible that animals, and in particular dogs, are exposed to Guinea worm infection by both foodborne and waterborne routes of transmission, or through some combination that amplifies infection in non-human hosts [19]. Although recent research efforts have focused on possible infection of dogs via consumption of raw or undercooked paratenic hosts infected with the parasite [15,20], targeted searches revealed a very low prevalence of infection among frogs and no Guinea worms detected in dissected fish [62]. This may point to waterborne transmission as the dominant route of infection in dogs [17]. This is especially true when comparing against the high infection rates among dogs in the villages in which the fish and frogs were obtained and the frequency of frog consumption among dogs. This hypothesis may also be supported by the observation of year-over-year clusters of worm emergence during short periods of time, due to staggered ingestion of infected paratenic hosts. Examining dog infection line lists may provide further clues and the continued evaluation of transmission routes could help refine or devise interventions [42]. Different approaches may also be required for different animal populations (e.g., domestic versus free-ranging dogs) and it will be important to identify risk factors to inform control efforts [19]. Community surveys about the presence of free-ranging or feral dogs, or wild dogs and cats, in endemic areas could also inform approaches and help to elucidate whether or to what extent these populations play a role in sustaining transmission.

Eradication of any infectious disease requires simple diagnostics, simple preventives and/or treatments, and political will. The growing scientific understanding of the zoonotic capacity of Guinea worm underscores the importance of diagnosis in non-human hosts. Diagnosis is key to enabling proper epidemiological understanding and to inform prevention and treatment decisions. At present, diagnosis in dogs is done in the same manner as for people (i.e., visual detection of the worm at the skin surface). This diagnostic approach allows for detection only at a very late stage of infection. A field-based rapid diagnostic assay such as antibody serology to assess pre-patent infection in dogs could support improved understanding of canine prevalence, and intervention decisions like proactive tethering. Hand-held ultrasound machines, frequently used in equine medicine, could also be used to detect the worms in advance of emergence. Identified infected dogs could then be prioritized by monitoring programs through routine checks for worm emergence. Some of the worms identified on ultrasound could potentially be removed surgically by qualified personnel, such as spay-neuter teams, where such resources are available. Improved diagnostics when combined with an interdisciplinary research and surveillance approach could shift the research paradigm toward a more comprehensive understanding of infection prevalence in other animals. For a less technical approach, routine spot-checks of dogs for signs of worm emergence, either conducted by program staff or owners, may increase early detection and containment of Guinea worms.

Similarly, new tools for environmental surveillance could be useful for targeting limited health education and surveillance resources toward communities and at highest risk. An assay developed to amplify Guinea worm DNA successfully identified larvae from infected copepods present in samples of pond water taken from Chad [63]. While such a tool could potentially shed light on the temporal and spatial distribution of larvae in the environment, a field-informed sampling strategy and a close collaboration with community health workers and water treatment teams would be needed to operationalize the results.

Community responses, participation in, and behavior change stemming from these activities should also be monitored [64], as such considerations will impact overall intervention effectiveness and could allow for eradication programs to tailor intervention strategies to specific sub-populations. For instance, monthly spot-checks of fish entrail burial sites have been conducted in villages under active surveillance in Chad since 2015, with consistent reports of high adherence [27,43,46]. If fish entrail burial is not associated with reductions in animal infections, further analysis of related human and animal behaviors may uncover alternate, more effective interventions, or suggest a different primary route of infection.

Beyond One Health, other aspects that require multisectoral approaches also challenge eradication efforts. For instance, conflict and migration present challenges for containing any infectious disease, but have notably hindered surveillance and control efforts for Guinea worm in both human and animal populations [12]. A new human case in Mali in 2020, the first in four years, may indicate conflict-related surveillance gaps [65]. In the Malian context, insecurity has also limited program operations in regions of the country where dogs are bred and become infected before being transported to other areas [36]. The Guinea Worm Eradication Program of South Sudan is taking action to address some of these challenges by tracking the migratory patterns of individuals associated with cattle camps, which characterized the Guinea worm cases in 2018 [59]. Similar efforts may prove beneficial in Chad, where dogs and humans seasonally migrate to fishing grounds, and where tracking these patterns may help identify new areas of endemicity.

5. Conclusions

The decades-long effort to eradicate GWD has been delayed as a result of contextual challenges but also because infections in non-human animal species are complicating control efforts. While existing strategies and interventions have achieved impressive decreases in human GWD cases, an apparent epidemiological shift occurred over the past decade whereby the largest burden of GWD shifted from human populations to animals. Although this shift likely reflects changes in surveillance and not novel transmission patterns in other species, it underscores the importance of embracing new approaches if the goal of eradicating GWD is to be realized. Accordingly, a One Health approach that seeks to improve surveillance efforts in human and animal populations, elucidate the burden of disease in animal populations, identify risk factors for transmission among human and animal populations, and foster horizontal and multidisciplinary interventions could represent one way to reach the elusive but attainable goal of eradicating GWD in humans and animals.

Author Contributions: Conceptualization, M.R.B. and C.J.S.; methodology, M.R.B, E.P.C., and C.J.S.; validation, E.P.C. and J.S.; resources, M.R.B. and E.P.C.; data curation, M.R.B. and J.S.; writing—original draft preparation, M.R.B., E.P.C.; writing—review and editing, M.R.B, E.P.C., J.S., and C.J.S.; visualization, M.R.B.; supervision, C.J.S. All authors have read and agreed to the published version of the manuscript.

References

1. Greenaway, C. Dracunculiasis (guinea worm disease). *CMAJ* **2004**, *170*, 495–500.
2. Beyene, H.B.; Bekele, A.; Shifara, A.; Ebstie, Y.A.; Desalegn, Z.; Kebede, Z.; Mulugeta, A.; Deribe, K.; Tadesse, Z.; Abebe, T.; et al. Elimination of Guinea Worm Disease in Ethiopia; Current Status of the Disease's, Eradication Strategies and Challenges to the End Game. *Ethiop. Med. J.* **2017**, *55*, 15–31. [PubMed]
3. Cairncross, S.; Muller, R.; Zagaria, N. Dracunculiasis (Guinea Worm Disease) and the Eradication Initiative. *Clin. Microbiol. Rev.* **2002**, *15*, 223–246. [CrossRef] [PubMed]
4. Biswas, G.; Sankara, D.P.; Agua-Agum, J.; Maiga, A. Dracunculiasis (guinea worm disease): Eradication without a drug or a vaccine. *Phil. Trans. R. Soc. B* **2013**, *368*, 20120146. [CrossRef] [PubMed]
5. Belcher, D. Opportunities for control of dracunculiasis: Transmission and epidemiology. In *Workshop on Opportunities for Control of Dracunculiasis*; National Academy Press: Washington, DC, USA, 1985; pp. 1–7.
6. Cook, G.; Zumla, A. *Manson's Tropical Diseases*, 22nd ed.; Elsevier: Philadelphia, PA, USA, 2009.
7. Muller, R. Guinea worm disease: Epidemiology, control, and treatment. *Bull. World Health Organ.* **1979**, *57*, 683.
8. Hopkins, D.R.; Ruiz-Tiben, E.; Eberhard, M.L.; Roy, S.L.; Weiss, A.J. Progress Toward Global Eradication of Dracunculiasis, January 2016–June 2017. *MMWR* **2017**, *66*, 1327–1331. [CrossRef]
9. World Health Organization. Dracunculiasis (Guinea-Worm Disease). Available online: https://www.who.int/dracunculiasis/portal/en/ (accessed on 12 March 2020).
10. Roberts, L. Battle to wipe out Guinea worm stumbles. *Nature* **2019**, *574*, 157–158. [CrossRef]
11. Galán-Puchades, M.T. WHO delays guinea-worm disease eradication to 2020: Are dogs the sole culprits? *Lancet* **2017**, *17*, 1124–1125. [CrossRef]
12. Hopkins, D.R.; Ruiz-Tiben, E.; Eberhard, M.L.; Roy, S.L. Progress toward Global Eradication of Dracunculiasis, January 2013–June 2014. *MMWR* **2014**, *63*, 1150–1154.
13. Thiele, E.A.; Eberhard, M.L.; Cotton, J.A.; Durrant, C.; Berg, J.; Hamm, K.; Ruiz-Tiben, E. Population genetic analysis of Chadian Guinea worms reveals that human and non-human hosts share common parasite populations. *PLoS Negl. Trop. Dis.* **2018**, *12*, e0006747. [CrossRef]
14. Callaway, E. Dogs thwart effort to eradicate Guinea worm. *Nature* **2016**, *529*, 10–11. [CrossRef]
15. Eberhard, M.L.; Ruiz-Tiben, E.; Hopkins, D.R.; Farrell, C.; Toe, F.; Weiss, A.; Withers, P.C., Jr.; Jenks, M.H.; Thiele, E.A.; Cotton, J.A.; et al. The Peculiar Epidemiology of Dracunculiasis in Chad. *Am. J. Trop. Med. Hyg.* **2014**, *90*, 61–70. [CrossRef] [PubMed]
16. Eberhard, M.L.; Cleveland, C.A.; Zirimwabagabo, H.; Yabsley, M.J.; Ouakou, P.T.; Ruiz-Tiben, E. Guinea Worm (*Dracunculus medinensis*) Infection in a Wild-Caught Frog, Chad. *Emerg. Infect. Dis.* **2016**, *22*, 1961–1962. [CrossRef]
17. Galán-Puchades, M.T. Dracunculiasis: Water-borne anthroponosis vs. food-borne zoonosis. *J. Helminthol.* **2019**, *94*. [CrossRef] [PubMed]

18. Hopkins, D.R.; Ruiz-Tiben, E.; Eberhard, M.L.; Weiss, A.; Withers, P.C., Jr.; Roy, S.L.; Sienko, D.G. Dracunculiasis Eradication: Are We There Yet? *Am. J. Trop. Med. Hyg.* **2018**, *99*, 388–395. [CrossRef]
19. McDonald, R.A.; Wilson-Aggarwal, J.K.; Swan, G.J.F.; Goodwin, C.E.D.; Moundai, T.; Sankara, D.; Biswas, G.; Zingeser, J.A. Ecology of domestic dogs Canis familiaris as an emerging reservoir of Guinea worm Dracunculus medinensis infection. *PLoS Negl. Trop. Dis.* **2020**, *14*, e0008170. [CrossRef]
20. Molyneux, D.; Sankara, D.P. Guinea worm eradication: Progress and challenges—Should we beware of the dog? *PLoS Negl. Trop. Dis.* **2017**, *11*, e0005495. [CrossRef] [PubMed]
21. Cleveland, C.A.; Eberhard, M.L.; Thompson, A.T.; Smith, S.J.; Zirimwabagabo, H.; Bringolf, R.; Yabsley, M.J. Possible Role of Fish as Transport Hosts for *Dracunculus* spp. Larvae. *Emerg. Infect. Dis.* **2017**, *23*, 1590–1592. [CrossRef]
22. Karesh, W.B.; Cook, R.A. The Human-Animal Link. *Foreign Aff.* **2005**, *84*, 38–50. [CrossRef]
23. Lee, K.; Brumme, Z.L. Operationalizing the One Health approach: The global governance challenges. *Health Policy Plan.* **2013**, *28*, 778–785. [CrossRef]
24. The Carter Center. Guinea Worm Wrap-Up. Available online: https://www.cartercenter.org/news/publications/health/guinea_worm_wrapup_english.html (accessed on 12 March 2020).
25. The Carter Center. *Guinea Worm Wrap-Up, #222*; The Carter Center: Atlanta, GA, USA, 2013; pp. 1–20.
26. The Carter Center. *Guinea Worm Wrap-Up, #223*; The Carter Center: Atlanta, GA, USA, 2014; pp. 1–8.
27. The Carter Center. *Guinea Worm Wrap-Up, #262*; The Carter Center: Atlanta, GA, USA, 2019; pp. 1–10.
28. The Carter Center. *Guinea Worm Wrap-Up, #238*; The Carter Center: Atlanta, GA, USA, 2016; pp. 1–12.
29. Wilson-Aggarwal, J.K.; Goodwin, C.E.D.; Swan, G.J.F.; Fielding, H.; Tadesse, Z.; Getahun, D.; Odiel, A.; Adam, A.; Marshall, H.H.; Bryant, J.; et al. Ecology of domestic dogs (*Canis familiaris*) as a host for Guinea worm (*Dracunculus medinensis*) infection in Ethiopia. *Transbound. Emerg. Dis.* **2020**. [CrossRef] [PubMed]
30. The Carter Center. *Guinea Worm Wrap-Up, #265*; The Carter Center: Atlanta, GA, USA, 2020; pp. 1–8.
31. The Carter Center. *Guinea Worm Wrap-Up, #263*; The Carter Center: Atlanta, GA, USA, 2019; pp. 1–13.
32. The Carter Center. *Guinea Worm Wrap-Up, #231*; The Carter Center: Atlanta, GA, USA, 2015; pp. 1–21.
33. The Carter Center. *Guinea Worm Wrap-Up, #235*; The Carter Center: Atlanta, GA, USA, 2015; pp. 1–16.
34. The Carter Center. *Guinea Worm Wrap-Up, #246*; The Carter Center: Atlanta, GA, USA, 2017; pp. 1–10.
35. The Carter Center. *Guinea Worm Wrap-Up, #252*; The Carter Center: Atlanta, GA, USA, 2018; pp. 1–18.
36. The Carter Center. *Guinea Worm Wrap-Up, #256*; The Carter Center: Atlanta, GA, USA, 2019; pp. 1–13.
37. Callahan, K.; Bolton, B.; Hopkins, D.R.; Ruiz-Tiben, E.; Withers, P.C.; Meagley, K. Contributions of the Guinea Worm Disease Eradication Campaign toward Achievement of the Millennium Development Goals. *PLoS Negl. Trop. Dis.* **2013**, *7*, e2160. [CrossRef]
38. The Carter Center. *Guinea Worm Wrap-up, #261*; The Carter Center: Atlanta, GA, USA, 2019; pp. 1–9.
39. Brieger, W.; Otusanya, S.; Adeniyi, D.; Tijani, J.; Banjoko, M. Eradicating guinea worm without wells: Unrealized hopes of the water decade. *Health Policy Plan.* **1997**, *12*, 354–362. [CrossRef] [PubMed]
40. Hopkins, D.R.; Ruiz-Tiben, E. Dracunculiasis (Guinea Worm Disease): Case Study of the Effort to Eradicate Guinea Worm. In *Water and Sanitation-Related Diseases and the Environment: Challenges, Interventions, and Preventive Measures*, 1st ed.; Selendy, J.M.H., Ed.; Wiley-Blackwell: Hoboken, NJ, USA, 2011; pp. 125–132.
41. Hopkins, D.R.; Ruiz-Tiben, E.; Eberhard, M.L.; Roy, S.L. Progress toward Global Eradication of Dracunculiasis, January 2014–June 2015. *MMWR* **2015**, *64*, 1161–1165. [CrossRef] [PubMed]
42. Garrett, K.B.; Box, E.K.; Cleveland, C.A.; Majewska, A.A.; Yabsley, M.J. Dogs and the classic route of Guinea Worm transmission: An evaluation of copepod ingestion. *Sci. Rep.* **2020**, *10*, 1430. [CrossRef]
43. The Carter Center. *Guinea Worm Wrap-Up, #257*; The Carter Center: Atlanta, GA, USA, 2018; pp. 1–16.
44. The Carter Center. *Guinea Worm Wrap-Up, #247*; The Carter Center: Atlanta, GA, USA, 2017; pp. 1–10.
45. The Carter Center. *Guinea Worm Wrap-Up, #259*; The Carter Center: Atlanta, GA, USA, 2019; pp. 1–13.
46. The Carter Center. *Guinea Worm Wrap-Up, #237*; The Carter Center: Atlanta, GA, USA, 2015; pp. 1–13.
47. The Carter Center. *Guinea Worm Wrap-Up, #244*; The Carter Center: Atlanta, GA, USA, 2016; pp. 1–13.
48. The Carter Center. *Guinea Worm Wrap-Up, #245*; The Carter Center: Atlanta, GA, USA, 2017; pp. 1–13.
49. The Carter Center. *Guinea Worm Wrap-Up, #254*; The Carter Center: Atlanta, GA, USA, 2018; pp. 1–9.
50. The Carter Center. *Guinea Worm Wrap-Up, #264*; The Carter Center: Atlanta, GA, USA, 2019; pp. 1–13.
51. Woolhouse, M.E.; Gowtage-Sequeria, S. Host range and emerging and reemerging pathogens. *Emerg. Infect. Dis.* **2005**, *11*, 1842–1847. [CrossRef]
52. Dowdle, W.R. The Principles of Disease Elimination and Eradication. *MMWR* **1999**, *48*, 23–27.

53. McGuinness, S.L.; Leder, K. Global burden of Toxocariasis: A common neglected infection of poverty. *Curr. Trop. Med. Rep.* **2014**, *1*, 52–61. [CrossRef]
54. Etheart, M.D.; Kligerman, M.; Augustin, P.D.; Blanton, J.D.; Monroe, B.; Fleurinord, L.; Millien, M.; Crowdis, K.; Fenelon, N.; Wallace, R.M. Effect of counselling on health-care-seeking behaviours and rabies vaccination adherence after dog bites in Haiti, 2014–2015: A retrospective follow-up survey. *Lancet Glob. Health* **2017**, *5*, e1017–e1025. [CrossRef]
55. Lushasi, K.; Steenson, R.; Bernard, J.; Changalucha, J.J.; Govella, N.J.; Haydon, D.T.; Hoffu, H.; Lankester, F.; Magoti, F.; Mpolya, E.A.; et al. One Health in Practice: Using Integrated Bite Case Management to Increase Detection of Rabid Animals in Tanzania. *Front. Public Health* **2020**, *8*, 13. [CrossRef]
56. World Health Organization. *Rabies: Rationale for Investing in the Global Elimination of Dog-Mediated Human Rabies*; World Health Organization: Geneva, Switzerland, 2015; pp. 1–30.
57. Cunningham, A.A.; Daszak, P.; Wood, J.L.N. One Health, emerging infectious diseases and wildlife: Two decades of progress? *Phil. Trans. R. Soc. B* **2017**, *372*, 20160167. [CrossRef] [PubMed]
58. Buyon, L.; Slaven, R.; Emerson, P.M.; King, J.; Debrah, O.; Aboe, A.; Ruiz-Tiben, E.; Callahan, E.K. Achieving the endgame: Integrated NTD case searches. *PLoS Negl. Trop. Dis.* **2018**, *12*, e0006623. [CrossRef]
59. The Carter Center. *Guinea Worm Wrap-Up, #260*; The Carter Center: Atlanta, GA, USA, 2019; pp. 1–12.
60. The Carter Center. *Guinea Worm Wrap-Up, #266*; The Carter Center: Atlanta, GA, USA, 2020; pp. 1–8.
61. Standley, C.; Boyce, M.R.; Klineberg, A.; Essix, G.; Katz, R. Organization of oversight for integrated control of neglected tropical diseases within Ministries of Health. *PLoS Negl. Trop. Dis.* **2018**, *12*, e0006929. [CrossRef] [PubMed]
62. Cleveland, C.A.; Eberhard, M.L.; Thompson, A.T.; Garrett, K.B.; Swanepoel, L.; Zirimwabagabo, H.; Moundai, T.; Ouakou, P.T.; Ruiz-Tiben, E.; Yabsley, M.J. A search for tiny dragons (*Dracunculus medinensis* third-stage larvae) in aquatic animals in Chad, Africa. *Sci. Rep.* **2019**, *9*, 375. [CrossRef] [PubMed]
63. Boonham, N.; Tomlinson, J.; Ostoja-Starzewska, S.; McDonald, R. A pond-side test for Guinea worm: Development of a loop-mediated isothermal amplification (LAMP) assay for detection of *Dracunculiasis medinensis*. *Exp. Parasitol.* **2020**, *217*, 107960. [CrossRef]
64. Bardosh, K. Global aspirations, local realities: The role of social science research in controlling neglected tropical diseases. *Infect. Dis. Poverty* **2014**, *3*, 35. [CrossRef] [PubMed]
65. The Carter Center. *Guinea Worm Wrap-Up, #268*; The Carter Center: Atlanta, GA, USA, 2020; pp. 1–12.

8

Lymphatic Filariasis in Mainland Southeast Asia: A Systematic Review and Meta-Analysis of Prevalence and Disease Burden

Benjamin F. R. Dickson [1,*], Patricia M. Graves [2] and William J. McBride [3]

1 College of Medicine & Dentistry, James Cook University, Cairns, QLD 4870, Australia
2 College of Public Health, Medical and Veterinary Sciences, James Cook University, Cairns, QLD 4870, Australia; patricia.graves@jcu.edu.au
3 College of Medicine & Dentistry, James Cook University, Cairns, QLD 4870, Australia; john.mcbride@jcu.edu.au
* Correspondence: benjamin.dickson@my.jcu.edu.au;

Abstract: Accurate prevalence data are essential for the elimination of lymphatic filariasis (LF) as a public health problem. Despite it bearing one of the highest burdens of disease globally, there remains limited reliable information on the current epidemiology of filariasis in mainland Southeast Asia. We conducted a systematic review and meta-analysis of available literature to assess the recent and current prevalence of infection and morbidity in the region. Fifty-seven journal articles and reports containing original prevalence data were identified, including over 512,010 participants. Data were summarised using percentage prevalence estimates and a subset combined using a random effects meta-analysis by country and year. Pooled estimates for microfilaraemia, immunochromatographic card positivity and combined morbidity were 2.64%, 4.48% and 1.34% respectively. Taking into account pooled country estimates, grey literature and the quality of available data, we conclude that Lao People's Democratic Republic (PDR), Myanmar and Northeast India demonstrate ongoing evidence of LF transmission that will require multiple further rounds of mass drug administration. Bangladesh, Malaysia, Thailand and Vietnam appear close to having eliminated LF, whilst Cambodia has already achieved elimination status. We estimate that the burden of morbidity is likely high in Thailand; moderate in Cambodia, Myanmar, and Northeast India; and low in Bangladesh. There was insufficient evidence to accurately estimate the disease burden in Lao PDR, Malaysia or Vietnam. The results of this study indicate that whilst considerable progress toward LF elimination has been made, there remains a significant filariasis burden in the region. The results of this study will assist policy makers to advocate and budget for future control programs.

Keywords: lymphatic filariasis; Southeast Asia; prevalence; infection; morbidity; lymphoedema; hydrocoele

1. Introduction

Lymphatic filariasis (LF) is a mosquito-borne tropical disease that affects 67.88 million people in 73 countries worldwide [1–3]. It is caused by infection with the nematodes *Wuchereria bancrofti (Wb)*, *Brugia malayi (Bm)* or *Brugia timori*. Chronic infection causes lymphatic dysfunction, resulting in severe morbidity from progressive, irreversible swelling of the limbs and genitals. LF is a significant cause of permanent disability worldwide, accounting for an estimated 19.43 million cases of hydrocoele, 16.68 million cases of lymphoedema and 2.02 million disability-adjusted life years lost [3,4].

In recognition of the significant worldwide burden of LF, the World Health Organization (WHO) established the Global Program to Eliminate LF (GPELF) calling for the elimination of LF by 2020 [1,5]. The program adopted a two-pronged approach: first, interrupt transmission through annual single-dose mass drug administration (MDA) of entire at-risk populations with albendazole in combination with either diethylcarbamazine (DEC) or ivermectin for a minimum of five years; and, second, alleviate the significant morbidity burden associated with the disease.

Numerous methods are currently used to diagnose LF infection. Traditionally, thick blood smears (TBS) were used to identify microfilaraemia (mf) in the peripheral circulation. TBS have now been largely superseded by more sensitive antigen-based tests but are still used as a measure of potential infectivity and ongoing transmission. Antigen tests include immunochromatographic card tests (ICT) and Og4C3 enzyme-linked immunosorbent assays (ELISA) which use monoclonal antibodies to detect the excretory-secretory antigens produced by adult filarial worm infection [6,7]. Because they detect a different stage of the life-cycle and do not require adult worms to be producing microfilariae, they are two- to fivefold more sensitive than TBS [8]. Antibody-based tests detect circulating IgG4 antibodies against Bm14 antigen (*B. malayi* and *W. bancrofti)* or BmR1 (*B. malayi* only) [9]. Whilst highly sensitive and specific, antibody prevalence cannot prove current infection because antibodies remain elevated for many years after treatment [9]. Urinary antibody tests have been trialled but are less sensitive than blood-based antibody tests [8,10]. PCR assays to detect LF DNA in humans are also available, but are not used routinely because they require advanced laboratory facilities and are less sensitive than other methods [8,10].

LF is endemic in all countries within mainland Southeast Asia [1,2,5]. The geographical region spans both the WHO Southeast Asia and Western Pacific regions and includes Cambodia, Lao People's Democratic Republic (PDR), Myanmar, Thailand, Vietnam and Malaysia. Emerging data suggest a possibly high prevalence of filariasis in Myanmar. Given the country's significant shared border with Northeast India and Bangladesh, both were also included.

The WHO Southeast Asia and Western Pacific regions account for 55.7% of the at-risk population, with 94.6% of reported lymphoedema cases and 85.2% of reported hydrocoele cases globally [2]. The areas considered here (mainland Southeast Asia plus Northeast India and Bangladesh) account for over a fifth of the population of these two regions. Elimination of LF in this area would therefore have a significant impact on the global disease burden. LF in these countries is caused by *W. Bancrofti* and *B. malayi*, and transmitted mainly by *Culex quinquefasciatus*, with some contribution by *Aedes* spp. and *Mansonia* spp. mosquitoes [11].

All countries in this review have commenced elimination programs. Elimination as a public health problem has been validated in Cambodia, whilst Bangladesh, Thailand and Vietnam have transitioned to post-MDA surveillance. The remaining countries are still conducting MDA [1,2,5].

WHO country validation of 'elimination of LF as a public health problem' requires a set of surveys and steps to determine whether the prevalence is below the target level (upper 95% CI of 2% in *Culex* spp. transmission areas such as Southeast Asia) [12]. One important milestone is the passing of three consecutive transmission assessment surveys (TAS) conducted on six- to seven-year-old children in each defined geographical evaluation unit (EU). The TAS survey sets critical cut-off values for the number of positive children that must not be exceeded for the EU to pass [13]. The sample sizes and critical cut-off values for the TAS in *Culex* spp. transmission areas are designed so that an EU has (1) at least a 75% chance of passing if the true prevalence of antigenaemia is 1.0% (half the target level); and (2) no more than a 5% chance of incorrectly passing if the true prevalence of antigenaemia is $\geq$2% [13].

Despite the significant LF burden in this region, there remain limited reliable data on the current prevalence of infection and morbidity. Whilst previous reviews have examined this topic, all are significantly out-dated or incomplete [14–16]. Reliable, current data on the prevalence of LF are required for the implementation and evaluation of elimination programs as well as future advocacy efforts. Accordingly, we conducted a systematic review and meta-analysis of publicly-available data in studies and grey literature to assess the recent (since the early 1990s) and current prevalence of LF infection and morbidity in mainland Southeast Asia, Bangladesh and Northeast India.

2. Materials and Methods

2.1. Protocol

This systematic review is reported using the Preferred Reporting Items for Systematic Reviews and Meta-Analysis (PRISMA) guidelines [17]. A review protocol was registered with PROSPERO international prospective register of systematic reviews, which can be viewed online [18].

2.2. Information Sources

Information was gathered through three sources: (1) a literature search of PubMed and MEDLINE databases; (2) a web-based search of the WHO library for relevant publications; and (3) direct contact with regional and national LF Program directors to obtain National LF Program reports [19]. Countries with National LF Programs submit annual reports to their respective WHO regional office outlining their MDA and surveying activities for the preceding year. A summary of the data is published annually in a regional WHO meeting report. Reference lists of all papers were screened to identify additional publications.

2.3. Search Strategy

A literature search was conducted for available publications on PubMed and MEDLINE via OvidSP up until 11 December 2016 by one investigator. The search strategy used for both databases was: (lymphatic filariasis or Wuchereria bancrofti or Brugia timori or Brugia malayi or lymphoedema or hydrocoele or elephantiasis or microfilariae or microfilaraemia) AND ((Myanmar or Burma or Thailand or Laos or Cambodia or Vietnam or Malaysia or Bangladesh) OR (India and Assam or Meghalaya or Nagaland or Manipur or Tripura or Mizoram or Arunachal Pradesh)). Combinations of the database search terms were used to search the WHO library.

2.4. Study Selection and Inclusion Criteria

The titles, abstracts and if indicated, full text of records from online databases and the WHO library (IRIS) were screened for eligibility. Published studies and reports with original prevalence data on LF infection or morbidity from identified countries were included. Where reports were not available, WHO publications referencing their data were used and recorded.

Only literature available in English and published from 1995 onward was included. There were no restrictions on age, study size, design or power. Any uncertainty regarding the inclusion of a paper was resolved through consensus discussion with other authors.

2.5. Data Collection Process

A standardised data collection form was used to record information from included publications. All data was then entered into a Microsoft Excel spreadsheet for analysis.

2.6. Data Items

Extracted data included study characteristics, sampling method and prevalence data. Data were extracted directly from text and tables within the publications.

Primary outcomes were the prevalence of infection (including measurement method and species) and chronic morbidity (lymphoedema or hydrocoele) in the given population.

Where interventional studies were included, the prevalence data that were most representative of the population were used. That is, when a whole area participated in MDA external to the study, the post-intervention data were used. When an intervention was implemented only on the study sample, baseline data were used.

2.7. *Risk of Bias Assessment*

A modified bias risk assessment tool was developed to evaluate included studies. It was based on the Crowe and GATE validated critical appraisal tools [20,21]. Risk of bias was assessed by one reviewer on the basis of five independent factors: total sample size (>1000, 300–1000 or <300), sampling of location (representative randomisation, not stated/unclear or non-representative), sampling of participants (representative randomisation, not stated/unclear or non-representative), assessment of infection (internationally accepted methodology, not stated/unclear or non-consensus methods) and assessment of morbidity (independently assessed, not stated/unclear or patient reported). A total risk of bias score was generated by allocating zero, one or two points for each factor. The quality assessment was used to interpret the reliability of each study's results. Because of the limited number and significant quality variation between studies, the bias assessment was not incorporated directly into the meta-analysis.

WHO filariasis publications are based on national LF programs annual reports. WHO Regional Program Review Groups (RPRG) assess annual national LF program surveillance reports during their consideration of the country's request for the donation of MDA drugs. Although general guidelines are provided by WHO, methodology within countries frequently varies substantially and may not be optimal due to poorly resourced programs and frequent personnel changes [22]. Independent assessments of data quality within programs are rarely done.

2.8. *Summary Measures and Synthesis of Results*

Available data were summarised using percentage prevalence estimates and presented in tables by country and region.

A meta-analysis of primary outcomes from studies was completed using the *metaprop* procedure in STATA version 12.1 to produce overall estimates with exact binomial confidence intervals. A subset meta-analysis of migrant workers in Thailand and India was also done. A random effects model was used to account for the variation in LF prevalence between and within studies.Weighting of studies was done using the method of DerSimonian and Laird [23]. The heterogeneity of data from each meta-analysis was measured using the I^2 statistic [24].

A map of baseline and most recent LF distribution was generated by combining government prevalence maps found in grey literature. Endemicity was classified at implementation unit level by all countries. Recent maps were available for all countries except Malaysia.

3. Results

3.1. *Study Selection*

The search protocol identified 629 papers (Figure 1). Of these, 554 clearly did not meet the inclusion criteria (i.e., were review articles or did not include original prevalence data on infection or morbidity published since 1995 from the identified areas). From the remaining 75 records, 17 were excluded because they did not contain original prevalence data, and one because the full text was not available after contacting the author. The included 57 papers comprised 38 peer-reviewed journal articles and 19 grey literature reports [5,25–79]. With the exception of Chansiri et al. [30], which contained only polymerase-chain reaction (PCR) infection data, all studies were included in the meta-analysis.

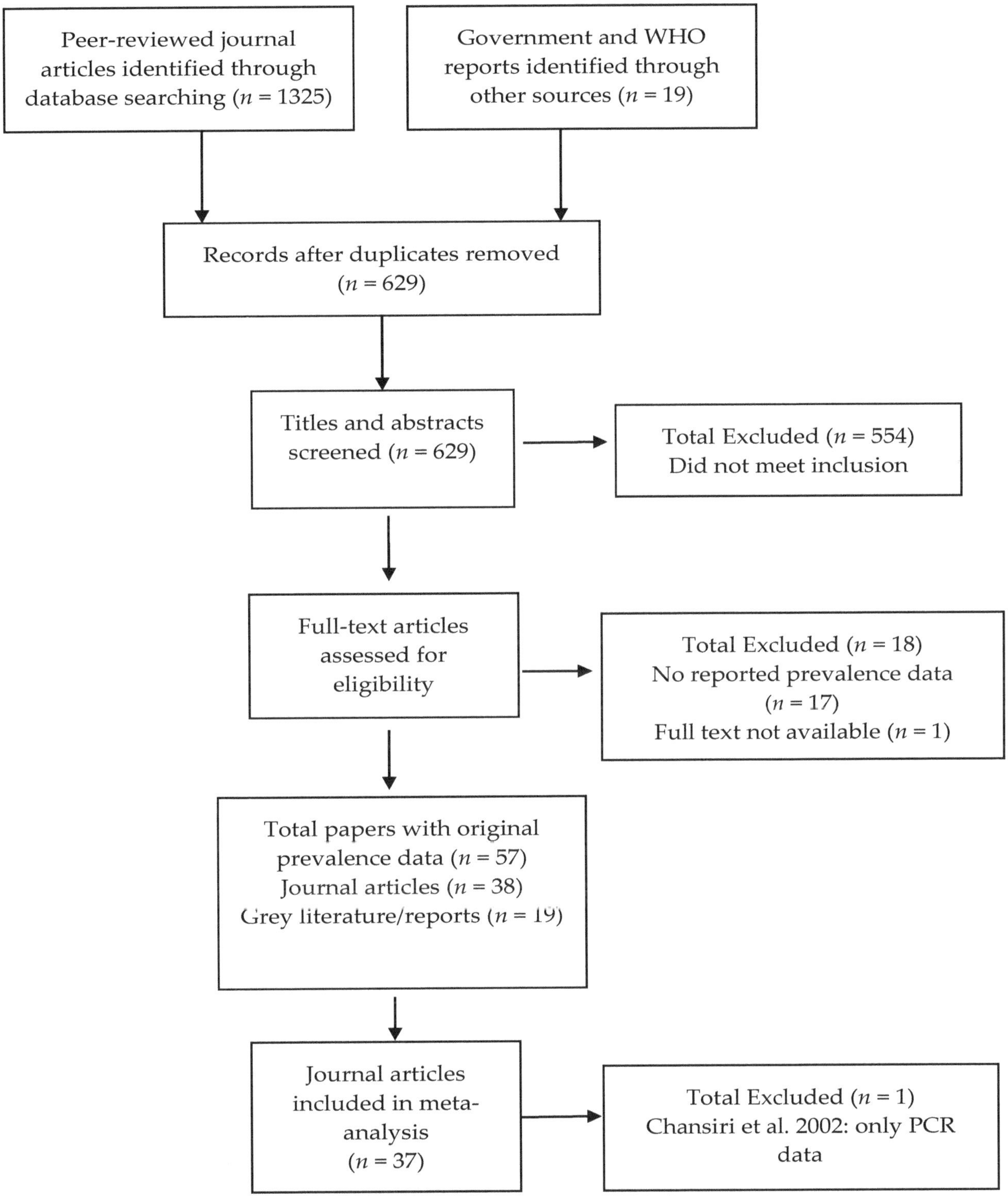

Figure 1. Study selection flow chart.

3.2. *Study Characteristics*

The characteristics of the 38 included journal articles are summarised by country in Table 1. This includes 17 from Thailand, eight each from Malaysia and Northeast India, three from Bangladesh and two from Cambodia. There were no studies included from Lao PDR, Myanmar or Vietnam.

All articles described primary studies, and included cross-sectional surveys (CSS) (25 studies, 66%), field diagnostic test evaluation studies (FDE) (8, 21%), field drug trials (FDT) (3, 8%) as well as a longitudinal observational and a retrospective cohort study. Publication year ranged from 1995 to 2016.

Together the included studies assessed 382,274 participants with wide variation in sampling unit and sample size (145 to 232,005). Two studies, Saha et al. (2011) and Krairittichai et al. (2012), contributed substantially to overall participant numbers with sample sizes of 232,005 and 102,090, respectively [44,55]. Eleven of the 17 studies from Thailand assessed Myanmar migrant populations, whilst seven of the eight papers from Northeast India examined those living in tea estates.

Studies most frequently assessed infection with the traditional thick blood smear (TBS) method (30 studies, 79%), followed by ICT (10, 26%), IgG4 antibody (10, 26%), Og4C3 ELISA (6, 16%) and PCR (3, 8%) tests. One study used urine rather than blood to detect IgG4 antibodies [56]. Almost half of the studies (16, 42%) used multiple methods. Sixteen studies assessed the prevalence of chronic LF morbidity. Of these, seven (44%) assessed both hydrocoele and lymphoedema.

Table 2 summarises the characteristics of the 19 included grey literature reports. These include 15 WHO publications, three annual national programmatic reports and a report from a non-governmental organisation.With the exception of one WHO report, all papers summarise data from government prevalence surveys conducted as part of their national MDA programs. Whilst only some sample sizes were reported, at least 129,736 individuals were surveyed. Baseline mapping and MDA surveillance surveys predominantly used TBS to diagnose infection, whilst post-MDA TASs used ICT.Some government morbidity information was available for all countries, but the data were very limited.

3.3. Risk of Bias within Studies

The risk of bias assessment of included studies is summarised in Table S1. Overall, study quality was suboptimal. Only seven studies (18%) used fully representative sampling methods and consensus data collection methods.

The sample sizes of published studies were overall acceptable, with 33 studies including greater than 300 participants. However, sample sizes were generally small relative to government surveys.

The sampling of study location introduced a significant risk of bias. Only ten (26%) studies adequately described the random site selection required for regionally representative data. Of the remaining studies, 21 (55%) did not describe the method/reason for study site selection, and seven (18%) intentionally selected study sites.

Participant sampling within study locations also contributed to risk of bias. Only 18 (47%) studies described random participant selection. Eighteen (47%) studies did not clearly state the method of selection, whilst the remaining two studies excluded those with recent diethylcarbamazine treatment.

With the exception of Chansiri et al., all studies used a consensus method for the detection of LF infection [30]. It is unclear whether the TBS samples in Krairittichai et al. were taken at night, which may have affected the sensitivity of their results [44].

Of the fifteen studies that assessed LF morbidity, only four (25%) described examination methods in detail. Of the remaining papers, eight (50%) provided some detail and four (25%) did not state the method used.

Table 1. Included peer-reviewed journal articles.

Study (Publication Date) [Study Period] [Ref.]	Study Design	Sampling Population/Unit (Age of Participants)	Sample Size	Diagnostic Method	
				Infection	Morbidity
		Bangladesh			
Hafiz et al. (2015) (2011) [33]	CSS [a]	Households in 30 villages (≥10)	1242	Mf, ICT	Hyd./Lymph. [h]
Saha et al. (2011) [NS [g]] [55]	CSS	Households in 19 unions (≥1)	232,005	-	Lymph.
Samad et al. (2013) [NS] [56]	FDE [d]	School children (5–10)	319	ICT, IgG4 [e]	-
		Cambodia			
Leang et al. (2004) (2000–2001) [45]	CSS	83 villages (≥1)	3468	Mf, ICT	Hyd./Lymph.
Priest et al. (2016) (2012) [52]	CSS	2200 households (women 15–39)	2150	IgG4	-
		Northeast India			
Dutta et al. (1995) (1992) [32]	CSS	Individuals in 1 tea estate (≥1)	1553	Mf	NS
Khan et al. (1999) [NS] Study 1 [37]	CSS	Individuals in 1 tea estate (≥1)	821	Mf	Hyd./Lymph.
Khan et al. (1999) [NS] Study 2 [40]	CSS	2 communities: tea workers and non-tea workers (≥1)	1446	Mf	NS
Khan et al. (1999) [NS] Study 3 [38]	CSS	1 weaving community (≥1)	446	Mf	-
Khan et al. (2004) [NS] [39]	CSS	Individuals in 1 tea estate (≥1)	656	Mf	Hyd./Lymph.
Khan et al. (2015) (2012–2013) [41]	CSS	Individuals in 1 tea estate (infection ≥2, morbidity ≥18)	634	Mf	Hyd./Lymph.
Medhi et al. (2006) (2002–2003) [47]	CSS	Households in 8 tea estates (≥1)	4016	Mf	Hyd./Lymph.
Prakash et al. (1998) (1994) [51]	CSS	Households in 1 tea estate (≥1)	1105	Mf	Hyd./Lymph.
		Malaysia			
Ahmad et al. (2014) [NS] [25]	CSS	Households/schools on 1 island (≥1)	298	Mf	-
Cox-Singh et al. (1999) [NS] [31]	CSS	2 districts (NS)	145	Mf, PCR	-
Hakim et al. (1995) (1992) [34]	FDT [c]	2 villages (≥6 months old)	499	Mf	-
Jamail et al. (2005) (2001–2002) [35]	FDE	7 districts(≥1)	2545	Mf, IgG4	-
Lim et al (2001) [NS] [46]	FDE	5 villages and 2 schools (≥1)	1134	Mf, IgG4	-
Rahmah et al. (2003) [NS] [53]	FDE	16 schools (7–12)	5138	IgG4	-
Rahmah et al. (2010) [NS] [54]	FDE	School children (6–10)	973	IgG4	-
Wan Omar et al. (2001) [NS] [62]	FDE	Migrant workers in palm oil estates (WA [i])	630	Mf	Lymph.

Table 1. *Cont.*

Study (Publication Date) [Study Period] [Ref.]	Study Design	Sampling Population/Unit (Age of Participants)	Sample Size	Diagnostic Method	
				Infection	Morbidity
		Thailand			
Bhumiratana et al. (2004) (2002) [28]	FDT	Myanmar workers (WA [i])	860	Mf, ICT, Og4C3	-
Bhumiratana et al. (2005) (1998–2001) [26]	CSS	Myanmars and Thais in multiple villages (≥1)	433	Mf, ICT, Og4C3	-
Bhumiratana et al. (1999) (1998) [27]	FDE	Multiple villages (≥1)	225	Mf, ICT	Hyd.
Bhumiratana et al (2002) (1999) [29]	CSS	1 village (≥1)	219	Mf, ICT	Hyd.
Chansiri et al. (2002) (1997–2001) [30]	CSS	Migrant workers in 4 provinces (WA [i])	1299	PCR	-
Jiraamonnimit et al. (2009) (2005 to 2006] [36]	LO [d]	3 provinces (≥7)	500	Mf, IgG4	Lymph.
Koyadun et al. (2003) (2001–2002) [43]	FDT	Myanmar migrants and Thais in 3 districts (≥15)	660	ICT	-
Koyadun et al. (2005) (2003) [42]	CSS	Myanmar workers (≥10)	904	Mf	-
Krairittichai et al. (2012) (2010) [44]	RCS [f]	Migrant workers at 1 hospital (WA [i])	102,090	Mf	-
Nuchprayoon et al. (2003) [NS] Study 1 [48]	FDE	Myanmar workers at 2 factories (WA [i])	337	Mf, ICT, Og4C3	Hyd.
Nuchprayoon et al. (2003) [NS] Study 2 [49]	CSS	2 villages (≥1)	433	Mf, Og4C3, IgG4	-
Nuchprayoon et al. (2001) [NS] [50]	CSS	1 sub-district (≥1)	196	Mf, Og4C3, PCR	-
Satimai et al. (2011) [NS] [57]	CSS	Myanmar migrants and Thais in 2 provinces (≥1)	1031	ICT, IgG4	-
Swaddiwudhipong et al. (1996) (1995) [58]	CSS	Myanmar workers and their families (≥1)	8377	Mf	NS
Triteeraprapab et al. (1999) [NS] [61]	CSS	Myanmar workers in 6 industrial plants (WA [i])	654	Mf	-
Triteeraprapab et al. (2001) [NS] Study 1 [59]	CSS	4 districts in 1 province (≥1)	2462	Mf	-
Triteeraprapab et al. (2001) (1999) Study 2 [60]	CSS	Myanmar migrants in 1 community (≥2)	371	Mf, Og4C3, IgG4	-

[a] Field diagnostic test evaluation. [b] Cross-sectional survey. [c] Field Drug trial. [d] Longitudinal observational study. [e] Urine IgG4. [f] Retrospective cohort study. [g] Not stated. [h] Hydrocoele/lymphoedema. [i] Working age.

Table 2. Included grey literature.

Reports [Ref.]	Year	Sample Size	Diagnostic Method	
			Infection	Morbidity
Annual Reports				
Myanmar Ministry of Health. National Program to Eliminate LF: Annual Reports [68–70]	2004	23,668	Mf	-
	2011	10,845	Mf	-
	2012	14,649	Mf	Hyd./Lymph. [c]
World Health Organization Reports				
WHO SEARO: Elimination of lymphatic filariasis in the Southeast Asia Region. Reports of the 1st, 7th, 8th, 9th, 10th Meeting of the Regional Program Review Group. [74–78]	2005 2010 2011 2012 2013	NS [b]	Mf (ICT) [a]	Hyd./Lymph.
WHO Regional Office for Southeast Asia: Elimination of lymphatic filariasis in the Southeast Asia Region. Reports of the 5th and 8th Meeting of the Regional Program Managers. [63,64]	2006 2011	NS	Mf (ICT) [a]	Hyd./Lymph.
WHO Regional Office for Southeast Asia: Towards eliminating lymphatic filariasis: Progress in the Southeast Asia Region (2001–2011). [5]	2013	NS	Mf	Hyd./Lymph.
WHO Regional Office for Southeast Asia: Regional Strategic Plan for Elimination of Lymphatic Filariasis (2004–2007). [71]	2004	NS	Mf	Hyd./Lymph.
WHO Western Pacific Region: First Mekong-Plus Program Managers Workshop on Lymphatic Filariasis and Other Helminthiasis. [66]	2009	Cambodia: 23,705 Lao PDR: 9286 Vietnam: 18,302	Mf/ICT	Hyd./Lymph.
WHO Regional Office for the Western Pacific. Reports of the 13th and 14th Meeting of the Western Pacific Regional Program Review Group on Neglected Tropical Diseases. [72,79]	2013 2014	NS	Mf/ICT	Hyd./Lymph.
WHO Malaysia Office. Country Cooperation Strategy 2009–2013. [67]	2010	NS	Mf	-
WHO: Meeting of the Neglected Tropical Disease Strategic and Technical Advisory Group's Monitoring and Evaluation Subgroup on Disease Specific Indicators. [80]	2014	NS	Mf	-
UNDP/World Bank/WHO/UNICEF. Research on rapid geographical assessment of Bancroftian filariasis. [73]	1997	7000	ICT	-
Non-Governmental Organization Reports				
Family Health International 360 and USAID: End Neglected Tropical Diseases in Asia Final Report. [65]	2015	Cambodia: 18,809 Lao PDR:3472 Vietnam: NS	Mf/ICT	Hyd./Lymph.

[a] ICT only used in one survey. [b] Not stated. [c] Hydrocoele/lymphoedema.

4. Prevalence Results and Discussion by Country

4.1. Overview

This systematic review and meta-analysis assessed the prevalence estimates for LF infection and morbidity in mainland Southeast Asia, Bangladesh and Northeast India. These estimates are important for the successful implementation and evaluation of elimination programs. Data on the prevalence and distribution of infection are needed to identify and prioritise regions for inclusion in MDA programs. MDA rounds aim to interrupt LF transmission to prevent new infections, eventuating in LF elimination. Prevalence data are then required following MDA rounds to evaluate their effectiveness and reassess the need for further rounds. However, even after transmission has ceased, those with previous infection may, or will have already developed chronic disease manifestations. National programs therefore require data on the morbidity burden in order to implement alleviation programs.

Prevalence data from included studies and grey literature are summarised by country and region in Tables S2–S3. Figure 2 illustrates the most recent distribution of LF compared to that at baseline (pre-MDA).

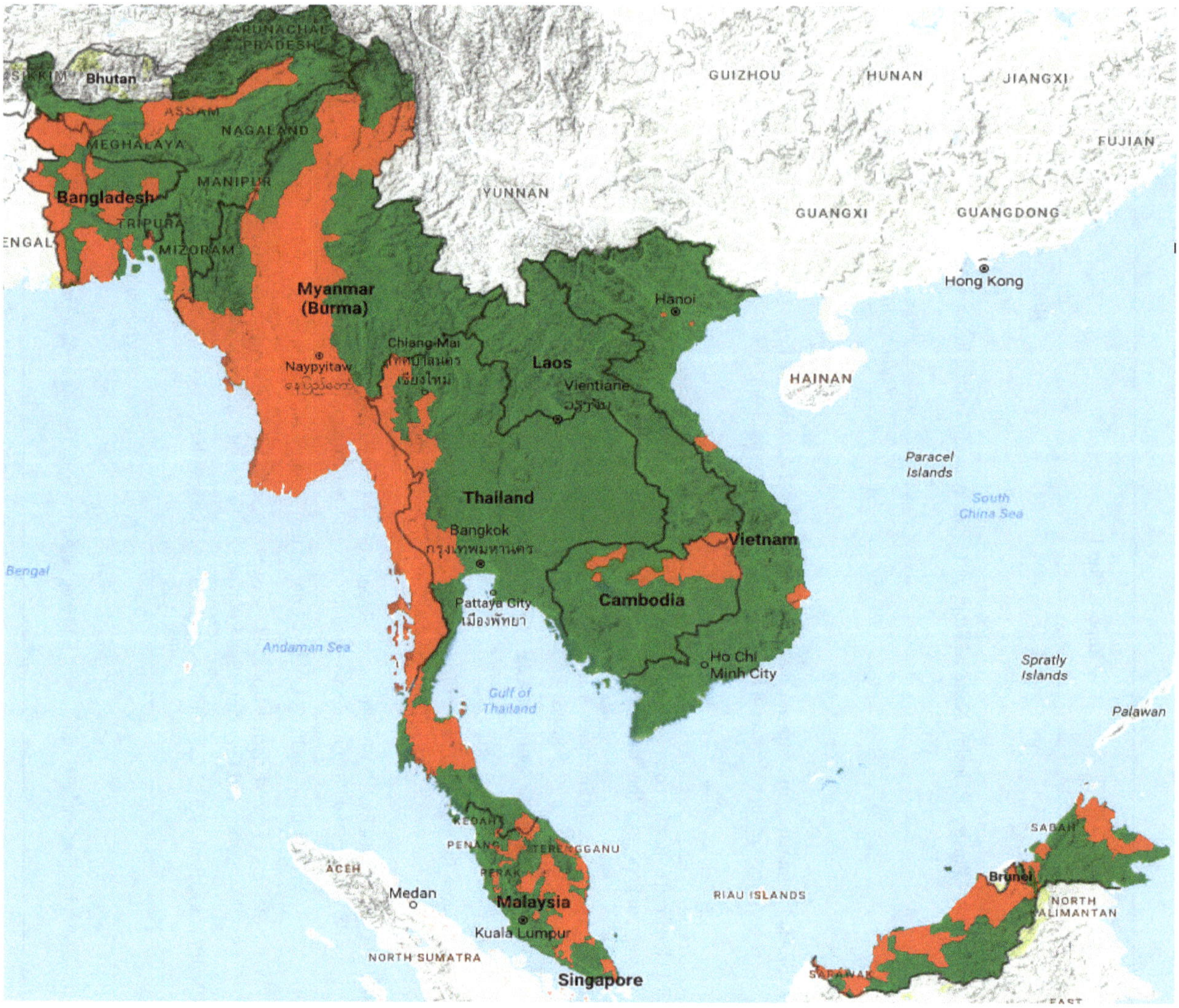

(a)

Figure 2. *Cont.*

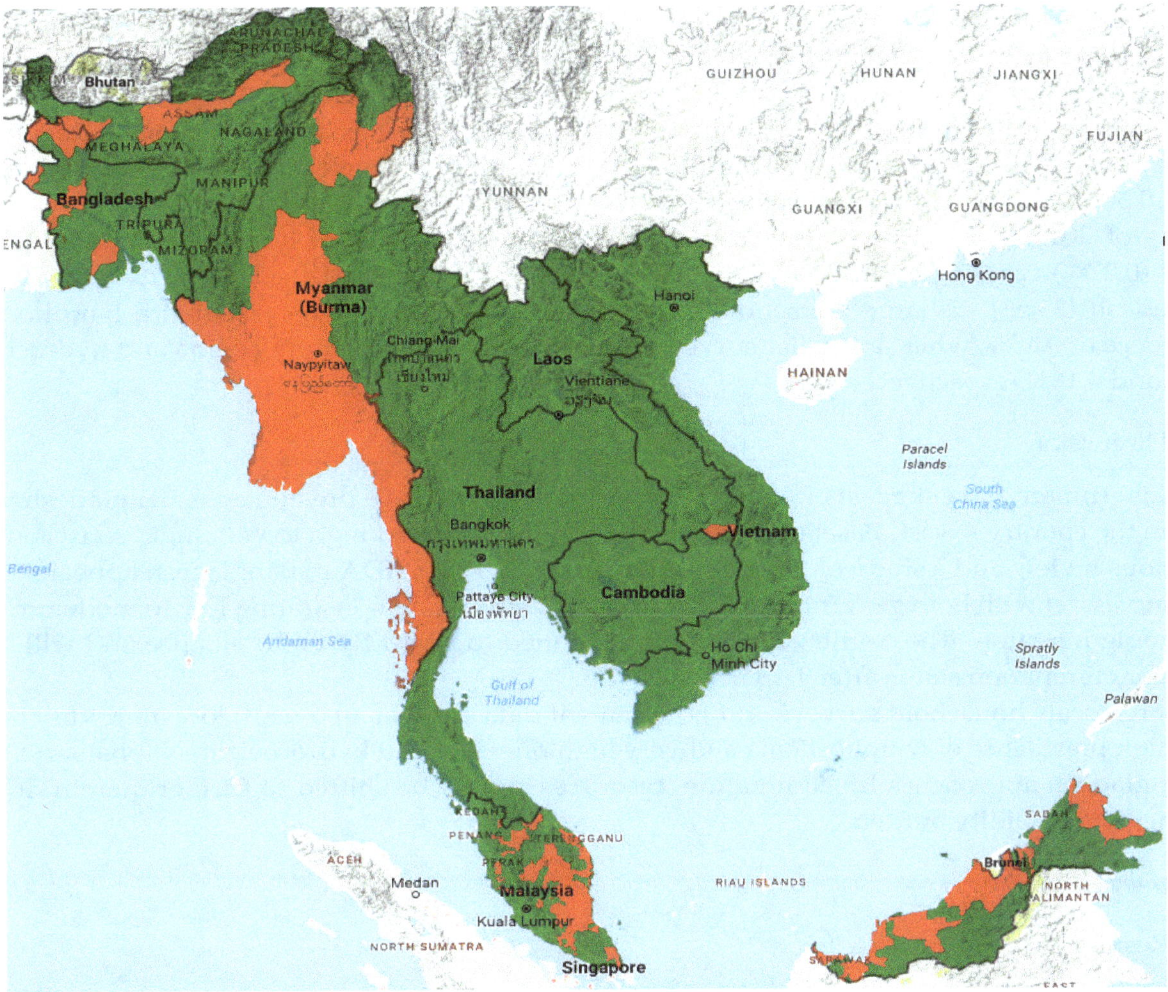

(**b**)

Figure 2. Distribution of LF endemic areas (red): (**a**) at baseline; and (**b**) based on most recent data.

Exact prevalence estimates cannot be calculated because of the nature of available data. However, we have attempted to estimate the current prevalence of infection and morbidity for each country through assessment of pooled country estimates, grey literature and the quality of available data.

Given the varied sensitivity of detection methods, we defined infection prevalence as low (Mf <0.5%, ICT/Og4C3 <1%, IgG4 <2%), medium (Mf 0.5–1.9%, ICT/Og4C3 1–3.9%, IgG4 2–7.9%), high (Mf 2–3.9%, ICT/Og4C3 4–7.9%, IgG4 8–15.9%) and very high (Mf ≥4%, ICT/IgG4 ≥8%, IgG4 ≥16%). For morbidity, we defined a prevalence of <0.5% as low, Mf 0.5–1.9% as medium, 2–3.9% as high and ≥4% as very high. Baseline prevalence refers to the level of infection prior to the commencement of the national elimination program.

4.2. Bangladesh

4.2.1. Results

Grey literature indicates that bancroftian filariasis was endemic in 34 of the 64 districts of Bangladesh during mapping between 2002 and 2004, with an estimated 75.96 million of the country's 148.77 million at risk [5,65,78]. Fifteen districts were considered low endemic with antigenaemia levels greater than 1% but microfilaraemia less than <0.6% [65,80]. They did not undergo MDA and have now passed two of three TAS, with the last to be completed in 2016 [65]. The remaining 19 districts had initial microfilaraemia prevalences of 0.2–16% [80]. These districts completed MDA rounds in

2014 and have now passed a TAS survey to determine whether MDA can be stopped, with a further TAS planned for 2017 to 2018. National infection prevalence estimates decreased from 1% in 2004 to 0% in 2010 [5].

Three studies from 2011–2013 have assessed infection prevalence in the northern endemic states of Nilphamari and Panchargarh [33,55,56]. They have found prevalences by Mf, ICT and IgG4 of 1.13%, 0.31–1.70% and 2.19%, respectively.

As of 2011, government surveys had identified 23,486 cases of lymphoedema (0.10%) and 65,320 (0.27%) cases of hydrocoele [76]. Two studies have assessed the morbidity prevalence in Bangladesh [33,55]. A large household survey of 232,005 participants reported a lymphoedema prevalence of 0.45%, whilst a smaller survey found a prevalence of lymphoedema and hydrocoele of 2.66% and 4.16% respectively

4.2.2. Discussion

Government data suggests *W. bancrofti* was historically widespread across Bangladesh with a focus in the country's west. Baseline infection prevalence appeared high to very high, consistent with a previous review and a study of Bangladeshi migrants [15,62]. MDA in Bangladesh appears to have been successful with both government data and recent studies demonstrating low to moderate levels of ongoing infection. The country has now transitioned to post-MDA surveillance and will aim to apply for elimination status after TAS in 2018.

Large-scale household surveys and government data suggest an overall low morbidity burden but a high prevalence of lymphoedema and very high prevalence of hydrocoele in Nilphamari District. As Bangladesh approaches LF elimination, resources should be shifted to further quantifying and tackling the morbidity burden.

4.3. Cambodia

4.3.1. Results

Government mapping in 2004 reported 18 endemic districts in four northern and northeastern provinces with 3.61% of the national population at risk (474 800) [5]. Government surveys reported a pre-MDA prevalence of 0.38–2.75% in these provinces (mixed ICT and TBS) [65]. A 2000–2001 study in these endemic provinces showed Mf and ICT prevalence ranging 0–1.13%, and 0–1.94%, respectively [45].

Five rounds of MDA were completed between 2005 and 2009. A post-MDA countrywide serological study in 2012 found a prevalence by IgG4 of 6.60% in this north region and 1.19–1.65% in the rest of the country [52]. All endemic districts passed required TAS by 2015 [65]. In 2016, Cambodia was validated by the WHO as having eliminated LF as a public health problem [2].

In 2001, the government reported 58 cases of LF-related morbidity (40 lymphoedema and 18 hydrocoele) in Cambodia [66]. The highest prevalence was in Stung Treng (10), Takeo (10) and Rattanakiri (9). A study from the same year found the prevalence of lymphoedema and hydrocoele in endemic provinces ranged from 0 to 0.44% and 0 to 2.97% respectively [45].

4.3.2. Discussion

Government baseline mapping indicated *W. bancrofti* and *B. malayi* were endemic at low to moderate levels in four provinces in northern Cambodia. Two representative studies and a prior review confirmed these findings [14]. Cambodia completed post-MDA surveillance in 2015 and WHO validated elimination of LF as a public health problem in 2016.

Whilst LF transmission has now ceased, an overall moderate combined morbidity burden remains in Cambodia. Although the government reported only 58 cases of morbidity in 2001, a representative survey from the same year found a low prevalence of lymphoedema (0.34%) and moderate prevalence of hydrocoele (1.64%) across the four endemic provinces. When the study's results are extrapolated using 1998 census population data [81], case estimates for lymphoedema and hydrocoele are 2800–17,382 and

8474–27,461 in the four provinces, respectively. Now that MDA is complete, efforts in Cambodia need to shift to assessing and alleviating the morbidity burden in the country.

4.4. Northeast India

4.4.1. Results

Filariasis is endemic in 250 districts across 20 states in India, with 617 million individuals at risk [78]. Assam is considered the only endemic state in Northeast India [5].

Baseline government mapping from 2004 illustrates a line of endemic districts from the Bangladesh to the Myanmar border with a prevalence of 0–5% [5].

Studies prior to the commencement of MDA in 2004 found a bancroftian Mf prevalence of 0.61–10.27% and 0.45–1.79% in tea-estate and non-tea-estate populations, respectively [32,37–40,51]. Sub-group meta-analysis showed a significantly higher Mf prevalence in populations living in tea-estates (6.11%, 95%CI 3.49–9.41%) compared to those who did not (0.88%, 0.3–1.54) ($p = 0.000$). A more recent study found persistent microfilaraemia of 7.41% in a tea-estate following six rounds of MDA [41]. The government reports that the national infection prevalence has decreased from 1.24% in 2004 to 0.35% in 2011 [5].

The prevalence of lymphoedema and hydrocoele found in tea-estate populations was 0.12–0.72% and 1.01–8.96%, respectively [32,37,39–41,51]. One study assessed morbidity in a non-tea-estate community and found no clinical cases [40].

4.4.2. Discussion

Available data indicate that Assam is the only LF-endemic state in Northeast India. Baseline mapping and studies demonstrated very high levels of *W. bancrofti* infection amongst those living in tea-estates and a moderate prevalence in non-tea-estate populations. Tea-estates are predominantly composed of workers who migrated from states such as Bengal, Bihar, Odisha, Uttar Pradesh, Madhya Pradesh, Tamil Nadu and Jharkhand as part of the British tea trade in the 19th and early 20th century. Whilst national infection prevalence has progressively declined since the commencement of the MDA program in 2004, a recent study found very high levels of persisting microfilaraemia in a tea-estate following six rounds of MDA [41]. Reports of missed MDA rounds in seven districts in 2009, as well as suboptimal drug coverage may account for the ongoing LF transmission in the region [63,74,75]. Further rounds of MDA with sufficient coverage and uptake are required.

Multiple representative studies have demonstrated an overall moderate burden of disease in the tea-estate population of Assam with a low prevalence of lymphoedema but very high prevalence of hydrocoele. Insufficient datawere available to assess the morbidity burden in the non-tea estate population. In addition to ongoing MDA, programmatic efforts should focus on assessing the morbidity burden in non-tea populations and implementing alleviation programs.

4.5. Lao PDR

4.5.1. Results

No studies on the prevalence of LF in Lao PDR were found.Grey literature indicates that *W. bancrofti* is only endemic in the southern Attapeu and Sekong Provinces of Lao PDR with 137,000 individuals at risk [65,66,72,79]. Mapping of the Attapeu's five districts in 2009 showed an antigenaemia prevalence ranging 1.9–27.4% [65]. MDA commenced in Attapeu in one district in 2008 and was expanded to all five in 2009. Only one village in Sekong Province is endemic with a prevalence of 6% [65]. Two rounds of focused MDA have been completed in this and surrounding villages.

Only one case of lymphoedema and no cases of hydrocoele have been reported in the country [66].

4.5.2. Discussion

Government data from Lao PDR suggest that *W. bancrofti* is focussed in Attapeu province (along the Cambodian border) and parts of the adjacent Sekong province. Infection prevalence was initially considered low to moderate as noted by previous reviews [1,11,14,15]. However, further baseline surveys in 2009 found very high levels of antigenaemia in Attapeu province. Since the commencement of widespread MDA, infection prevalence appears to have decreased to low to moderate levels, however no independent studies are available to validate government data.

Insufficient dataare available to assess the morbidity burden in Lao PDR. Given the infection prevalence in Attapeu and morbidity burden in neighbouring Cambodia, numerous cases would be expected. Further studies are urgently needed to validate government data and assess the morbidity burden in Lao PDR.

4.6. *Malaysia*

4.6.1. Results

WHO reports indicate that 116 of the 994 implementation units (subdistricts and districts) are endemic across Peninsular Malaysia, Sabah and Sarawak with 1.12 million people at risk [72,79]. Subperiodic *B. malayi* accounts for the majority of cases, with 2% caused by *W. bancrofti*. Government data suggest Mf prevalence had decreased from 1% to 0.2% in Peninsular Malaysia and 5.5% to 1.5% in Sabah and Sarawak from the 1980s until the commencement of the National MDA Program in 2004 [66,67].

Pre-MDA studies of the local population in Peninsular Malaysia, Sabah and Sarawak found a prevalence of *B. malayi* Mf of 0.26–23.85%, 20.69% and 0.90%, respectively [31,34,35,46,53].

Since 2004, Malaysia has completed five rounds of MDA in Peninsular Malaysia and seven rounds in Sabah and Sarawak. As of 2014, only five IUs were still conducting MDA rounds with the remainder commencing TAS [79]. More recent studies in Peninsular Malaysia have found a prevalence of Mf and IgG4 of 0 and 2.16% respectively [25,54].

No data on the prevalence of LF-associated morbidity in the local Malaysian population were found.

4.6.2. Discussion

Brugia malayi (and to a lesser extent *W. bancrofti*) was widely endemic across Peninsular Malaysia, Sabah and Sarawak. Government surveys reported a low to moderate baseline infection prevalence. Whilst pre-MDA studies showed greater levels of infection than government data, most were not representative. These studies likely reflected the presence of highly-endemic foci in parts of Peninsular Malaysia and Sabah, rather than a high baseline prevalence. More recent surveys suggest infection levels are declining in Malaysia, although one study was conducted in a known low-endemic area [54]. Whilst recent government data are lacking, a 2016 xenomonitoring survey across five states in Peninsular Malaysia and Sabah found no active transmission [82], suggesting a likely low level of infection and supporting Malaysia's progress toward LF elimination. Further studies are required to assess current infection prevalence and the need for ongoing MDA.

Although there are no data on the morbidity prevalence in the local Malay population, a significant burden of lymphoedema is expected given the previously highly endemic foci of *B. malayi* infection. Studies assessing the morbidity burden are needed to fill this knowledge gap.

4.7. *Myanmar*

4.7.1. Results

Bancroftian filariasis is endemic in 45 of the 65 districts of Myanmar with 85.5% of the population at risk [5]. No published prevalence studies on Myanmar were found. One study described in a WHO report assessed filarial antigenaemia prevalence in 1997 [73]. One hundred individuals were tested by

ICT from seventy randomly selected townships across 14 districts. The central and western dry zone was highly endemic (20–30%) with the northern, eastern and southern areas less endemic or free from filariasis. Most recent government microfilaraemia prevalence data for the western Sagaing, Magway, Rakhine and Chin regions range from 0–65% [68–70]. Prevalence in Mandalay, Kayin and Yangon regions ranges from 0–2% [68–70]. Mean national prevalence has reduced from 7.1% in 2001 to 2.7% in 2011 [5]. Myanmar commenced its MDA Program in 2001. As of 2014, the program had been scaled-up to 22 of the 24 endemic districts.

One government survey assessed self-reported morbidity in 280 000 individuals in Sagaing region in 2004 and identified 520 cases of lymphoedema (0.19%) and 827 cases of hydrocoele (0.59%) [68].

4.7.2. Discussion

Baseline surveys suggest that *W. bancrofti* were widely endemic in the low-lying parts of Myanmar with over 85% of the population at risk. They suggested very high baseline levels of infection in the central and western dry zones, consistent with that seen in Myanmar migrants in Thailand. Meanwhile, the northern, eastern and southern areas were less endemic or free from filariasis. Government data suggest declining levels of infection in Mandalay, Kayin and Yangon states since the commencement of MDA, but very high rates of persisting infection in the western states of Sagaing, Magway, Rakhine and Chin. As Myanmar continues to expand its MDA program, independent studies are required to validate government prevalence data.

The only morbidity survey found low levels of self-reported lymphoedema and moderate levels of hydrocoele in Sagaing region [68]. However, morbidity self-reporting questionnaires are not a sensitive or specific indicator of clinical disease [45,83]. The significant morbidity found in Myanmar migrants in Thailand suggests that the true morbidity prevalence is likely much higher. Representative prevalence studies are required to elucidate the morbidity burden in Myanmar.

4.8. Thailand

4.8.1. Results

Baseline government mapping in 2001 found filariasis to be endemic in two foci in Thailand with 160,000 individuals at risk [5]. *Wuchereria bancrofti* was present in five provinces along the Thai-Myanmar border, whilst *B. malayi* was endemic along the southern Thai peninsula. Studies in provinces along the Myanmar border between 1998 and 2003 found an infection prevalence of 1.01–10.20%, 13.3–26.42%, 21.89–36.79% and 53.93% by TBS, ICT, Og4C3 and IgG4, respectively [26,27, 29,49,50]. Meanwhile, studies conducted along the Thai peninsula between 2001 and 2006 reported a prevalence of *B. malayi* infection of 0–2.00% and 8.00–23.67% by TBS and IgG4 [36,43,59].

The 11 studies which assessed infection in Myanmar migrants living in Thailand found a prevalence of 0–5.83%, 0.2–13.57%, 4.0–23.98%, and 2.73–42.32% by TBS, ICT, Og4C3 and IgG4, respectively [26,28,29,42,43,48,57,58,60,61].

Thailand commenced an elimination program in 2002. Mass drug administration was completed in 2007 in all provinces except Narathiwatt, which extended rounds until 2011. Thailand commenced the process of verifying LF elimination in 2012 after all areas passed TAS. National mean data suggest infection prevalence has decreased from 0.77% in 2003 to 0.09% in 2010 [5]. No post-MDA prevalence studies on the local population were identified.

Available studies have found the prevalence of lymphoedema and hydrocoele in the local population in endemic areas was 1.2% and 0–8.15% [27,29,36]. Studies of Myanmar migrants found a prevalence of hydrocoele of 8.62–16.13% [29,48]. As of 2011, the government had 200 identified cases of lymphoedema [77].

4.8.2. Discussion

Two highly endemic LF foci previously existed in Thailand. *W. bancrofti* was present along the Thai-Myanmar border, whilst *B. malayi* was endemic along the southern Thai peninsula. Government surveys suggest that LF transmission has ceased following MDA, but no studies have independently verified this.

The influx of LF-infected Myanmar migrants into Thailand, combined with a documented ability of Thai *Culex quinquefasciatus* mosquitoes to transmit the Myanmar strain of *W. bancrofti* has raised concerns regarding the potential for re-introduction of transmission [84,85]. The Thai government has acknowledged this and expanded its MDA program to include registered migrant workers from Myanmar and Laos [57,86]. However, the considerable number of unregistered migrants still poses a threat to elimination efforts.

Whilst the government had only identified 200 cases of lymphoedema in 2011, available studies suggest a potentially moderate prevalence of lymphoedema and very high prevalence of hydrocoele in previously endemic areas. However the representativeness of these surveys is uncertain, indicating the need for further studies to establish the true disease burden in these areas.

4.9. Vietnam

4.9.1. Results

No peer-reviewed studies from Vietnam were identified. Government data suggest filariasis was endemic in six of Vietnam's eight regions during 1960–2000 [66]. However, by the start of the National Elimination Program in 2003, only the Red River delta, north-central coast and central-southern coast regions remained endemic despite no MDA [65,66]. Within these regions, 12 districts were considered endemic and six selected for MDA with a total population at-risk of 675,000. *Brugia malayi* predominates in the north with *W. bancrofti* in the south [65,66].

Baseline prevalence in endemic districts in 2002 ranged from 0 to 3.6% [65,66]. Vietnam completed its MDA program in 2011 and passed TAS in all districts in 2015. It has subsequently applied to the WHO for LF elimination confirmation [65].

A government clinical survey in 2002 in 77 districts reported 570 cases of limb morbidity and 47 cases of hydrocoele [66]. A later survey in 2012 identified 489 morbidity cases in five provinces [65].

4.9.2. Discussion

Filariasis was historically widespread in Vietnam with *Brugia malayi* predominating in the north and *W. bancrofti* in the south. However by the commencement of the MDA Program, it had become confined to the Red River delta, north-central coast and central-southern coast regions. These findings are consistent with those found in prior reviews [14–16]. It has been suggested that the reduction in infection prevalence prior to MDA was likely the result of improvements in housing and living conditions, man-made ecological changes, the use of bed-nets and individual case treatment [16,65]. These changes appear to have resulted in low baseline infection prevalence levels by the start of the MDA with the exception of Khanh Vinh and Ninh Hoa districts, where prevalence remained high. Government data suggest that since MDA, LF transmission has now ceased, although no independent studies have yet validated this.

Whilst government surveys suggest a relatively few cases of morbidity, the number of participants surveyed is unknown, and therefore prevalence estimates cannot be made. Given filariasis was historically widespread with some highly endemic foci, the true morbidity burden may be higher [16]. As Vietnam approaches LF elimination, studies are needed to validate government progress and assess the morbidity burden in the country.

4.10. Overall Prevalence Estimates for Mainland Southeast Asia

4.10.1. Meta-Analysis Results

A random effects meta-analysis of available infection and morbidity data was completed. Figures 3–7 and Figures S1–S9 show the point estimates with 95% exact binomial confidence intervals (95% CI) for each meta-analysis ordered by country and study date. Substantial heterogeneity between surveys was demonstrated by I^2 values, between 83.57% and 98.74%.

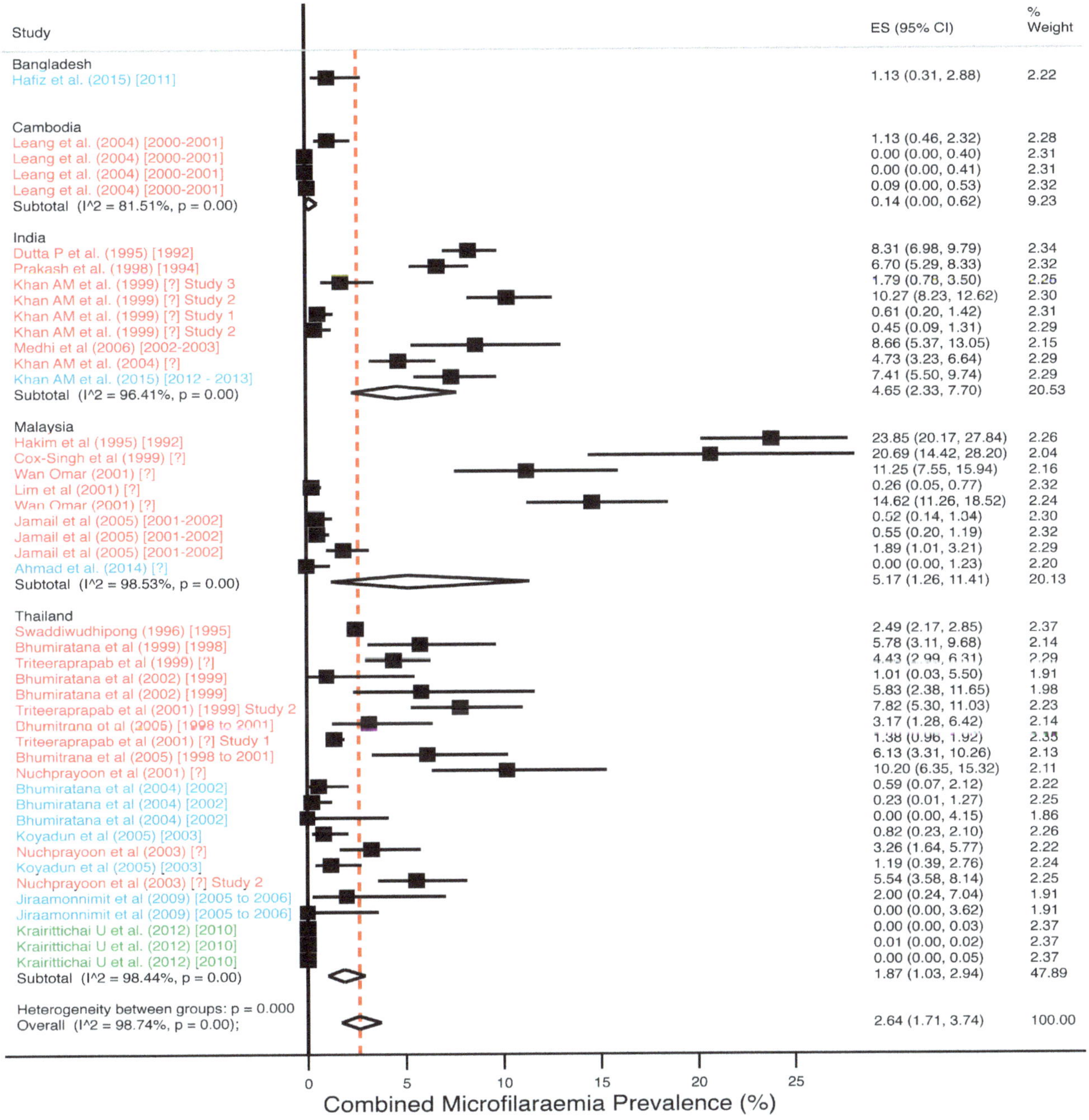

Figure 3. Percentage estimates of combined microfilaraemia prevalence by country and year. ES: prevalence estimate. Red-dashed line: overall estimate. Diamond: subgroup estimate. Horizontal line: 95% CI. Red study: pre-MDA, blue study: mid-MDA, green study: post-MDA.

For microfilaraemia, 30 studies testing 133,747 individuals estimated a pooled prevalence of *W. bancrofti* Mf of 1.77% (1.00–2.74%), *B. malayi* Mf of 0.36% (0.07–0.82%) and combined Mf of 2.64%

(1.71–3.74%). For ICT antigenaemia, 10 studies testing 7237 individuals estimated a pooled prevalence of 4.48% (1.97–7.87%). For IgG4 antibodies, 10 studies testing 14,339 individuals estimated a pooled prevalence of 7.08% (3.63–11.54%).

For combined morbidity, 16 studies testing 256,591 individuals estimated a pooled prevalence of 1.34% (0.81–1.97%). For hydrocoele, nine studies testing 4179 estimated a pooled prevalence of 3.84% (2.11–6.03%). For lymphoedema, nine studies testing 240,987 individuals estimated a pooled prevalence of 0.49% (0.24–0.80%).

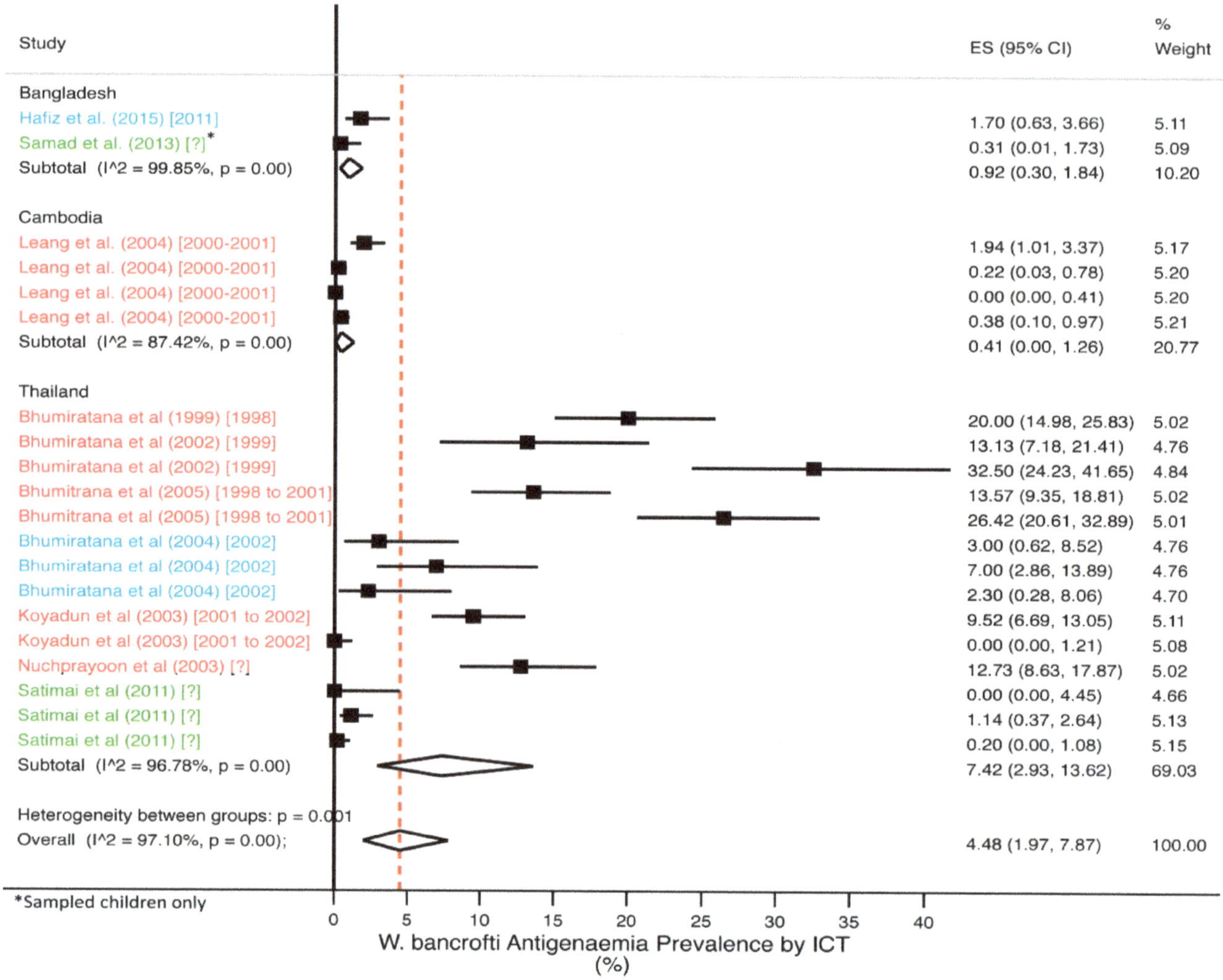

Figure 4. Percentage estimates of ICT antigenaemia prevalence by country and year. ES: prevalence estimate. Red-dotted line: overall estimate. Blue diamond: sub-group estimate. Horizontal line: 95% CI. Red study: pre-MDA, blue study: mid-MDA, green study: post-MDA.

4.10.2. Discussion

Meta-analysis showed an overall high prevalence of infection (Mf: 2.64%, antigenaemia: 4.48%) and moderate burden of morbidity (1.34%) in the region. However, pooled estimates and sub-group analyses by country are biased by the significant differences in location, time, design, diagnosis method, sampling unit and representativeness of the included studies, and should therefore be interpreted with caution. Despite this, meta-analyses show a general decline in infection prevalence with time and a higher prevalence of hydrocoele compared to lymphoedema across all countries (overall hydrocoele:lymphoedema ratio of 7.84:1).

In the context of pooled country estimates, grey literature and the quality of available data, we conclude that Lao PDR, Myanmar and Northeast India demonstrate ongoing evidence of LF transmission that will require multiple further rounds of MDA. Bangladesh, Malaysia, Thailand and Vietnam appear close to having eliminated LF, whilst Cambodia has already achieved elimination status. We estimated that the burden of morbidity is likely high in Thailand, moderate in Cambodia, Myanmar, and Northeast India, and low in Bangladesh. There was insufficient evidence to accurately estimate the disease burden in Lao PDR, Malaysia or Vietnam.

These results indicate that whilst considerable progress toward LF elimination has been made, there remains a significant filariasis burden in the region. The results will assist policy makers to advocate and budget for future MDA and morbidity control programs.

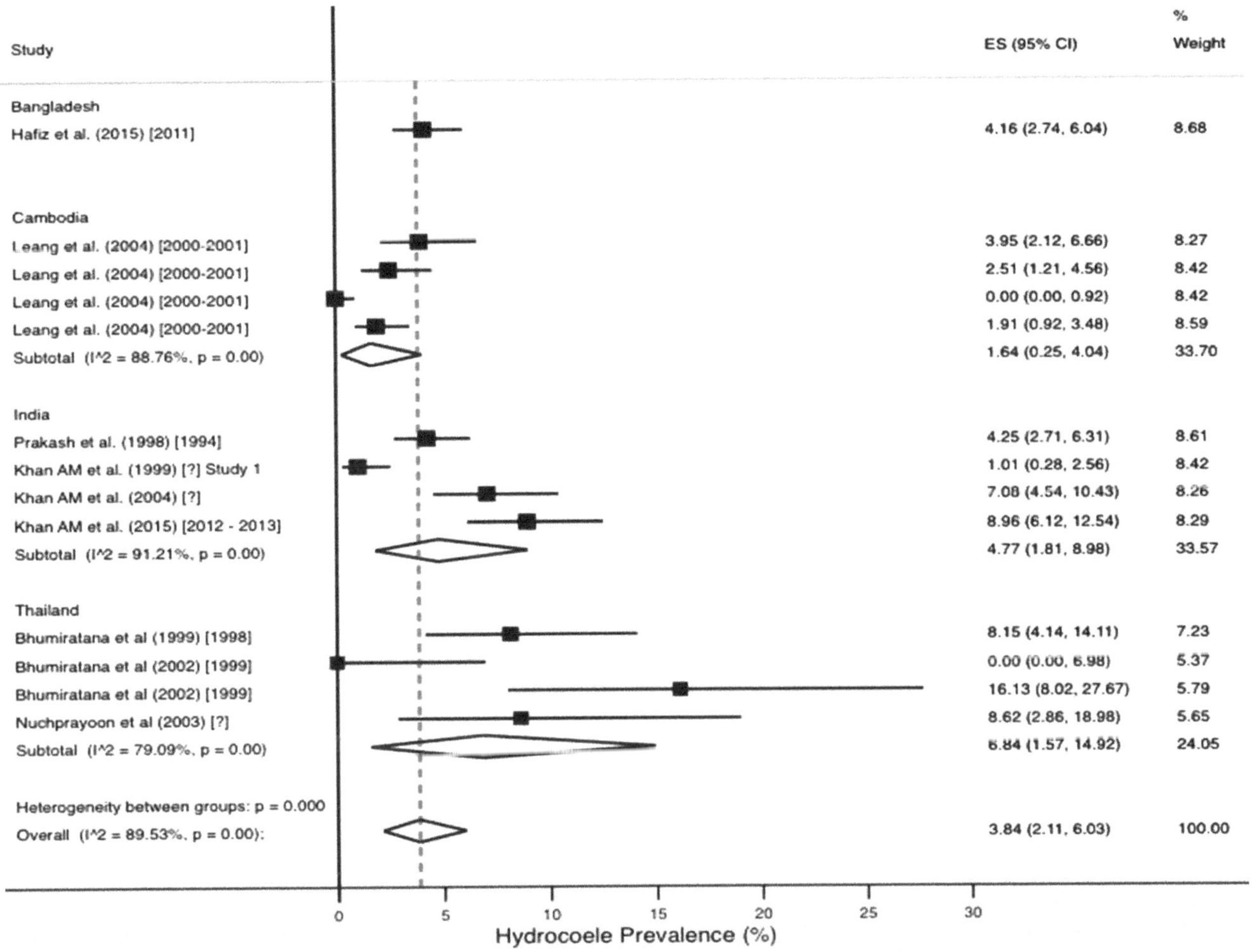

Figure 5. Percentage estimates of hydrocoele prevalence by country and year. ES: prevalence estimate. Red-dotted line: overall estimate. Diamond: sub-group estimate. Horizontal line: 95% CI.

4.11. Limitations

This systematic review was hindered by limitations at the study and review level. The overall quality of primary studies was suboptimal. Only 18% of studies used fully representative sampling methods and consensus data collection methods. Some of the studies were out-dated because one or more MDA rounds had occurred since data collection. The quality of grey literature further hindered data analysis. Available reports frequently omitted sample sizes or gave prevalence data in percentage ranges, making further analysis difficult.The uncertain methodology of government surveys further complicated grey literature assessment. Whilst national programs follow the WHO guidelines, there is often considerable variation in sampling and data collection practices in the field [22]. No published studies were available from Lao PDR, Myanmar or Vietnam to compare with government data.

Incomplete literature retrieval led to limitations at the review level. Original copies of government annual reports were obtained only from Myanmar, although use of WHO reports alleviated this deficiency to some extent. Retrieval of these data would provide a more complete picture of filariasis prevalence in these countries.

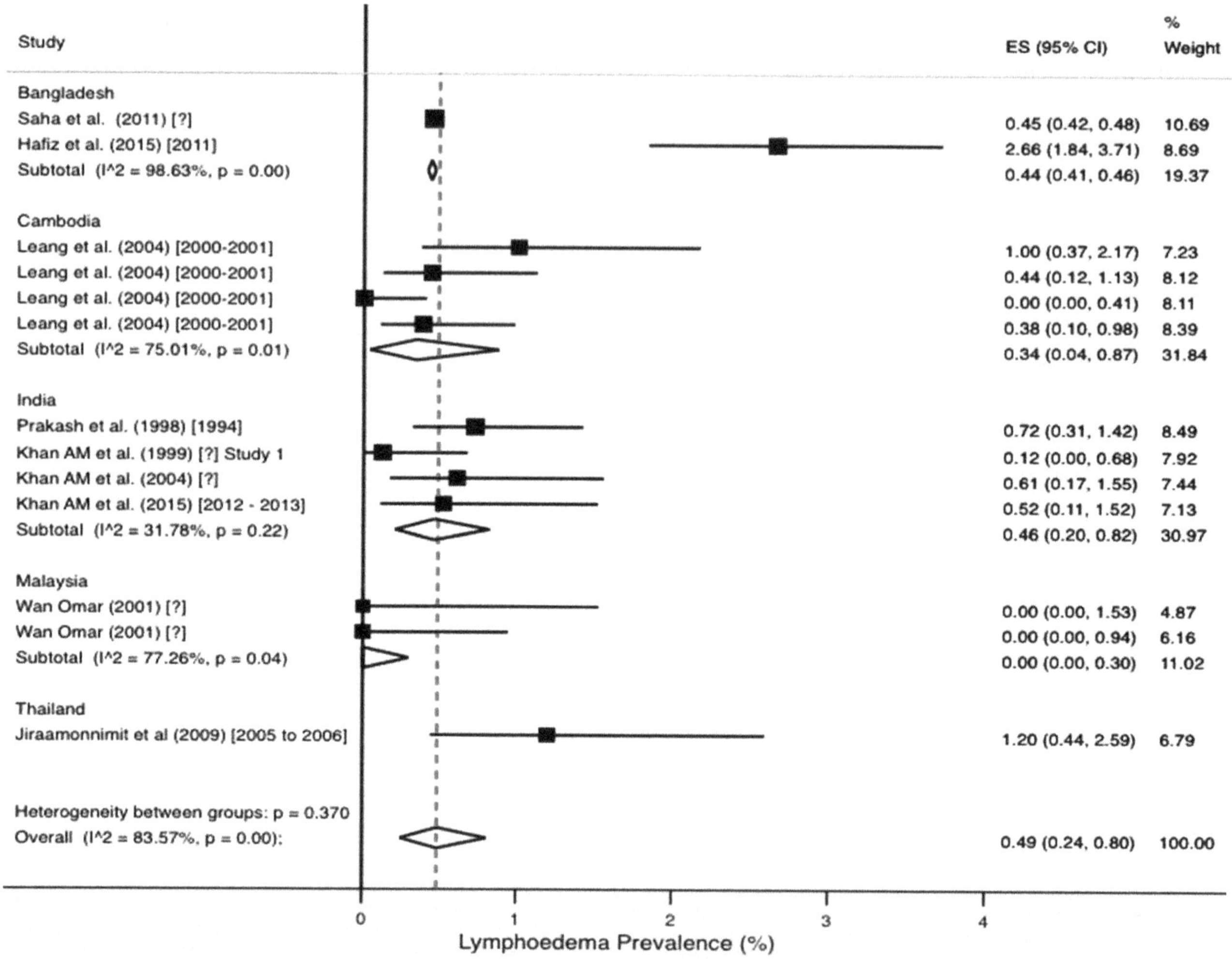

Figure 6. Percentage estimates of lymphoedema prevalence by country and year. ES: prevalence estimate. Red-dotted line: overall estimate. Diamond: sub-group estimate. Horizontal line: 95% CI.

The lack of representative and recent studies in many of the countries placed reliance on government sources for current prevalence data. Whilst sufficient information on infection was available to produce country estimates, data on the morbidity burden are notably lacking. This indicates the substantial need for further studies, with a particular focus on morbidity, to more accurately assess the current LF prevalence in the region.

It is important to note that the findings and conclusions in this paper are based solely on published prevalence data. It is therefore possible that they may not truly reflect the actual situation in these countries.

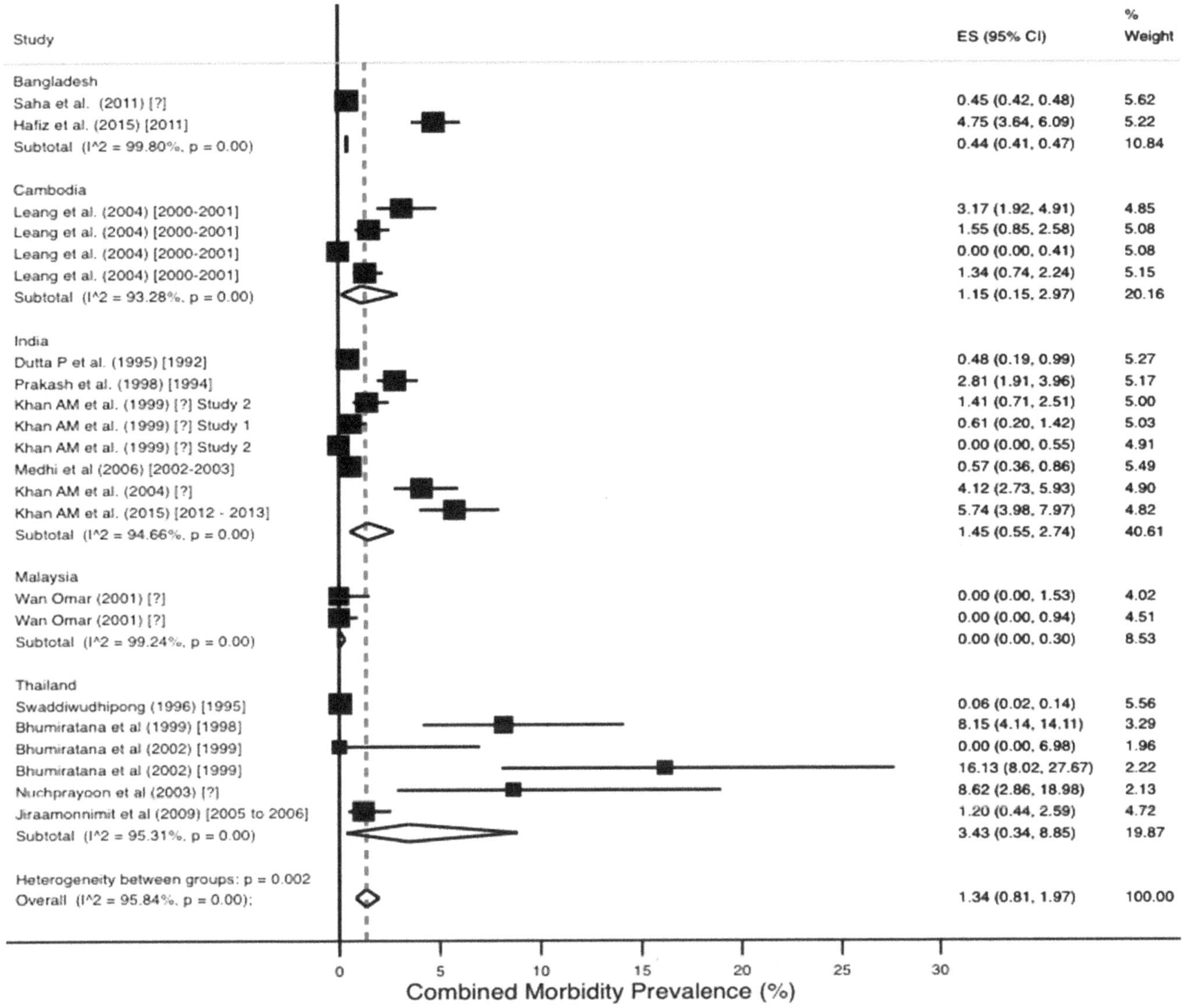

Figure 7. Percentage estimates of combined morbidity prevalence by country and year. ES: prevalence estimate. Red-dotted line: overall estimate. Diamond: sub-group estimate. Horizontal line: 95% CI.

5. Conclusions

Considerable progress has been made toward the LF elimination in mainland Southeast Asia, Bangladesh and Northeast India. Five of the eight countries reviewed are close to eliminating, or have eliminated, LF infection. The remaining three countries will require increasing support if they are to achieve LF elimination by 2020. The significant morbidity burden in the region requires increasing and urgent attention. Further studies are needed to more accurately assess the morbidity prevalence and implement desperately needed alleviation programs.

Supplementary Materials:
Quality Assessment of Included Peer-Reviewed Journal Articles; Table S2: Infection and Morbidity Prevalence by Country and Region in Peer-Reviewed Journals; Table S3: Infection and Morbidity Prevalence by Country and Region in Grey Literature; Figure S1: Percentage estimates of *W. bancrofti* microfilaraemia prevalence by country and year; Figure S2: Percentage estimates of *B. malayi* microfilaraemia prevalence by country and year; Figure S3: Percentage estimates of Og4C3 antigenaemia prevalence by country and year; Figure S4: Percentage estimates of IgG4 antibody prevalence by country and year; Figure S5: Percentage estimates of combined microfilaraemia prevalence in Northeast India; Figure S6: Percentage estimates of combined microfilaraemia prevalence in Thailand; Figure S7: Percentage estimates of ICT antigenaemia prevalence in Thailand; Figure S8: Percentage

estimates of hydrocoele prevalence in Thailand; Figure S9: Percentage estimates of combined morbidity prevalence in Thailand. Figure S10: PRISMA checklist.

Acknowledgments: The authors would like to thank Mohamed Jamsheed (WHO SEARO), Krongthong Thimasarn (WHO Myanmar), Gawrie Galappaththy (WHO Myanmar), San San Win (WHO Myanmar), Md. Kamar Rezwan (WHO Bangladesh), Kapa Ramaiah (consultant to WHO WPRO), Ni Ni Aye (VBDC Program, Myanmar Ministry of Health) and Aya Yajima (WHO WPRO) for information, collaboration and reports. We would also like to thank James Cook University for funding this research.

Author Contributions: B.F.R.D., P.M.G. and W.J.M. designed the study. B.F.R.D. collected the data. B.F.R.D. and P.M.G. analysed the data. B.F.R.D. and P.M.G. wrote the paper with input from W.J.M. All authors reviewed the final manuscript.

References

1. World Health Organization. *WHO Global Programme to Eliminate Lymphatic Filariasis: Progress Report for 2000–2009 and Strategic Plan 2010–2020*; World Health Organization: Geneva, Switzerland, 2010.
2. World Health Organization. Global programme to eliminate lymphatic filariasis: Progress report, 2015. *Wkly. Epidemiol. Record* **2016**, *91*, 441–460.
3. Ramaiah, K.; Ottesen, E.A. Progress and impact of 13 years of the global programme to eliminate lymphatic filariasis on reducing the burden of filarial disease. *PLoS Negl. Trop. Dis.* **2014**, *8*, e3319. [CrossRef] [PubMed]
4. Murray, C.J.; Barber, R.M.; Foreman, K.J.; Ozgoren, A.A.; Abd-Allah, F.; Abera, S.F.; Aboyans, V.; Abraham, J.P.; Abubakar, I.; Abu-Raddad, L.J. Global, regional, and national disability-adjusted life years (DALYs) for 306 diseases and injuries and healthy life expectancy (HALE) for 188 countries, 1990–2013: Quantifying the epidemiological transition. *Lancet* **2015**, *386*, 2145–2191. [CrossRef]
5. World Health Organization: Regional Office for South-East Asia. *Towards Eliminating Lymphatic Filariasis: Progress in the South-East.Region. (2001–2011)*; World Health Organization Regional Office for South-East Asia: New Delhi, India, 2013.
6. Weil, G.J.; Jain, D.C.; Santhanam, S.; Malhotra, A.; Kumar, H.; Sethumadhavan, K.V.P.; Liftis, F.; Ghosh, T.K. A monoclonal antibody-based enzyme immunoassay for detecting parasite antigenemia in bancroftian filariasis. *J. Infect. Dis.* **1987**, *156*, 350–355. [CrossRef] [PubMed]
7. Weil, G.J.; Lammie, P.J.; Weiss, N. The ICT filariasis test: A rapid-format antigen test for diagnosis of bancroftian filariasis. *Parasitol. Today* **1997**, *13*, 401–404. [CrossRef]
8. Gass, K.; de Rochars, M.V.B.; Boakye, D.; Bradley, M.; Fischer, P.U.; Gyapong, J.; Itoh, M.; Ituaso-Conway, N.; Joseph, H.; Kyelem, D. A multicenter evaluation of diagnostic tools to define endpoints for programs to eliminate bancroftian filariasis. *PLoS Negl. Trop. Dis.* **2012**, *6*, e1479. [CrossRef] [PubMed]
9. Lammie, P.J.; Weil, G.; Noordin, R.; Kaliraj, P.; Steel, C.; Goodman, D.; Lakshmikanthan, V.B.; Ottesen, E. Recombinant antigen-based antibody assays for the diagnosis and surveillance of lymphatic filariasis—A multicenter trial. *Filaria J.* **2004**, *3*, 9. [CrossRef] [PubMed]
10. Rebollo, M.P.; Bockarie, M.J. Shrinking the lymphatic filariasis map: Update on diagnostic tools for mapping and transmission monitoring. *Parasitology* **2014**, *141*, 1912–1917. [CrossRef] [PubMed]
11. World Health Organization. *WHO Global Programme to Eliminate Lymphatic Filariasis: Practical Entomology*; World Health Organization: Geneva, Switzerland, 2013.
12. World Health Organization. *Validation of Elimination of Lymphatic Filariasis as A Public Health Problem*; World Health Organization: Geneva, Switzerland, 2017.
13. World Health Organization. *Transmission Assessment Surveys in the Global Programme to Eliminate Lymphatic Filariasis: WHO Position Statement*; World Health Organization: Geneva, Switzerland, 2012.
14. Sudomo, M.; Chayabejara, S.; Duong, S.; Hernandez, L.; Wu, W.P.; Bergquist, R. Elimination of lymphatic filariasis in Southeast Asia. *Adv. Parasitol.* **2010**, *72*, 205–233. [PubMed]
15. Michael, E.; Bundy, D.A.P.; Grenfell, B.T. Re-assessing the global prevalence and distribution of lymphatic filariasis. *Parasitology* **1996**, *112*, 409–428. [CrossRef] [PubMed]
16. Meyrowitsch, D.W.; Nguyen, D.T.; Hoang, T.H.; Nguyen, T.D.; Michael, E. A review of the present status of lymphatic filariasis in Vietnam. *Acta Trop.* **1998**, *70*, 335–347. [CrossRef]

17. Moher, D.; Liberati, A.; Tetzlaff, J.; Altman, D.G. Preferred reporting items for systematic reviews and meta-analyses: The PRISMA statement. *Ann. Intern. Med.* **2009**, *151*, 264–269. [CrossRef] [PubMed]
18. PROSPERO Registered Study Protocol. Available online: http://www.crd.york.ac.uk/PROSPERO/display_record.asp?ID=CRD42014013070#.VAihrWSSxBA (accessed on 11 December 2016).
19. World Health Organization. *Institutional Repository of Information Sharing*. Available online: http://apps.who.int/iris/ (accessed on 11 December 2016).
20. Crowe, M. *Crowe Critical Appraisal Tool (CCAT) User Guide*; Conchra House: Scotland, UK, 2013.
21. Jackson, R.; Ameratunga, S.; Broad, J.; Connor, J.; Lethaby, A.; Robb, G.; Wells, S.; Glasziou, P.; Heneghan, C. The GATE frame: Critical appraisal with pictures. *Evid. Based Nurs.* **2006**, *9*, 68–71. [CrossRef] [PubMed]
22. World Health Organization. *Monitoring and Epidemiological Assessment of the Programme to Eliminate Lymphatic Filariasis at Implementation Unit Level*; World Health Organization: Geneva, Switzerland, 2005.
23. DerSimonian, R.; Laird, N. Meta-analysis in clinical trials. *Controll. Clin. Trials* **1986**, *7*, 177–188. [CrossRef]
24. Higgins, J.; Thompson, S.G.; Deeks, J.J.; Altman, D.G. Measuring inconsistency in meta-analyses. *BMJ* **2003**, *327*, 557–560. [CrossRef] [PubMed]
25. Ahmad, A.F.; Ngui, R.; Muhammad Aidil, R.; Lim, Y.A.; Rohela, M. Current status of parasitic infections among Pangkor Island community in Peninsular Malaysia. *Trop. Biomed.* **2014**, *31*, 836–843. [PubMed]
26. Bhumiratana, A.; Koyadun, S.; Srisuphanunt, M.; Satitvipawee, P.; Limpairojn, N.; Gaewchaiyo, G. Border and imported bancroftian filariases: Baseline seroprevalence in sentinel populations exposed to infections with *Wuchereria bancrofti* and concomitant HIV at the start of diethylcarbamazine mass treatment in Thailand. *Southeast Asian J. Trop. Med. Public Health* **2005**, *36*, 390–407. [PubMed]
27. Bhumiratana, A.; Koyadun, S.; Suvannadabba, S.; Karnjanopas, K.; Rojanapremsuk, J.; Buddhirakkul, P.; Tantiwattanasup, W. Field trial of the ICT filariasis for diagnosis of *Wuchereria bancrofti* infections in an endemic population of Thailand. *Southeast Asian J. Trop. Med. Public Health* **1999**, *30*, 562–568. [PubMed]
28. Bhumiratana, A.; Siriaut, C.; Koyadun, S.; Satitvipawee, P. Evaluation of a single oral dose of diethylcarbamazine 300 mg as provocative test and simultaneous treatment in Myanmar migrant workers with *Wuchereria bancrofti* infection in Thailand. *Southeast Asian J. Trop. Med. Public Health* **2004**, *35*, 591–598. [PubMed]
29. Bhumiratana, A.; Wattanakull, B.; Koyadun, S.; Suvannadabba, S.; Rojanapremsuk, J.; Tantiwattanasup, W. Relationship between male hydrocele and infection prevalences in clustered communities with uncertain transmission of *Wuchereria bancrofti* on the Thailand-Myanmar border. *Southeast Asian J. Trop. Med. Public Health* **2002**, *33*, 7–17. [PubMed]
30. Chansiri, K.; Phantana, S. A polymerase chain reaction assay for the survey of bancroftian filariasis. *Southeast Asian J. Trop. Med. Public Health* **2002**, *33*, 504–508. [PubMed]
31. Cox-Singh, J.; Pomrehn, A.S.; Rahman, H.A.; Zakaria, R.; Miller, A.O.; Singh, B. Simple blood-spot sampling with nested polymerase chain reaction detection for epidemiology studies on Brugia malayi. *Int. J. Parasitol.* **1999**, *29*, 717–721. [CrossRef]
32. Dutta, P.; Gogoi, B.K.; Chelleng, P.K.; Bhattacharyya, D.R.; Khan, S.A.; Goswami, B.K.; Mahanta, J. Filariasis in the labour population of a tea estate in Upper Assam. *Indian J. Med. Res.* **1995**, *101*, 245–246. [PubMed]
33. Hafiz, I.; Graves, P.; Haq, R.; Flora, M.S.; Kelly-Hope, L.A. Clinical case estimates of lymphatic filariasis in an endemic district of Bangladesh after a decade of mass drug administration. *Trans. R. Soc. Trop. Med. Hyg.* **2015**, *109*, 700–709. [CrossRef] [PubMed]
34. Hakim, S.L.; Vythilingam, I.; Marzukhi, M.I.; Mak, J.W. Single-dose diethylcarbamazine in the control of periodic brugian filariasis in Peninsular Malaysia. *Trans. R. Soc. Trop. Med. Hyg.* **1995**, *89*, 686–689. [CrossRef]
35. Jamail, M.; Andrew, K.; Junaidi, D.; Krishnan, A.K.; Faizal, M.; Rahmah, N. Field validation of sensitivity and specificity of rapid test for detection of Brugia malayi infection. *Trop. Med. Int. Health* **2005**, *10*, 99–104. [CrossRef] [PubMed]
36. Jiraamonnimit, C.; Wongkamchai, S.; Boitano, J.; Nochot, H.; Loymek, S.; Chujun, S.; Yodmek, S. A cohort study on anti-filarial IgG4 and its assessment in good and uncertain MDA-compliant subjects in brugian filariasis endemic areas in southern Thailand. *J. Helminthol.* **2009**, *83*, 351–360. [CrossRef] [PubMed]
37. Khan, A.M.; Dutta, P.; Khan, S.A.; Baruah, N.K.; Sarma, C.K.; Mahanta, J. Prevalence of bancroftian filariasis in a foot-hill tea garden of upper Assam. *J. Commun. Dis.* **1999**, *31*, 145–146. [PubMed]
38. Khan, A.M.; Dutta, P.; Khan, S.A.; Baruah, N.K.; Sharma, C.K.; Mahanta, J. Bancroftian filariasis in a weaving community of lower Assam. *J. Commun. Dis.* **1999**, *31*, 61–62. [PubMed]

39. Khan, A.M.; Dutta, P.; Khan, S.A.; Mahanta, J. A focus of lymphatic filariasis in a tea garden worker community of central Assam. *J. Environ. Biol.* **2004**, *25*, 437–440. [PubMed]
40. Khan, A.M.; Dutta, P.; Khan, S.A.; Mohapatra, P.K.; Baruah, N.K.; Sharma, C.K.; Mahanta, A.J. Lymphatic filariasis in two distinct communities of upper Assam. *J. Commun. Dis.* **1999**, *31*, 101–106. [PubMed]
41. Khan, A.M.; Dutta, P.; Sarmah, C.K.; Baruah, N.K.; Das, S.; Pathak, A.K.; Sarmah, P.; Hussain, M.E.; Mahanta, J. Prevalence of lymphatic filariasis in a tea garden worker population of Dibrugarh (Assam), India after six rounds of mass drug administration. *J. Vector Borne Dis.* **2015**, *52*, 314–320. [PubMed]
42. Koyadun, S.; Bhumiratana, A. Surveillance of imported bancroftian filariasis after two-year multiple-dose diethylcarbamazine treatment. *Southeast Asian J. Trop. Med. Public Health* **2005**, *36*, 822–831. [PubMed]
43. Koyadun, S.; Bhumiratana, A.; Prikchu, P. *Wuchereria bancrofti* antigenemia clearance among Myanmar migrants after biannual mass treatments with diethylcarbamazine, 300 mg oral-dose FILADEC tablet, in Southern Thailand. *Southeast Asian J. Trop. Med. Public Health* **2003**, *34*, 758–767. [PubMed]
44. Krairittichai, U.; Pungprakiet, D.; Boonthongtho, K.; Arsayot, K. Prevalence of infectious diseases of immigrant workers receiving health examinations at Rajavithi Hospital. *J. Med. Assoc. Thail.* **2012**, *95* (Suppl. 3), S1–S6.
45. Leang, R.; Socheat, D.; Bin, B.; Bunkea, T.; Odermatt, P. Assessment of disease and infection of lymphatic filariasis in Northeastern Cambodia. *Trop. Med. Int. Health* **2004**, *9*, 1115–1120. [CrossRef] [PubMed]
46. Lim, B.H.; Rahmah, N.; Afifi, S.A.; Ramli, A.; Mehdi, R. Comparison of Brugia-ELISA and thick blood smear examination in a prevalence study of brugian filariasis in Setiu, Terengganu, Malaysia. *Med. J. Malays.* **2001**, *56*, 491–496.
47. Medhi, G.K.; Hazarika, N.C.; Shah, B.; Mahanta, J. Study of health problems and nutritional status of tea garden population of Assam. *Indian J. Med. Sci.* **2006**, *60*, 496–505. [PubMed]
48. Nuchprayoon, S.; Porksakorn, C.; Junpee, A.; Sanprasert, V.; Poovorawan, Y. Comparative assessment of an Og4C3 ELISA and an ICT filariasis test: A study of Myanmar migrants in Thailand. *Asian Pac. J. Allergy Immunol.* **2003**, *21*, 253–257. [PubMed]
49. Nuchprayoon, S.; Sanprasert, V.; Porksakorn, C.; Nuchprayoon, I. Prevalence of bancroftian filariasis on the Thai-Myanmar border. *Asian Pac. J. Allergy Immunol.* **2003**, *21*, 179–188. [PubMed]
50. Nuchprayoon, S.; Yentakam, S.; Sangprakarn, S.; Junpee, A. Endemic bancroftian filariasis in Thailand: detection by Og4C3 antigen capture ELISA and the polymerase chain reaction. *J. Med. Assoc. Thail.* **2001**, *84*, 1300–1307.
51. Prakash, A.; Mohapatra, P.K.; Das, H.K.; Sharma, R.K.; Mahanta, J. Bancroftian filariasis in Namrup tea estate, district Dibrugarh, Assam. *Indian J. Public Health* **1998**, *42*, 103–107. [PubMed]
52. Priest, J.W.; Jenks, M.H.; Moss, D.M.; Mao, B.; Buth, S.; Wannemuehler, K.; Soeung, S.C.; Lucchi, N.W.; Udhayakumar, V.; Gregory, C.J. Integration of multiplex bead assays for parasitic diseases into a national, population-based serosurvey of women 15–39 years of age in Cambodia. *PLoS Negl. Trop. Dis.* **2016**, *10*, e0004699. [CrossRef] [PubMed]
53. Rahmah, N.; Lim, B.H.; Azian, H.; Ramelah, T.S.; Rohana, A.R. Short communication: Use of a recombinant antigen-based ELISA to determine prevalence of brugian filariasis among Malaysian schoolchildren near Pasir Mas, Kelantan-Thailand border. *Trop. Med. Int. Health* **2003**, *8*, 158–163. [CrossRef] [PubMed]
54. Rahmah, N.; Nurulhasanah, O.; Norhayati, S.; Zulkarnain, I.; Norizan, M. Comparison of conventional versus real-time PCR detection of *Brugia malayi* DNA from dried blood spots from school children in a low endemic area. *Trop. Biomed.* **2010**, *27*, 54–59. [PubMed]
55. Saha, A.K.; Mohanta, M.K. Bancroftian elephantiasis in Nilphamari, Bangladesh. *Mymensingh Med. J. MMJ* **2011**, *20*, 40–44. [PubMed]
56. Samad, M.S.; Itoh, M.; Moji, K.; Hossain, M.; Mondal, D.; Alam, M.S.; Kimura, E. Enzyme-linked immunosorbent assay for the diagnosis of *Wuchereria bancrofti* infection using urine samples and its application in Bangladesh. *J. Parasitol. Res.* **2013**, *62*, 564–567. [CrossRef] [PubMed]
57. Satimai, W.; Jiraamonnimit, C.; Thammapalo, S.; Choochote, W.; Luenee, P.; Boitano, J.J.; Wongkamchai, S. The impact of a national program to eliminate lymphatic filariasis in selected Myanmar immigrant communities in Bangkok and Ranong Province, Thailand. *Southeast Asian J. Trop. Med. Public Health* **2011**, *42*, 1054–1064. [PubMed]
58. Swaddiwudhipong, W.; Tatip, Y.; Meethong, M.; Preecha, P.; Kobasa, T. Potential transmission of bancroftian filariasis in urban Thailand. *Southeast Asian J. Trop. Med. Public Health* **1996**, *27*, 847–849. [PubMed]

59. Triteeraprapab, S.; Karnjanopas, K.; Porksakorn, C.; Sai-Ngam, A.; Yentakam, S.; Loymak, S. Lymphatic filariasis caused by *Brugia malayi* in an endemic area of Narathiwat Province, southern of Thailand. *J. Med. Assoc. Thail.* **2001**, *84* (Suppl. S1), S182–S188.
60. Triteeraprapab, S.; Nuchprayoon, I.; Porksakorn, C.; Poovorawan, Y.; Scott, A.L. High prevalence of *Wuchereria bancrofti* infection among Myanmar migrants in Thailand. *Ann. Trop. Med. Parasitol.* **2001**, *95*, 535–538. [CrossRef] [PubMed]
61. Triteeraprapab, S.; Songtrus, J. High prevalence of bancroftian filariasis in Myanmar-migrant workers: A study in Mae Sot district, Tak province, Thailand. *J. Med. Assoc. Thail.* **1999**, *82*, 735–739.
62. Wan Omar, A.; Sulaiman, O.; Yusof, S.; Ismail, G.; Fatmah, M.S.; Rahmah, N.; Khairul, A.A. Epidemiological screening of lymphatic filariasis among immigrants using dipstick colloidal dye immunoassay. *Malays. J. Med. Sci.* **2001**, *8*, 19–24. [PubMed]
63. World Health Organization: Regional Office for South-East Asia. *Elimination of Lymphatic Filariasis in the South-East Asia Region: Report of the Eighth Meeting of National National Programme Managers*; WHO Regional Office for South-East Asia: New Delhi, India, 2011.
64. World Health Organization: Regional Office for South-East Asia. *Elimination of Lymphatic Filariasis in the South-East Asia Region: Report of the Fifth Meeting of National National Programme Managers*; WHO Regional Office for South-East Asia: New Delhi, India, 2006.
65. United States Agency for International Development. *FHI360/USAID. End Neglected Tropical Diseases in Asia: Final Report*; USAID: Washington, DC, USA, 2015.
66. World Health Organization: Regional Office for the Western Pacific. *First Mekong-Plus Programme Managers Workshop on Lymphatic Filariasis and Other Helminthiasis, Phnom Penh, Cambodia, 23–26 March 2009*; WHO Regional Office for the Western Pacific: Manila, Philippines, 2009.
67. World Health Organization: Regional Office for the Western Pacific. *Malaysia: Country Cooperation Strategy 2009–2013*; WHO Regional Office for the Western Pacific: Manila, Philippines, 2010.
68. Myanmar Ministry of Health. *Myanmar National Programme to Eliminate Lymphatic Filariasis: Annual Report (2005)*; Myanmar Ministry of Health: Naypyitaw, Myanmar, 2005.
69. Myanmar Ministry of Health. *Myanmar National Programme to Eliminate Lymphatic Filariasis: Annual Report (2011)*; Myanmar Ministry of Health: Naypyitaw, Myanmar, 2011.
70. Myanmar Ministry of Health. *Myanmar National Programme to Eliminate Lymphatic Filariasis: Annual Report (2012)*; Myanmar Ministry of Health: Naypyitaw, Myanmar, 2012.
71. World Health Organization: Regional Office for South-East Asia. *Regional Stategic Plan. for Elimination of Lymphatic Filariasis (2004–2007)*; WHO Regional Office for South-East Asia: New Delhi, India, 2004.
72. World Health Organization: Regional Office for the Western Pacific. *Report of the Thirteenth Meeting of the Western Pacific Regional Programme Review Group on Neglected Tropical Diseases*; WHO Regional Office for the Western Pacific: Manila, Philippines, 2013.
73. World Health Organization. *UNDP-World Bank-WHO Special Programme for Research and Training in Tropical Diseases WHO-UNICEF Joint Programme for Health Mapping World Health Organization: Division of Tropical Diseases. Research on Rapid Geographical Assessment of Bancroftian Filariasis*; World Health Organization: Geneva, Switzerland, 1998.
74. World Health Organization: Regional Office for South-East Asia. *South-East Asia Regional Programme Review Group of Elimination of Lymphatic Filariasis: Report of the Eight Meeting*; WHO Regional Office for South-East Asia: New Delhi, India, 2011.
75. World Health Organization: Regional Office for South-East Asia. *South.-East. Asia Regional Programme Review Group of Elimination of Lymphatic Filariasis: Report of the First Meeting*; WHO Regional Office for South-East Asia: New Delhi, India, 2005.
76. World Health Organization: Regional Office for South-East Asia. *South.-East. Asia Regional Programme Review Group of Elimination of Lymphatic Filariasis: Report of the Ninth Meeting*; WHO Regional Office for South-East Asia: New Delhi, India, 2012.
77. World Health Organization: Regional Office for South-East Asia. *South.-East. Asia Regional Programme Review Group of Elimination of Lymphatic Filariasis: Report of the Seventh Meeting*; WHO Regional Office for South-East Asia: New Delhi, India, 2010.

78. World Health Organization: Regional Office for South-East Asia. *South.-East. Asia Regional Programme Review Group of Elimination of Lymphatic Filariasis: Report of the Tenth Meeting*; WHO Regional Office for South-East Asia: New Delhi, India, 2013.
79. World Health Organization: Regional Office for the Western Pacific. *Report of the Fourteenth Meeting of the Western Pacific Regional Programme Review Group on Neglected Tropical Diseases*; WHO Regional Office for the Western Pacific: Manila, Philippines, 2014.
80. World Health Organization. *Strengthening the Assessment of Lymphatic Filariasis Transmission and Documenting the Achievement of Elimination*; World Health Organization: Geneva, Switzerland, 2016.
81. Cambodia Ministry of Planning. *General Population Census of Cambodia 1998: Final Results*, 2nd ed.; Cambodia Ministry of Planning: Phnom Penh, Cambodia, 2002.
82. Beng, T.S.; Ahmad, R.; Hisam, R.S.R.; Heng, S.K.; Leaburi, J.; Ismail, Z.; Sulaiman, L.H.; Soyoti, R.F.H.M.; Lim, L.H. Molecular xenomonitoring of filarial infection in Malaysian mosquitoes under the National Program for Elimination of Lymphatic Filariasis. *Southeast Asian J. Trop. Med. Public Health* **2016**, *47*, 617–624.
83. Mathieu, E.; Amann, J.; Eigege, A.; Richards, F.; Sodahlon, Y. Collecting baseline information for national morbidity alleviation programs: Different methods to estimate lymphatic filariasis morbidity prevalence. *Am. J. Trop. Med. Hyg.* **2008**, *78*, 153–158. [PubMed]
84. Triteeraprapab, S.; Kanjanopas, K.; Suwannadabba, S.; Sangprakarn, S.; Poovorawan, Y.; Scott, A.L. Transmission of the nocturnal periodic strain of *Wuchereria bancrofti* by *Culex quinquefasciatus*: Establishing the potential for urban filariasis in Thailand. *Epidemiol. Infect.* **2000**, *125*, 207–212. [CrossRef] [PubMed]
85. Bhumiratana, A.; Intarapuk, A.; Koyadun, S.; Maneekan, P.; Sorosjinda-Nunthawarasilp, P. Current bancroftian filariasis elimination on Thailand-Myanmar border: Public Health Challenges toward Postgenomic MDA Evaluation. *ISRN Trop. Med.* **2013**, *2013*. [CrossRef]
86. Toothong, T.; Tipayamongkholgul, M.; Suwannapong, N.; Suvannadabba, S. Evaluation of mass drug administration in the program to control imported lymphatic filariasis in Thailand. *BMC Public Health* **2015**, *15*, 975. [CrossRef] [PubMed]

9

Soil-Transmitted Helminths in Tropical Australia and Asia

Catherine A. Gordon [1,*], Johanna Kurscheid [2], Malcolm K. Jones [3], Darren J. Gray [2] and Donald P. McManus [1]

1 QIMR Berghofer Medical Research Institute, Molecular Parasitology Laboratory, Queensland 4006, Australia; Don.McManus@qimrberghofer.edu.au
2 Australian National University, Department of Global Health, Research School of Population Health, Australian Capital Territory 2601, Australia; Johanna.Kurscheid@anu.edu.au (J.K.); darren.gray@anu.edu.au (D.J.G.)
3 School of Veterinary Science, University of Queensland, Brisbane, QLD 4067, Australia; m.jones@uq.edu.au
* Correspondence: Catherine.Gordon@qimrberghofer.edu.au;

Abstract: Soil-transmitted helminths (STH) infect 2 billion people worldwide including significant numbers in South-East Asia (SEA). In Australia, STH are of less concern; however, indigenous communities are endemic for STH, including *Strongyloides stercoralis*, as well as for serious clinical infections due to other helminths such as *Toxocara* spp. The zoonotic hookworm *Ancylostoma ceylanicum* is also present in Australia and SEA, and may contribute to human infections particularly among pet owners. High human immigration rates to Australia from SEA, which is highly endemic for STH *Strongyloides* and *Toxocara*, has resulted in a high prevalence of these helminthic infections in immigrant communities, particularly since such individuals are not screened for worm infections upon entry. In this review, we consider the current state of STH infections in Australia and SEA.

Keywords: soil-transmitted helminths; *Trichuris trichiura*; *Ascaris lumbricoides*; hookworm; *Ancylostoma ceylanicum*; *Strongyloides stercoralis*; South East Asia; Australia

1. Introduction

Soil-transmitted helminths (STH) are estimated to infect 2 billion people worldwide. Many of these infections occur in South-East Asia (SEA) [1,2]. Species included in the term STH are the human hookworm species *Ancylostoma duodenale* and *Necator americanus*, the human roundworm *Ascaris lumbricoides*, and the human whipworm *Trichuris trichiura* [3]. Hookworm and *Trichuris* have zoonotic counterparts (*A. caninum*, *A. ceylanicum*, *T. suis*, and *T. vulpis*) [4–14]. *A. lumbricoides* itself is a zoonosis as the previously-identified pig roundworm, *A. suum*, has been found through molecular characterisation to be nearly identical to *A. lumbricoides*, and instead represents a haplotype of *A. lumbricoides* [6,15]. *Toxocara canis* and *Strongyloides stercoralis* are additional important nematode species of dogs that can also infect humans and are included in this review. *Strongyloides* is estimated to infect 30–100 million people [16,17], while the seroprevalence (2–5% in urban areas, 14.2–37% in rural areas) of *Toxocara* in developed countries indicates that the number of people at risk of infection may be in the millions [18]. While *Toxocara* and *Strongyloides* have low prevalences in Australia, our closest neighbours in SEA, as well as many countries from which refugees and immigrants originate, are highly endemic for these parasites. These helminths are also considered neglected tropical diseases (NTD) due to their occurrence in low socio-economic regions and have thus not received as much attention as other diseases occurring in developed countries. Primarily, these helminthic infections are endemic in tropical and subtropical areas due to the requirements for warm moist soil for egg or larval development.

Another potential reason for their status as NTDs is the chronic rather than acute nature of the infections they cause. Symptoms are similar between the causative species and are generally non-specific; namely nausea and/or vomiting, diarrhoea, abdominal pain, and fever. In adults the impact can be seen as lower ability to work. As such, the impact of these parasites should be examined by considering the disability adjusted life years (DALYs) to measure disease burden. According to the WHO definition, one DALY is one year of life quality lost compared to a healthy individual, and the sum of these DALYs across a population is a measurement of the gap between current health status and an ideal health situation [19].

As of 2010 there were an estimated 438.9 million people infected globally with hookworm, 819.0 million with *A. lumbricoides*, and 464.4 million with *T. trichiura* [20]. It was calculated that STH contributed to 4.98 million years lived with disability (YLDs), with 65% attributed to hookworm, 22% to *A. lumbricoides*, and 13% to *T. trichiura* [20]. The DALYs for intestinal helminths (including only *A. lumbricoides*, *T. trichiura*, and hookworm) have been reduced from 170 per 100,000 (94–290) in 1990 to 75 per 100,000 (43–128) in 2010 and 69.4 per 100,000 (43.3–106.4) in 2013 [21,22]. DALYs are not considered a good measurement of the burden of disease for *S. stercoralis* since the majority of infections cause limited clinical symptoms; the most common complaint and symptom is stomachache. Poor diagnostics for *S. stercoralis* also result in the true prevalence being underestimated [23].

Infection with hookworm or hyper-infection with *S. stercoralis* can result in anaemia, and hookworm can also present with cutaneous rash from larval migration. *Ascaris*, *Strongyloides* and hookworm larvae migrate to the lungs to be coughed up and swallowed, thus entering the gut where they mature. Lung-stage infection by *Ascaris* can cause pneumonia, called Loeffler's pneumonia, while disseminated *Strongyloides* can also cause pneumonia and pulmonary haemorrhage; hookworm-associated pneumonia, 'eosinophilic pneumonia', is a rare manifestation [24–26]. *Toxocara* infections can result in a range of symptoms depending on where the larvae migrate. The migrating larvae themselves, much like in *Strongyloides* and hookworm infections, can result in a rash, or larval tracks, due to inflammation. In the eye, *Toxocara* can cause partial or total retinal detachment leading to blindness and may result in neurological symptoms if the larvae are present in the brain [18,27].

Strongyloides stercoralis, which is endemic in aboriginal communities of Australia, can be a serious roundworm infection with severe health implications due to autoinfection and dissemination. Infection in immunocompromised individuals is particularly serious, and can be fatal. Autoinfection with *S. stercoralis* occurs when the larvae produced by the adult worms cause reinfection without ever having to leave the body. In such instances there is no immune response against the migrating larvae and this can lead to hyperinfection and dissemination. Continuous reinfection with *S. stercoralis* through autoinfection can also lead to persistent infections lasting many years (Figure 1). Infections in immigrants in Australia have been found more than 20 years after moving away from an endemic area (Table 1). Disseminated strongyloidiasis occurs when the parasite is distributed throughout the body and is more commonly seen in people with impaired immune systems [28]. It can lead to abdominal pain and swelling, pulmonary and neurological complications and meningitis, depending on where the parasite is located, as well as septicaemia, a leading cause of death in *S. stercoralis* infection [28,29]. Septicaemia occurs due to migration of larvae through the gastrointestinal wall. While generally considered as a human parasite, *S. stercoralis* has also been found in non-human primates and dogs [30–32]. There are also haplotypes identified for this species, and grouping of haplotypes from humans with haplotypes from canids and indicates potential zoonotic transmission [33,34]. Sequencing of isolates found in dogs and humans in Cambodia found two haplotypes of *S. stercoralis* in dogs, one of which was indistinguishable from that found in humans, again indicating the potential for zoonotic transmission [30]. Dogs are an important reservoir for zoonotic infections in terms of transmission as they live in close contact with humans, increasing the likelihood of transmission when compared with other potential zoonotic hosts such as non-human primates, which have a far more limited association with humans. Australia has a high pet ownership, particularly dogs and cats, with many also living inside homes, thus providing clear potential for transmission [35].

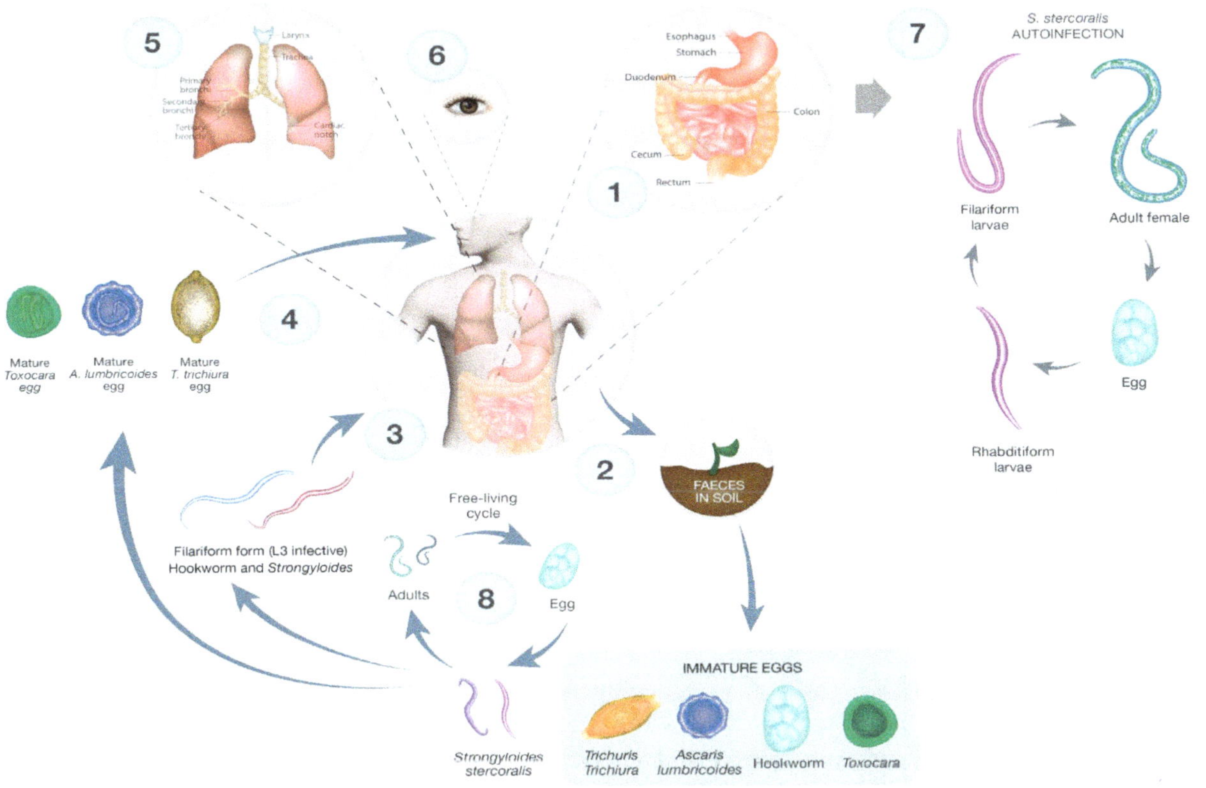

Figure 1. Lifecycles of soil-transmitted helminths (STH), *S. sterocoralis*, and *Toxocara*. **1.** Adult worms reside in the gastrointestinal tract (GIT). Hookworm, *A. lumbricoides*, and *S. stercoralis* adults reside in the small intestine while *T. trichiura* adults reside in the cecum and ascending colon. Female worms produce eggs which are passed in the stool of an infected person. **2.** *T. trichiura*, *Toxocara*, and *A. lumbricoides* eggs mature in soil but do not hatch. Hookworm eggs hatch in soil and mature into L3 hookworm larvae. *S. stercoralis* eggs hatch into rhabditiform larvae in the gut, which are then excreted via the faeces. Rhabditiform larvae then mature into infective filariform larvae or free-living adults. **3.** Infectious L3 filariform larvae of hookworm and *S. stercoralis* penetrate the skin directly, enter the circulation and migrate to the GIT after passing into the lumen of the lungs. **4.** Mature eggs of *Toxocara*, *A. lumbricoides*, and *T. trichiura* are swallowed by the host. The eggs hatch, releasing larvae in the GIT. *T. trichiura* larvae hatch in the small intestine and mature into adults in the colon while *Toxocara* and *A. lumbricoides* larvae penetrate the gut. *Toxocara* larvae are carried by the circulation to a variety of tissue types while *A. lumbricoides* larvae are carried to the lungs. **5.** Hookworm and *A. lumbricoides* larvae penetrate the alveolar walls and ascend the bronchial tree to the throat and are swallowed. Once they reach the small intestine the larvae mature into adults. *S. stercoralis* can also follow bronchial migration, or they can penetrate straight to the GIT. **6.** *Toxocara* larvae can be carried to any tissue type. As humans are dead-end hosts the larvae do not undergo further development once they reach these sites, they can cause local reactions, known as the disease toxocariasis. Ocular toxocariasis, where the larvae penetrate the eye, can result in blindness. **7.** *S. stercoralis* can also undergo autoinfection, where the rhabditiform larvae become infective filarial form larvae in the small intestine and penetrate the gut or perianal region. The filariform larvae can then disseminate to throughout the body. **8.** *Strongyloides* rhabditiform larvae develop into free-living adults that produce eggs from which rhabditidorm larvae hatch. Rhabditiform larvae then develop into infectious filariform larvae and penetrate a human host. The free-living cycle exists for one generation cycle only.

Table 1. Prevalence of soil-transmitted helminths diagnosed in immigrants, refugees, ADF[#] personnel, and returned travellers in Australia since 2000.

Years Sampled	Reference	Status	Country of Origin	Parasite Species	Prevalence	Diagnostics
2000, 2002	[36]	Immigrant	East Africa Cambodia	*S. stercoralis* *T. trichiura* *S. stercoralis* Hookworm spp.	11% (n = 124) 4% (n = 124) 42% (n = 230) 1.96% (n = 230)	Faecal samples (method unclear) Serology (method unclear)
7–20 years after resettlement	[37]	Immigrant	Laos	*S. stercoralis*	24.21% (n = 95)	Faecal microscopy Strongyloides serology
2–52 years after resettlement 1998–2005	[38] *	Immigrant	Fiji (1), SEA (5), China (1), Sri Lanka (1), India (2), Seychelles (2), Ethiopia (2), Russia (1), Italy (1), Greece (1)	*S. stercoralis*	100% (n = 17) *	Faecal microscopy Strongyloides serology
1998–2005	[38]*	Returned travellers	Papua New Guinea (1), Vanuatu (1), SEA (7), Africa (2)	*S. stercoralis*	100% (n = 11) *	Faecal microscopy Strongyloides serology
2004	[39]	Returned ADF [#] member	Solomon Islands	*A. ceylanicum*	100% (n = 1)	Harada-Mori culture, direct faecal smear
Served 1962–1975 2010	[40]	ADF veterans	Vietnam	*S. stercoralis*	11.6% (n = 249)	Faecal microscopy ELISA
2006–2007	[41]	RAMSI personnel ***	Solomon Islands	*S. stercoralis*	100% (n = 14) *	Faecal microscopy, Serology (ELISA)

Table 1. *Cont.*

Years Sampled	Reference	Status	Country of Origin	Parasite Species	Prevalence	Diagnostics
2002–2012	[42]	Residents Northern Territory	Australia	*T. trichiura*	0.65% (n = 63,668) **	Wet mount microscopy, Concentration method
2002–2011	[43]	Residents Northern Territory	Australia	Hookworm	0.17% (n = 64,691) **	Wet mount microscopy, Concentration method
2004–2008	[44]	Immigrants	Burma	*S. stercoralis*	26% (n = 156)	Serology
2002	[45]	Immigrants	Cambodia	*S. stercoralis*	36% (n = 234) *	ELISA, faecal microscopy
2010–2011	[46]	Residents Northern Territory	Australia	*S. stercoralis*	16.5% (n = 124) pre-treatment 12% (n = 30) post-treatment	Serology (NIE ELISA, NIE-DBS-ELISA)
2000–2006	[29]	Residents	Australia	*S. stercoralis*	100% (n = 18) *	Faecal microscopy, serology
1994–1996	[47]	Residents	Australia	*T. canis* *S. stercoralis* *S. stercoralis*	21% (n = 29) 28% (n = 29) 19% (n = 314)	Serology Serology Formol-ether
	[48]	Immigrant	Laos	*S. stercoralis*	Single patient	Larvae in sputum
2010–2011	[49]	Immigrants Residents Residents	Australia	*N. americanus* *A. ceylanicum* *A. duodenale*	(n = 5/227) **** (n = 2/227) (n = 4/227)	PCR Sequencing

Australian Defence Force (ADF); * retrospective review of positive cases; ** faecal samples; *** Regional Assistance Mission to Solomon Islands; **** faecal samples from individuals with a documented history of gastrointestinal disorders.

Recent molecular analysis of hookworm species has been important for speciation and shows a different epidemiological pattern than previously thought, including a much higher prevalence of *A. ceylanicum,* which had been considered to be only a rare infection in humans [4,11,50–53]. This is due in part to the morphological similarity of eggs and larval stages between hookworm species leading to misdiagnosis, and partly due to initial erroneous assumptions of their epidemiology [53]. While dogs are thought to be the primary source of zoonotic *A. ceylanicum,* there is evidence that human–human transmission can occur [11]. Two haplotypes have been identified, with the zoonotic haplotype also identified in cats [11,54]. This has public health implications, since dogs and cats will act as reservoir hosts and will thus need to be taken into consideration for control. Dogs are also the main host for *A. caninum,* which can cause gastric enteritis in humans, and *Toxocara canis* which can cause serious eye disease often resulting in blindness, as well as neurological symptoms depending on where the parasite migrates to in the body. *T. cati,* found in cats, can also cause similar pathology.

We review the STH, *Strongyloides* and *Toxocara* in SEA and Australia, considering their lifecycles; prevalence in SE Asia and Australia; diagnosis; and treatment and control. In addition, their zoonotic potential will be further explored.

2. Lifecycles

The lifecycles of the STH are shown in Figure 1, illustrating key differences in infection strategy and migration pathways. Adults of all STH species and *S. stercoralis* live in the gastrointestinal tract (GIT) and produce eggs that are excreted into the environment via the stool. STH and *S. stercoralis* require moist, warm soil to develop, largely restricting these parasites to tropical areas. Hookworm eggs hatch in the faecal mass and moult from L1 to infective L3 larvae. The L3 larvae then migrate onto vegetation, penetrate the skin, are carried via the blood to the lungs where they undergo tracheal migration, pass through to the small intestine, mature into adults and attach to the gut wall [55]. For both *T. trichiura* and *A. lumbricoides,* eggs are passed unembryonated and mature to an infectious stage after 15 days. The now infectious eggs are ingested, often due to poor hygiene and contaminated food, and hatch in the small intestine. Larvae of *T. trichiura* then mature in the small intestine into adults [56]. *A. lumbricoides* larvae penetrate the gut and undergo tracheal migration similar to hookworm larvae, and develop into mature adults once in the small intestine (Figure 1) [57].

The lifecycle of *S. stercoralis* is more complicated than other STH since it has a free-living stage in addition to the parasitic lifecycle [58]. Adults in the gut produce eggs that hatch into first-stage larvae, which have a distinctive oesophageal appearance that gives rise to the descriptive term 'rhabditiform larva'. This first stage larva will moult to become either free-living, a dioecious adult or an infectious larva, the filariform larva. Free-living adults produce eggs that hatch as rhabditiform larvae that moult twice to become 3rd stage filariform larvae. Filariform larvae then penetrate the skin, much like hookworm L3 larvae, and migrate to the gut – this can be via the lungs and they are coughed up as occurs in the hookworm lifecycle, or direct travel to the gut. Autoinfection occurs when eggs from adult parasites hatch into rhabditiform larvae that become filariform larvae while still in the gut. The filariform larvae can complete the lifecycle in the gut, or disseminate, migrating to other organs and tissues (Figure 1). The free-living cycle for *S. stercoralis* only persists for one generation, not indefinitely as in *Parastrongyloides sp.* [59,60].

Humans are accidental hosts of *Toxocara* spp. and become infected by ingesting eggs in contaminated soil [61]. The eggs hatch in the gut and the larvae penetrate the gut and are carried by the blood to different organs where they can promote a local reaction, which is the cause of toxocariasis. Visceral and ocular migrans are the most common presentations. There is also a suggested link between seropositivity for toxocariasis and epilepsy [62].

3. STH and *Strongyloides* in SEA

STH infections are common in SEA, where approximately one-third of global STH cases occur, with active, stable transmission occurring in all countries of the region [63–65] (Figure 2). Risk factors for infection include poverty, lack of access to clean water and toilets, as well as unhygienic practices such as not washing hands [64].

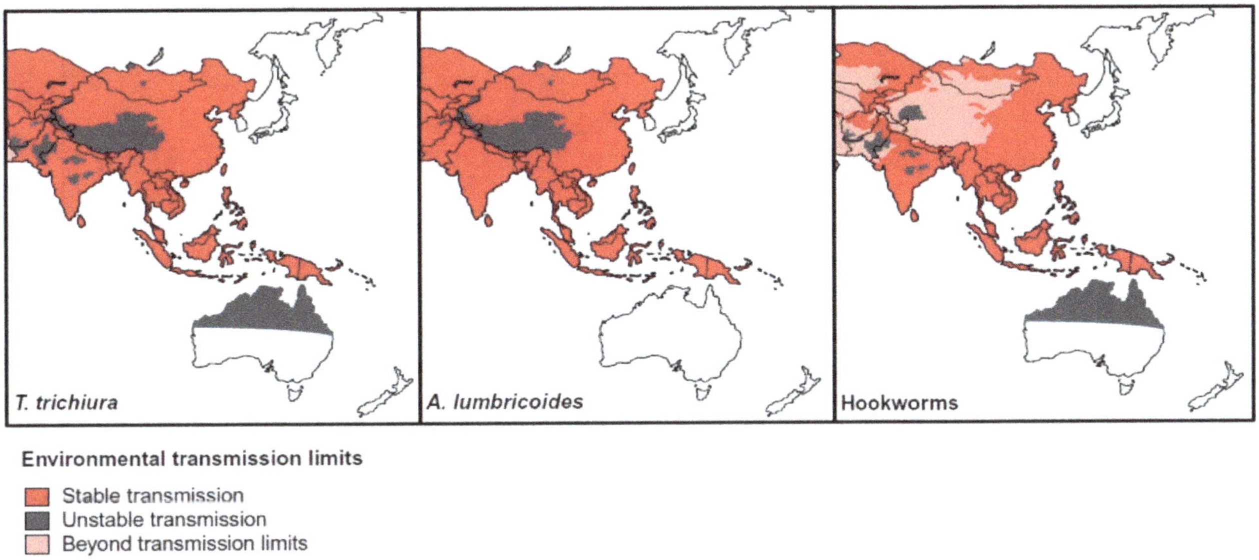

Figure 2. Distribution of STH in South-East Asia and Australia, modified from Brooker et al., [64].

T. trichiura, *A. lumbricoides* and hookworm are the most prevalent STH and infected individuals are often found with co-infections. Polyparasitism with STH is very common in SEA, mainly due to the shared geographical locations in tropical areas, where these worms are endemic. Additionally, the infection pathways of the STH are similar (Figure 1). Polyparasitism with STH is more likely than mono-infection in endemic areas, where co-infection with other helminths and protozoan parasites is also very high [66–71]. Because STH endemicity is quite low in Australia, data for polyparasitism is limited, although it may occur in remote Aboriginal communities [42].

Co-infections with parasites have been identified with increased disease status, and synergism between parasite infections. Infection intensity of helminths in co-infections also seems to differ, with hookworm infection intensity significantly increased with multiple infections [72]. Maternal infection with STH may also increase susceptibility of the unborn child to infection with STH, but it is unclear if this is due to shared environmental factors [73,74]. Co-infections may necessitate combination chemotherapy depending on drug efficacy for the infecting species.

The precise global prevalence of *Strongyloides* is unknown although it is estimated to infect 30–100 million people worldwide [75]. There are also issues with diagnosis because serology can return negative results, particularly in early infections, and may not pick up disseminated cases [16]. Eggs are rarely seen in the stool; rather the rhabditiform larvae are present instead, although often in low numbers. Both copro-culture, which can be laborious, and direct smears, can be used to identify larvae [76]. Other methods include the formalin ethyl acetate sedimentation method, which has low sensitivity, immunodiagnostics, and molecular methods [77]. Molecular methods, specifically PCR, have been used to sensitively diagnose *Strongyloides* [78,79]. *Strongyloides* is endemic in SEA and there are a number of reports from countries in the region using an array of different diagnostic techniques [80–83]. A comprehensive review is available of its global distribution based on community, hospital, and refugee and immigrant surveys [84] (Figure 3). Depending on the diagnostic method used, the prevalence of *S. stercoralis* given in Figure 3 may be an underestimate due to the low sensitivity of many of the procedures used, and the low number of larvae that are excreted, even in heavy infections [77,79,84].

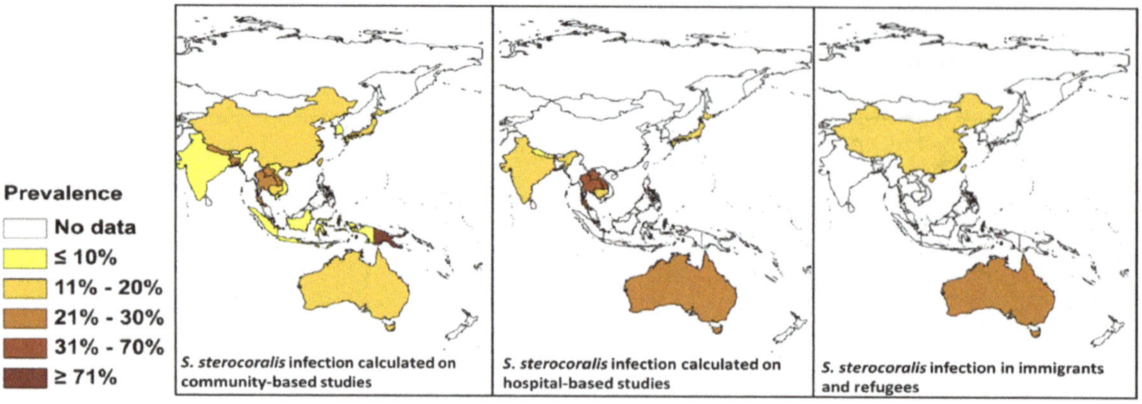

Figure 3. Prevalence of *S. stercoralis* in Asia and Australia based on community-based studies, hospital-based studies, and prevalence in immigrants and refugees. Modified from Schäret al., [84].

4. STH and *Strongyloides* in Australia

Australia has a low number of STH cases, largely because these worm infections can be readily controlled by good hygiene, access to safe, clean water, and the use of toilets. The overall prevalence of hookworm and *T. trichiura* in the Australian Northern Territory is quite low at 0.17% and 0.65%, respectively (Table 1), based on hospital data collected between 2002 and 2012 [42,43]. These cases were primarily detected in people admitted to hospital for reasons other than hookworm or *Trichuris* infection; thus the true prevalence may be much higher, and may follow a more focal intensity that would not be accounted for by recording state-wide or country-wide prevalence. For both species the prevalence has been reduced; with *T. trichiura,* there was a drop from 123.1 cases per 100,000 in 2002 to 35.8 cases per 100,000 in 2012 [42]. The zoonotic STHs, particularly *A. caninum* and *A. ceylanicum,* are of importance in Australia since they are found in domestic and wild canids (Table 2) [85,86]. Intestinal parasites of pigs in Australia also include *T. suis* and *A. suum,* which can infect humans, although the extent of human disease is unclear [4,87].

In 1918, hookworm was considered such a serious problem in North Queensland that a five-year campaign to eradicate the disease was instigated and although considered successful, hookworm infection continued to be a problem in Aboriginal communities [53,88]. The majority of published papers on STH in Australia are relatively old, with very few published in the last 10 years. Prociv and Luke [88] provide a solid review of the early history of hookworm infections in Australia. *Ascaris* spp. infection has never been very prevalent despite the requisite tropical climate and moist soil existing in Australia [89].

S. stercoralis appears to be more prevalent in Australia than the other STH, or at least, there are more published data available (Table 1) (Figure 2). The parasite is endemic in tropical regions of Australia including Queensland, the Northern Territory, Western Australia, as well as Northern NSW. It is primarily found among Aboriginal people living in remote communities, with a prevalence of >60% recorded (Table 1) [90–94]. This worm has persisted due to lack of attention to the disease it causes, despite the potential for high morbidity and mortality in immunosuppressed individuals [94]. Its true prevalence is unknown in Australia, and probably globally. As reported by Speare *et al* – "if you don't look, you won't find" [94]. As a human-only parasite, it can be readily treated with ivermectin and eliminated from the community. A retrospective study examined indigenous Australians in Central Australia who were positive for *S. stercoralis* infection and who may also have been positive for human T cell lymphotropic virus type I (HTLV-I). This virus invades adult T cells, thereby reducing the effectiveness of the immune system [29]. Of these subjects, eleven (n = 18) were tested for HTLV-I, of which seven were positive. Of those who tested positive for HTLV-I, four were never treated for *Strongyloides*, and of those who were treated, many were not treated at initial diagnosis and infection status was not checked on subsequent visits [29]. Of these eighteen patients, fifteen died from sepsis.

Table 2. Reported prevalences of *A. ceylanicum* human and animal infections in studies conducted in Australia and Asia since 2000.

Ref	Year	Country *	Human/Animal	Prevalence % (Total no.)	Species	Diagnostic
[95]	-	Taiwan	Human	Single patient	*A. ceylanicum*	Morphology
[69]	2009	Laos	Human	17.6% (n = 17) 82.4% (n = 17)	*A. ceylanicum* *N. americanus*	Nested PCR
[96]	2012	Cambodia	Human	51.6% (n = 124) 51.6% (n = 124) 3.2% (n = 124)	*A. ceylanicum* *N. americanus* *A. duodenale*	Microscopy, PCR
			Dog	94.4% (n = 90) 8.9% (n = 90) 1.1% (n = 90)	*A. ceylanicum* *A. caninum* *N. americanus*	Microscopy, PCR
[49] [#]	2010–2011	Australia	Human	0.88% (n = 227) 1.76% (n = 227) 1.76% (n = 227)	*A. ceylanicum* *A. duodenale* *N. americanus* [a]	PCR
[97]	-	China	Dog Cat Human	3 (n = 254) 5 (n = 102) 14 (n = 14)	*A. ceylanicum*	PCR sequencing
[98]	-	Malaysia	Dog	52% (n = 224) 48% (n = 224)	*A. ceylanicum* *A. caninum*	FECT, PCR
[99]	2007–2010	Malaysia	Cat	29.5% (n = 543)	*A. ceylanicum*	Microscopy
[100]	2009–2011	Malaysia	Human	87.2 (n = 47) 23.4 (n = 47)	*N. americanus* *A. ceylanicum*	Microscopy, PCR
[101]	2013	Malaysia (Chinese)	Human	Single patient	*A. ceylanicum*	Microscopy
[11]	2009–2011	Malaysia	Human	12.8% (n = 634) 76.6% (n = 634) 10.6% (n = 634)	*A. ceylanicum* *N. americanus* *Both species*	Microscopy, PCR
			Cats and dogs	52% (n = 105) 46% (n = 105)	*A. caninum* *A. ceylanicum*	Microscopy, PCR
[102]	-	Myanmar	Human	72.72% (n = 11) 27.27% (n = 11)	*N. americanus* *A. ceylanicum*	PCR sequencing
[103]	2004–2005	Australia	Dog	6.5% (n = 92) 70.7% (n = 92) 4.3% (n = 92) 2.2% (n = 92)	*A. ceylanicum* *A. caninum* *A. caninum + A. ceylanicum* *A. caninum + U. stenocephala*	Microscopy, PCR-RFLP
			Cat	30% (n = 10)	*A. caninum*	

Table 2. *Cont.*

Ref	Year	Country *	Human/Animal	Prevalence % (Total no.)	Species	Diagnostic
[12]	2011–2013	Thailand	Human	60% (n = 10) 30% (n = 10) 10% (n = 10)	*N. americanus* *A. ceylanicum* *A. duodenale*	PCR sequencing
[86]	>2007	Australia	Wild dog	100% (n = 26) 11.5% (n = 26)	*A. caninum* *A. ceylanicum* + *A. caninum*	Microscopy, PCR
			Dog scat	65.31% (n = 89) 71.43% (n = 89) 38.78% (n = 89)	*A. ceylanicum* *A. caninum* *A. caninum* + *A. ceylanicum*	
[39]	2004	Australia (Solomon Islands)	Human	Single patient	*A. ceylanicum*	Microscopy
[51]	2004–2005	Thailand	Dog	77% (n = 229) 9% (n = 229) 14% (n = 229)	*A. ceylanicum* *A. caninum* Both species	PCR
			Human	71.43% (n = 204) 28.57% (n = 204)	*N. americanus* *A. ceylanicum*	
[104]	2008	India	Dog	50.46% (n = 325) 51.92% (n = 104) 33.65% (n = 104) 15.38% (n = 104)	Hookworm spp. *A. caninum* *A. ceylanicum* *A. caninum* + *A. ceylanicum*	Microscopy, PCR-RFLP
[105]	2000	India	Dog	36% (n = 101) 38% (n = 101)	*A. caninum* *A. caninum* + *A. braziliense*	Microscopy, PCR-RFLP + sequencing
[85]	2011	Australia	Dog	96.4% (n = 84) 16.67%(n = 84) 14.0% (n = 84)	*A. caninum* *A. ceylanicum* *A. caninum* + *A. ceylanicum*	Microscopy, PCR
[106]	2013–2014	Malaysia	Dog Soil samples Cat	29.6% (n = 227) 6.6% (n = 227) 14.3% (n = 126) 2.4% (n = 126) 29.6% (n = 152) 6.6% (n = 152)	*A. ceylanicum* *A. caninum* *A. ceylanicum* *A. caninum* *A. ceylanicum* *A. caninum*	FECT, PCR
[107]	2015	Japan (Lao)	Human	Single patient	*A. ceylanicum*	Microscopy, PCR

Table 2. *Cont.*

Ref	Year	Country *	Human/Animal	Prevalence % (Total no.)	Species	Diagnostic
[108]	2013–2015	India	Human	100% (n = 143) 16.8% (n = 143) 8.4% (n = 143)	*N. americanus* *A. caninum* *A. duodenale*	PCR-RFLP
			Dog	27.9% 76.4%	*A. ceylanicum* *A. caninum*	
			Soil samples	60.2% (n = 78) 29.4% (n = 78) 16.6% (n = 78) 1.4% (n = 78)	*A. ceylanicum* *A. caninum* *A. duodenale* *N. americanus*	
[109]	2014	Thailand	Dog Cat	33.0% (n = 197) 58.46% (n = 180)	*A. ceylanicum*	Microscopy, PCR
[110]	2014	France (Myanmar)	Human	Single patient	*A. ceylanicum*	Microscopy, PCR
[111]	2014	Vietnam	Dog	54.3% (n = 94) 33% (n = 94) 12.7% (n = 94)	*A. ceylanicum* *A. caninum* *Both species*	PCR-RFLP, PCR (cox1)
[112]	2014	China	Cat	40.8% (n = 112) 59.2% (n = 112) 20.4% (n = 112)	*A. ceylanicum* *A. caninum* *Both species*	Microscopy, PCR
[113]	-	India	Human	95% 15% 5%	*N. americanus* *A. duodenale* *A. ceylanicum*	PCR-RFLP
[114]	2005	Thailand	Human	92% 4% 2% 2%	*N. americanus* *A. ceylanicum* *A. duodenale* *N. americanus* + *A. ceylanicum*	KK, PCR
[115]	2008	Lao	Human	5.91% 2.46% 1.48% 0.49%	*N. americanus* *A. duodenale* *A. caninum* *A. ceylanicum*	KK, PCR
[99]	2007–2010	Malaysia	Feral cats	29.5% (n = 251)	*A. ceylanicum*	Microscopy of adults (staining paracarmine)
[116]	-	Lao	Feral cats	69% (n = 55)	*A. ceylanicum*	Microscopy of adults (staining Mayers carmine)
[117]	-	Taiwan	Human	Single patient	*A. ceylanicum*	Method unclear. Adult identification.

* Origin of infection in brackets if not the same as the country of detection; # faecal samples from individuals with a documented history of gastrointestinal disorders; [a] individuals infected with *N. americanus* were refugees from Sierra Leone and Sudan, likely to be acquired in those countries.

A complication of disseminated strongyloidiasis is secondary bacterial infection that can become systemic, and has likely contributed to mortality in at least four cases. Further studies have found high prevalence of HTLV-I in Aboriginal communities (33.6% n = 889), which may lead to more cases of hyperinfection with *S. stercoralis* in the future [118,119]. Along with immune suppression due to infection with HIV or HTLV-I, and immunosuppression due to organ transplantation, treatment with steroid drugs suppresses the inflammatory response and can also result in hyperinfection [29,119–124]. There is a clear need to increase knowledge of physicians in endemic areas, perhaps as part of a database for NTDs. Speare et al [93] advocated that *S. stercoralis* be added to the national notifiable diseases surveillance system in Australia to help combat this sadly neglected disease. Notification would bring with it greater oversight and available information to physicians, which would help lead to better management of cases, including the provision of effective treatment. To date this has not occurred and, indeed, there are no helminth diseases on the list; malaria is the sole parasite infection listed.

5. Immigration Screening in Australia

Outside remote communities, it is primarily in immigrants from developing nations and returning travellers that STH cases occur in Australia (Table 1) (Figure 2). Current health screening for immigrants does not include testing for parasites and focuses on notifiable diseases such as tuberculosis and HIV/AIDS. Since STH infections are not notifiable, it is possible that there are autochthonous and returned traveller cases occurring in Australia that are not identified or reported.

Cross-sectional surveys have been performed on recent (1997–2000) and long-term immigrants to Australia in the East African and Cambodian communities in 2000 and 2002, and long-term immigrants from Cambodia [36] (Table 1). *S. stercoralis* and *T. trichiura* were identified in the East African cohort, with only *S. stercoralis* present in the Cambodian cohort. Despite having been in Australia for some years and subject to immigration screening, the high prevalence recorded, particularly in the Cambodian cohort (42%, Table 1), indicates a need to include NTDs such as STH in pre-immigration screening. *Entamoeba histolytica*, *Hymenolepis nana*, *Schistosoma* spp. (East African cohort), and *Dientamoeba fragilis* were also identified [36]. Far from being an isolated occurrence, there is a history of STH found in resettled immigrants (Table 1). An earlier study on immigrants from Laos, who had been resettled in Australia for at least 12 years prior to the survey, found *S. stercoralis* in 24% of participants (23/95) [37]. *Strongyloides* is the most commonly reported helminth infection in immigrants (Table 1). Generally *S. stercoralis* infections are asymptomatic. More severe complications from infection include eosinophilic pneumonia, malnutrition, and disseminated strongyloidiasis.

While screening for helminth and protozoan parasites does not occur upon entry to Australia, the government does provide reimbursement for GPs who perform heath assessments within 12 months of arrival [125]. There are also state-funded refugee services in most states and territories [126–130]. In theory, these services could include parasitological identification. As of June 2016, 28.5% of Australians were born overseas, with five of the top 10 countries of birth in SEA (China, India, the Philippines, Vietnam, Malaysia) [131], countries with high STH endemicity. A global distribution map for STH [64] shows stable transmission occurring in SEA and Africa, origins of many immigrants coming to Australia (Figures 2 and 3).

6. Returned Service Personnel

Another cohort for Australian STH infections are Australian army veterans, including older veterans who served in STH-endemic areas from World War II onwards (Table 2) [39–41,132]. *Strongyloides* is the most commonly identified helminth infection in this cohort, possibly the only STH actually considered. In Vietnam veterans, 11.6% had positive serology in 2013 for *Strongyloides*, despite serving between 1962 and 1975 [40]. This shows that the adult worms can persist for many years, as highlighted earlier for immigrants who had been long-term residents in Australia still testing positive for this disease.

7. Diagnostics

Microscopy

Stool-based microscopy remains the most common diagnostic method for STH, including in Australia, with the formol ethyl acetate sedimentation technique most commonly employed [133,134]. For *S. stercoralis*, serology is recommended, due to low and irregular numbers of larvae excreted in the stool even in heavy infections, with stool microscopy used to rule out other infections [133,135]. Diagnosis of STH in Australia is largely done on a case-by-case basis rather than by case detection. Case detection, involving diagnostic sweeps of a community, is more likely to occur as part of a research program in endemic countries. The diagnostic method used will vary. Case-by-case studies are likely to use more sensitive, albeit more laborious, diagnostics than prevalence surveys, which examine a large number or individuals and usually necessitating faster, cheaper diagnostics such as the Kato-Katz (KK) method.

In Asia, a number of different diagnostics have been employed, often as part of specific research projects or for assessing government control programs. The main diagnostic employed is the KK method, a tool also used for diagnosis of schistosomiasis and STH in the Philippines and China. The KK procedure is cheap and easy to perform, particularly under field conditions, which are the reasons it is generally used in large-scale studies. However, the KK is known to lack sensitivity, particularly in low prevalence/intensity infections, and particularly for *Strongyloides* [136–138]. Additionally, hookworm eggs hatch rapidly after stool deposition, with the result that KK slides need to be prepared and examined quickly before eggs lyse [139,140]. FLOTAC is another microscopic, albeit more recent, technique that has been used in STH diagnostics, and has a higher sensitivity than the KK procedure [136,137,141–144]. The main disadvantage of FLOTAC is the length of time it takes to implement, with a single FLOTAC taking around 30 minutes to produce a result [145]. Other methods include the Baermann technique, which is based on the movement of larvae out of stool, the formalin-ether concentration technique (FECT), and coproculture [136]. *Strongyloides* has low sensitivity on stool examination so either multiple stool samples need to be examined or serology undertaken, which is the recommended diagnostic approach [77]. Other methods such as PCR, agar plate culture, and Baermann sedimentation can also be performed on stool samples, and have a higher sensitivity than microscopy [77]. Both agar plate and the Baermann technique can be time consuming. While PCR is more expensive than microscopy, agar plate, or Baermann, it achieves higher sensitivity than all of these techniques [78].

8. Immunodiagnostics

As indicated, serology is often used in Australia for diagnosis of *S. stercoralis* [133], with microscopy employed for the other STH. In general, this holds true for Asia as well. For hookworms, which as discussed earlier, have fragile eggs, immunodiagnostics can be a more sensitive detection method than faecal microscopy. However, lack of specificity, cross-reactivity, and the inability to distinguish between past and current infections are limitations of many immunodiagnostic tests. The most common immunodiagnostic methods used for STH detection are enzyme-linked immunosorbent assays (ELISAs), western blots, and ELISPOT [14,146,147]. Dipstick assays are rapid diagnostics that usually detect antibodies in blood to a target parasite. A dipstick developed for *S. stercoralis*, which is no longer available, had a similar sensitivity (91%) to the ELISA assays it was compared to and a specificity of 97.7% [148]. While serology is recommended for strongyloidiasis due to the poor sensitivity of stool examination, serology can also miss heavy infections as demonstrated by a recent fatal case from Israel of hyperinfection with *S. stercoralis* that was ELISA-negative [23]. An assortment of immunodiagnostics are available for *Strongyloides*, which have a range of sensitivities and specificities [149].

Dried blood spot (DBS) testing occurs by blotting blood samples onto filter paper. Samples can be collected and stored for later analysis, allowing for large numbers of samples to be collected but without requiring large amounts of storage space, and allows relative ease of collection because only a drop from a fingerprick is required. Dried blood spots have been used for molecular diagnostic tests, but can also be used for immunodiagnostics [46]. Most recently, the application of DBS was utilised in serology to diagnose *S. stercoralis* in a remote community in Northern Australia [46].

9. Molecular Diagnostics

There is a range of molecular diagnostic tests available that offer higher sensitivity than microscopy-based diagnostics, albeit with a higher price tag, and these have been reviewed elsewhere [150]. The main benefit of molecular methods is the ability to multiplex assays, that is, identify multiple species using a single assay. However, as well as being more costly than microscopy techniques, they also require specialised equipment. An exception is loop-mediated isothermal amplification (LAMP), which can be performed in the field due to much reduced equipment requirements [151,152]. However LAMP does not allow for multiplexing and to date, of the STH, has only been used to detect hookworm infections [152].

Molecular methods with multiplexing capabilities include conventional polymerase chain reaction (cPCR), real-time PCR (qPCR), multiparallel and tandem qPCR, and digital droplet PCR (ddPCR). Both cPCR and ddPCR are endpoint PCRs, which rely on designing primers that produce amplicons of different lengths to distinguish individual parasite species. ddPCR also uses fluorescent dyes, while real-time PCR reactions utilise fluorescent probes to distinguish between amplicons; the use of taqman probes can increase the sensitivity and specificity of an assay. Of these methods only ddPCR has yet to be used to diagnose STH infections, although it has been utilised for other parasites such as *Schistosoma* spp., detecting cell-free DNA (cfDNA) in a range of body fluids (stool, serum, urine, saliva) [153,154]. The assay provides absolute quantification and can detect very low levels of target DNA; it is also more sensitive than qPCR. While currently only providing for two channels, it is possible to multiplex the reactions for four targets by utilising different size amplicons, much as for a conventional PCR multiplex, because targets can be separated based on size. While schistosomes are blood parasites, and are thus in contact with host blood and tissues, the STH live in the gut and the potential for detection of parasite cfDNA in body fluids such as blood, urine, and saliva would likely be reduced. However, since hookworm is a blood feeder it does gain access to the host blood stream and it is possible that hookworm cfDNA would be detectable in sera. Likewise, the larvae of hookworm and *Ascaris* penetrate the alveolae of the lungs to be coughed up and swallowed, thereby reaching the gut. It is therefore possible that a saliva or sputum sample would yield cfDNA or the larvae themselves. Regardless, the use of ddPCR on stool samples will readily amplify target parasite genes with very high sensitivity. Because it confers absolute quantification and by partitioning the PCR mix (containing master mix, primers, and DNA) into ~20,000 droplets pre-amplification, it effectively means that each sample has ~20,000 technical replicates. Therefore there is no need to run samples in duplicate or triplicate for ddPCR as there is for qPCR. This can save on costs, although in practice the cost of ddPCR and qPCR is similar.

10. Costs of Diagnostics

The cost of a single KK slide, excluding personnel costs and stool collection costs, is US$0.30 [155]. The total cost for single and duplicate KK slides have been estimated to be $US1.73 and US$2.06, respectively, while the FLOTAC costs $2.35 [145]. In comparison, a multiplex qPCR costs $7.68. For qPCR the major costs result from DNA extraction as the qPCR assay itself costs $1.68 per sample in triplicate. A multiparallel qPCR has been costed at $1 per sample, excluding DNA extraction costs [156].

11. Treatment and Mass Drug Administration (MDA) of STH Infections

Mass drug administration (MDA) is a hallmark of many control programs aimed at controlling STH infections. The benzimidazoles (albendazole and mebendazole) are the most commonly used drugs for STH infection in humans, and are recommended for MDA. In the Philippines there is an annual deworming program among school-aged children. In 2003 the prevalence of STH in pre-school children was 66%, after which the Philippines Department of Health introduced the national school deworming program, The Integrated Helminth Control Program (IHCP) [157], with albendazole or mebendazole being recommended for use. The program has been successful in reducing overall prevalence at least in some areas, although MDA coverage can vary. Chemotherapy does not prevent re-infection, and once out of the school program there is no mandated MDA for STH treatment in adults. Fear of birth defects has also been recorded as a reason for refusing STH treatment by pregnant women in the Philippines [158]. School-based MDA has a compliance of >75% while community wide MDAs tend toward low compliance (25–65%) [158,159]. In some cases this is due to poor community involvement, but also because of concerns with possible side effects of the drugs. In the IHCP school deworming program, there was an increase in STH in at least one city (46.05% in 2007 to 56.60% in 2011), and the overall prevalence remained high at 45% as of 2011 [160]. Assuming 100% coverage, the problem of STH will still exist, since re-infection can occur very quickly after treatment, and STH eggs/larvae can live in the environment for several weeks to months, remaining viable for infection. Another issue is drug efficacy. While most available drugs for STH are highly efficacious for *A. lumbricoides*, there are varying efficacies for hookworm, *Strongyloides* spp. and *Trichuris* spp. Efficacy varies depending on the drug given, whether the drug is given as a single or multiple dose, and the amount given. Most programs of MDA rely on a single dose, being easier and not relying on individuals returning for treatment on multiple days. Drug efficacy for hookworm species can be difficult to untangle, as many studies do not speciate the infecting worms. There are documented differences in drug efficacy between *A. duodenale* and *N. americanus*, with mebendazole less effective against *N. americanus*, and pyrantel pamoate less effective against *A. duodenale* [161]. For all STH, drug efficacy likely varies on a regional level depending on parasite populations and treatment programs, particularly those involving MDA.

A World Health Organization (WHO) report [162] showed a range of efficacies against STH for mebendazole, albendazole, pyrantel, levamisole, and ivermectin. For *A. lumbricoides*, efficacy was up to 100% for all drugs except ivermectin. For hookworm the highest efficacy, in terms of cure rate (CR), was achieved with levamisole (66%–100%), and for *T. trichiura* with mebendazole (45%–100%). In the same report comparing differing single doses of albendazole and mebendazole (recommended by the WHO for STH control and treatment) with multiple doses of mebendazole, multiple doses resulted in a higher CR for both hookworm and *Trichuris* spp., albeit the median CR was still around 80% [162]. However, the WHO also recommends periodic worming with albendazole or mebendazole where prevalence is >20% [163]. The aim of the WHO with regards to STH control is to carry out preventative worming in endemic countries with a prevalence of >20%. However if drug efficacy is low, particularly for hookworm and *Trichuris* spp., this approach is unlikely to decrease prevalence in the long term.

Of relevance to treatment of STH cases in Australia and SEA, a study on immigrant populations (in Canada) found an overall reduction in intestinal parasites (STH and *Giardia*) 6 years after resettlement and treatment with thiabendazole, from 63.7% down to 21.9%; however the prevalence of *S. stercoralis* remained relatively high with a reduction from 15% to 11% [37,164]. However, since that report, ivermectin has been designated the drug of choice for *Strongyloides* spp. infection because this has a high efficacy given singly as a 200 mcg/kg dose (96% CR) or as a split 400 mcg/kg dose (98% CR) [165]. This highlights the need for combined chemotherapy when treating individuals infected with more than one species of STH.

Cure rates may be lower than reported due to insensitive diagnostics used in many drug efficacy trials, primarily stool microscopy, and variation in CR given by the same drug regimens in different trials may be due to the methods used to assess treatment success or failure. The sensitivity of diagnosis varies considerably with the more traditional microscopic diagnostics, such as the Kato-Katz procedure, lacking the sensitivity of more recently developed techniques such as real-time PCR-based diagnostics. Serological diagnosis measuring antibodies should not be used to assess CR since they will detect antibodies from previous infections for several months post-treatment, assuming 100% efficacy. Antigen-based tests are more specific but many detected antigens tend to break down quickly in the body.

In an interesting development, the bacterium *Bacillus subtilis* has been engineered to express the anthelmintic protein Cry5B, which proved lethal to *Caenorhabditis elegans* and experimental *A. ceylanicum* hookworm infections in hamsters [166]. This approach could be used by modifying 'good' bacteria that are safe for human ingestion. There are numerous probiotics on the market, of which the most common bacterial species are *Lactobacillus acidophilus, L. casei, Bifidobacterium lactis, B. bifidum,* and *Bacillus subtilis*.

Resistance to anthelmintics continues to be a concern. Currently, resistance has been reported for the human helminth, *Onchocerca volvulus* against ivermectin [167]. *N. americanus* eggs heterozygous for a β-tubulin mutation associated with resistance to benzimidazoles (albendazole, mebendazole) in *A. caninum* were recovered from a small number of individuals (n = 28) in Haiti [168]; homozygous eggs were not identified, but may be present. This raises the possibility of emerging benzimidazole resistance in human hookworm infections, as it has in veterinary hookworm. Drug resistance is common in helminths of veterinary importance where resistance has been reported against not only benzimidazoles but also levamisole, avermectins, and milbemycins (which include ivermectin) [169,170]. Resistance has not been reported for any of the zoonotic helminths. With the increase of MDA programs in STH-endemic areas, there is increasing evolutionary pressure on parasite populations, which may lead to resistance. To rigorously assess resistance, however, sensitive diagnostics will be required, and research needs to be undertaken in the search for alleles conferring resistance. Wolstenholme *et al* [170] have provided an excellent overview of drug resistance in veterinary helminths, while Vercruysse *et al* [171] consider the potential of resistance to currently-available drugs developing in human helminths.

12. Control Programs

STH reinfections can largely be controlled with appropriate hygiene, including washing hands after defecation, and using a toilet, as augmentation to treatment. There are several programs operating in Asia that seek to combat STH infection by using educational interventions. These include the 'Magic Glasses' program in China [172,173], which has now been extended to the Philippines, and the WASH (water, sanitation, and hygiene) program, which aims to provide clean water, toilets, and promoting good hygiene practices, implemented, for example, in Timor-Leste [174,175]. Helminth infection is of lesser concern in developed countries, where toilets and clean running water are available. While STH chemotherapy is effective, it does not prevent re-infections that can happen very quickly after treatment [176]. The aim of currently applied interventions is to prevent re-infection, and thus reduce the overall prevalence and eventually eliminate STH from a community.

The Magic Glasses program targets school aged children in China to reduce prevalence of STH and to increase knowledge of STH parasites to reduce re-infections occurring [172]. The focal point of the intervention is a cartoon, produced along with other teaching aids, to teach children about STH and what they can do personally and in their homes to prevent infection, including washing hands after defecation, only using a toilet, covering food, and wearing shoes. In some schools, water tanks were provided outside toilets to facilitate handwashing. Parasite prevalence and intensity levels were assessed pre-intervention and a year later post-intervention; knowledge was also tested at these times using a questionnaire and quiz. The project was highly successful in reducing re-infection and increasing knowledge in Hunan province [172], and has been further trialled in Yunnan province. It is ongoing in the Philippines, where a new video was created to match local popular cartoons, culture and language. The program has the potential to be modified for many different cultures and areas, including Australia.

WASH for WORMS has been implemented in Timor-Leste as part of a trial where intervention villages had WASH implemented alongside mass drug administration (MDA) using albendazole, while control villages only received MDA [174,175]. Intervention villages were provided with access to clean water, the building of latrines and improving hygiene, particularly handwashing. Results of this intervention and the Magic Glasses trial in Yunnan and the Philippines are currently being formulated.

In both these types of interventions community involvement was crucial. With the Magic Glasses, one of the key components was to increase STH knowledge, focusing on school children whereas the WASH program was community-wide. Targeting only children, or any one group, may not significantly impact transmission in a community, but educational interventions in schools can be delivered by teachers, with the children and teachers taking the lessons learnt back to their families, thereby increasing community knowledge and practice [177]. Paradoxically, children often have the highest helminth infection prevalence in a community [178].

13. Zoonotic Roundworms

Zoonotic Hookworms

Ancylostoma duodenale and *N. americanus* are responsible for the majority of human hookworm infections. However, there are two prominent zoonotic hookworm species, *A. ceylanicum* and *A. caninum*, which can also infect humans. *A. ceylanicum*, particularly, is gaining prominence since many cases originally identified as *A. duodenale* may actually be due to *A. ceylanicum* [51]. Both *A. caninum* and *A. ceylanicum* are found in dogs, and *A. ceylanicum* infects cats (Table 2). *A. caninum* has been identified in cats, although this is uncommon (Table 2). While human infections with *A. ceylanicum* do occur, there is some discussion around whether infection with this species produces hookworm disease and morbidity (Table 1) [50,179]. Table 1 shows recent cases of *A. ceylanicum* infection in humans and animals since 2000. Conlan *et al* [179] provide a review of the historical perspective of *A. ceylanicum*. Infection with *A. ceylanicum* was confirmed by molecular methods using PCR, PCR-RFLP, sequencing, or microscopy. In Australia there have been only two recent studies, including one case study of a returned peacekeeper, identifying human infection with *A. ceylanicum*. Studies in dogs have shown that this species is present in Australia, but to a much lesser degree than *A. caninum*. In the Asia-Pacific, the main hookworm species identified is *N. americanus* (81.8%), while 18.18% harboured *A. ceylanicum*, including one individual who harboured both species [132]. An equal prevalence of *A. ceylanicum* and *N. americanus* was found in Cambodia (51.6%) [96,132]. Prevalence of hookworm in animals in Asia is also high, with dual infections of *A. ceylanicum* and *A. caninum* also occurring (Table 2). Certainly, therefore, the presence of *A. ceylanicum* in animals in Asia and Australia poses a risk to human health.

Pets or companion animals are increasingly popular and a potential source of zoonotic hookworms. Observing good hygiene practices, wearing footwear, and regular worming of pets will help prevent transmission of zoonotic hookworms to humans. However, studies on pets and their owners in Europe, which presents a similar socio-economic situation as Australia where handwashing practices, access to clean water and toilets, are similar, have shown that pet owners do not always wash their hands after handling their pets [180]. Only 15% of dog owners and 8% of cat owners stated that they always washed their hands. The same studies have also found *Toxocara* eggs on the fur of the study animals (both cats and dogs) [180–184]. Cats pose a particular risk for egg contamination because cat litter trays reside inside the house and are cleaned by the owner, while dog owners may also be required to pick up after their animals as well.

The rate of pet ownership in Australia is very high. As of 2016, an estimated 62% of households had at least one pet, with dogs the most popular (39%) followed by cats (29%) [35]. Handwashing among Australia children was examined, with only 41% reported to always or mostly wash their hands after playing with animals, indicating that this is an issue in Australia as with comparable countries in Europe [185]. Pet ownership data are also available for China (25% dogs, 10% cats), South Korea (20% dogs, 6% cats), Japan (7% dogs, 14% cats) and Hong Kong (14% dogs, 10% cats) [35].

There have been few human infections in Australia and Asia identified as *A. caninum*, with the two most recent reports of human infection with this species both coming from Asia (Laos and India)

(Table 2). In Australia, *A. caninum* has historically been associated with eosinophilic enteritis [186–192], although there are limited reports on this condition since the mid-1990s.

14. Toxocara

Toxocariasis is caused by the migration of *Toxocara* larvae to various tissues, causing visceral larva migrans. Traditionally the species involved are *T. canis* and *T. cati* nematodes of dogs and cats respectively, with the latter most likely to be involved in human disease [193]. Other *Toxocara* species may also cause infection such as *T. malaysiensis,* which is found in Malaysia, Vietnam, and China, although its potential to infect humans at this point is unknown [193–195]. *Toxocara malaysiensis* also infects cats. Stray dogs and cats are a primary source of infection in developing countries, while high pet ownership in developed countries means that pets are the main source of infection there. Soil samples taken from playgrounds in Malaysia found that 95.7% of samples tested had *Toxocara* eggs, and 88.3% had hookworm, showing very high contamination of the local soil with parasite eggs infectious to humans [196].

The most serious result of infection with *Toxocara* is ocular toxocariasis, which can lead to blindness. Humans are dead-end hosts; the parasite larvae migrate to many tissues, and while they do not develop further they can cause granulomas and inflammation in the tissues they reside in [197].

In Australia *T. canis* has long been known to exist with high prevalence found in dogs and in environmental samples [198,199]. There are very few reports of recent surveys of animals, environmental samples, or humans in Australia. In the 1990s the *T. canis* prevalence in the general population of Australia was 5.7% while in Aboriginal communities it ranged from 11.1%–43% [47]. Historical infections reported included serological examination of patients with ocular symptoms in Victoria (3.86% n = 621) [200]; 7% (n = 660) seroprevalence was recorded in healthy blood donors from the Australia Capital Territory [201]. More recently 21% (n = 29) prevalence was reported in a remote Aboriginal community in the Northern Territory [47].

15. *Ascaris suum*

It was originally thought that *A. suum* infected humans only rarely, but molecular tools have shown that the two species (*A. lumbricoides* and *A. suum*), which are morphologically identical, may in fact be one species and *A. suum* represents a haplotype of *A. lumbricoides*. It has been recognised that the haplotype, *A. suum,* can cause human infections; and has also been found in non-human primates [15,202]. A study in Japan sequenced the ITS1 region of *Ascaris* derived from humans and pigs, finding that 3 of 9 isolates derived from humans were identical to those derived from pigs [6]. A phylogeny study performed in China utilising the mitochondrial genes *cox1* and *nad1,* and found a high level of gene flow between human- and pig-derived *Ascaris,* as well as indicating the presence of 20 haplotypes based on the *cox1* gene and 26 based on the *nad1* [203]. There is also evidence from China of hybrid forms of *Ascaris* [204]. In India PCR-RFLP was performed on dog stools identifying the presence of *A. lumbricoides* eggs [205].

A. suum has been identified in pigs in Australia; however, limited molecular work has been done to characterise the genotypes. Due to control measures in pigs it is estimated that only 3% of pigs in Australia harbour *Ascaris* [206]. There is also limited information on *A. suum* human infections in Australia. Two cases of *Ascaris* infection in Tasmania were thought to be *A. suum* based on morphology of mouthparts, and based on history of contact with pigs; no molecular tools were utilised [207].

Worldwide, 800 million people are estimated to be infected with *Ascaris.* A number of prevalence studies have been done in developing countries using both microscopy, primarily KK, and molecular techniques [66,208–210]. Speciation, or the presence of haplotypes, is rarely looked for in prevalence studies; it is therefore difficult to calculate the number of *Ascaris* infections due to pig-derived worms.

16. *Trichuris suis* and *T. vulpis*

Pigs and canines are the primary hosts of *T. suis* and *T. vulpis*, respectively. Human infections with both species have been recorded, as have hybrids of *T. suis* and the human species *T. trichiura* [5,9,10,13]. In Thailand, both dogs and humans harbour *T. vulpis* and *T. trichiura*, indicating the likelihood of zoonotic transmission occurring for both species [5]. However, dogs in India appear to only carry *T. trichiura*, while further human infections with *T. vulpis* have occurred in North America and Africa [13,205,211].

Genetic analysis of *Trichuris* species in humans, pigs, and non-human primates indicates that there may be several genotypes of *Trichuris* circulating in humans and animals [212–214]. Sequencing of pig and human derived *Trichuris* indicates that they are separate species [215], unlike *A. suum* discussed above, which is considered to be the same species as *A. lumbricoides*. Experimental infections of humans with *T. suis* documented the previously undocumented symptoms of infection which included flatulence, diarrhoea, and upper abdominal pain, although these symptoms regressed over time, after repeated exposure to eggs, to subclinical symptoms [216].

17. Helminth Therapy

While not all STH have as severe consequences as *Strongyloides*, it is clear that treatment of STH is needed in infected individuals. However, it has also been suggested that intestinal worms may actually be beneficial to human health, particularly to bowel health and diseases of hypersensitivity. This is usually described as part of the hygiene hypothesis, linking 'cleaner' living conditions with higher levels of allergic disease, and now extended to inflammatory disorders such as inflammatory bowel disease (IBD) [217]. Helminth parasites are known to modulate the host immune system and it is thought that by doing so for self-benefit, this may cause a bystander effect on other immune-related diseases [218,219].

There have been clinical trials with hookworm and *Trichuris* for treatment of a range of syndromes, including coeliac disease, asthma, allergies, and psoriasis [220]. Hookworm and *Trichuris* eggs are available online through companies such as Wormswell [221], which provides *N. americanus* eggs, and Tanawisa, which provides *T. suis* (porcine *Trichuris* species) (TSO) [222] eggs. The link between asthma regulation and helminths has been studied for some time, although concrete significance in trials has yet to eventuate, and exact mechanisms of action are unclear [223]. Recent trials for asthma, where individuals were experimentally infected with hookworm, indicated some improvement between groups with hookworm and those without, but the results were not significant [220]. A study in Uganda showed maternal hookworm infections decreased the risk of childhood eczema [224]. Australian studies of hookworm therapy largely focus on coeliac disease, which has had mixed results with null or positive associations; any causal link between allergies and parasite infection has not been shown [225,226]. Gut microbiota may also play a role, although it is still unclear how parasites and the microbiota interact with each other [227]. While *T. suis* is primarily a parasite of pigs, it can establish patent infections in humans [9,10,228] and treatment with TSO has been linked to improvement of psoriasis [229].

So, whereas STH and *Strongyloides* are generally thought to be detrimental to health, the presence of a few worms might be beneficial, although more research needs to be performed to confirm this. Because of the risk of self-infection with helminth eggs, most current work aimed at clinical trials is focused on the isolation of particular components in worm secretions that provide beneficial protection or immune modulation of IBD diseases [230,231].

18. Discussion and Conclusion

While STH infections are generally low in Australia, they are still endemic and of significant health importance in remote Aboriginal communities, particularly *S. stercoralis*, which can be fatal in immunocompromised people. Limited data are available for hyperinfection and mortality due to strongyloidiasis in the Asia-Pacific area, but in Australia, infection has led to fatalities, which, in such a resource-rich country, is alarming and unacceptable. Part of the problem may be due to a general lack of awareness of worm infections, which have a low prevalence in the country as a whole. A physician in an urban area may never see, diagnose or treat a helminthiasis case [93,94]. In Aboriginal communities, where the prevalence of strongyloidiasis can be quite high (0.25%–59.5%) [90–92,94,232,233], the very high cost of healthcare delivery limits available services, and physicians may only be resident for a short time so that knowledge about STH and *S. stercoralis,* in particular, may not be being passed on or recorded in the hospital system. Adding STH, particularly especially *S. stercoralis,* to the national notifiable disease system would help increase knowledge and provide access to more information about the appropriate handling of these parasitic worm infections.

High prevalence of STH in refugees and immigrants from endemic areas, particularly the Asia-Pacific, where the majority of immigrants to Australia now originate, highlights a need for better and more comprehensive health screenings of these groups that include parasite diagnosis and treatment. This holds true for army veterans and current members who have served, or are serving, in STH-endemic areas, including long-term follow-ups in case of poor drug efficacy or ongoing autoinfection in the case of *S. stercoralis*. The Asia-Pacific area has particularly high endemicity for STH and, with so much movement between Asia-Pacific and Australia, better understanding and treatment of STH infections are key from a public health perspective.

Author Contributions: CAG wrote the first draft of the manuscript, CAG, DPM, MJ, JK, and DJG contributed to editing and rewrites. All authors have read and approved the final paper.

List of Abbreviations

STH	soil transmitted helminths
SEA	South-East Asia
DNA	deoxyribonucleic acid
qPCR	quantitative real-time polymerase chain reaction
cPCR	conventional polymerase chain reaction
ddPCR	digital droplet polymerase chain reaction
RFLP-PCR	restriction fragment length polymorphism polymerase chain reaction
Cox 1	cytochrome oxidase 1
LAMP	Loop-mediated isothermal amplification
GIT	gastrointestinal tract
WASH	water, sanitation, and hygiene
MDA	mass drug administration
NTDs	neglected tropical diseases
DALYs	disability adjusted life years
YLDs	years lived with disability
HTLV-I	human T cell lymphotropic virus type I
CR	cure rate
IHCP	the integrated helminth control program
WHO	World Health Organization
IBD	inflammatory bowel disease
KK	Kato-Katz
ELISA	enzyme linked immunosorbent assay
DBS	dried blood spot
TOS	*Trichuris suis* eggs

References

1. Bethony, J.; Brooker, S.; Alboico, M.; Geirger, S.M.; Loukas, A.; Diemart, D.; Hotez, P.J. Soil-transmitted helminth infections: Ascariasis, trichuriasis, and hookworm. *Lancet* **2006**, *367*, 1521–1532. [CrossRef]
2. Utzinger, J.; Keiser, J. Schistosomiasis and soil-transmitted helminthiasis: Common drugs for treatment and control. *Expert Opin. Pharmacother.* **2004**, *5*, 263–285. [CrossRef] [PubMed]
3. WHO; UNICEF. *Prevention and Control of Schistosomiasis and Soil-Transmitted Helminthiasis*; WHO: Geneva, Switzerland, 2004.
4. Gordon, C.A.; McManus, D.P.; Jones, M.K.; Gray, D.J.; Gobert, G.N. The increase of exotic zoonotic helminth infections: The impact of urbanization, climate change and globalization. *Adv. Parasitol.* **2016**, *91*, 311–397. [PubMed]
5. Areekul, P.; Putaporntip, C.; Pattanawong, U.; Sitthicharoenchai, P.; Jongwutiwes, S. *Trichuris vulpis* and *T. trichiura* infections among schoolchildren of a rural community in northwestern Thailand: The possible role of dogs in disease transmission. *Asian Biomed.* **2010**, *4*, 49–60.
6. Arizono, N.; Yoshimura, Y.; Tohzaka, N.; Yamada, M.; Tegoshi, T.; Onishi, K.; Uchikawa, R. Ascariasis in Japan: Is pig-derived *Ascaris* infecting humans? *Jpn. J. Infect. Dis.* **2010**, *63*, 447–448. [PubMed]
7. Betson, M.; Nejsum, P.; Bendall, R.P.; Deb, R.M.; Stothard, J.R. Molecular epidemiology of ascariasis: A global perspective on the transmission dynamics of *Ascaris* in people and pigs. *J. Infect. Dis.* **2014**, *210*, 932–941. [CrossRef] [PubMed]
8. Dutto, M.; Petrosillo, N. Hybrid *ascaris suum/lumbricoides* (ascarididae) infestation in a pig farmer: A rare case of zoonotic ascariasis. *Cent. Eur. J. Public Health* **2013**, *21*, 224–226. [PubMed]
9. Cutillas, C.; Callejon, R.; de Rojas, M.; Tewes, B.; Ubeda, J.M.; Ariza, C.; Guevara, D.C. *Trichuris suis* and *Trichuris trichiura* are different nematode species. *Acta Trop.* **2009**, *111*, 299–307. [CrossRef] [PubMed]
10. Nissen, S.; Al-Jubury, A.; Hansen, T.V.; Olsen, A.; Christensen, H.; Thamsborg, S.M.; Nejsum, P. Genetic analysis of *Trichuris suis* and *Trichuris trichiura* recovered from humans and pigs in a sympatric setting in Uganda. *Vet. Parasitol.* **2012**, *188*, 68–77. [CrossRef] [PubMed]
11. Ngui, R.; Lim, Y.A.; Traub, R.; Mahmud, R.; Mistam, M.S. Epidemiological and genetic data supporting the transmission of *Ancylostoma ceylanicum* among human and domestic animals. *PLoS Negl. Trop. Dis.* **2012**, *6*, e1522. [CrossRef] [PubMed]
12. Phosuk, I.; Intapan, P.M.; Thanchomnang, T.; Sanpool, O.; Janwan, P.; Laummaunwai, P.; Aamnart, W.; Morakote, N.; Maleewong, W. Molecular detection of *Ancylostoma duodenale, Ancylostoma ceylanicum,* and *Necator americanus* in humans in northeastern and southern Thailand. *Korean J. Parasitol.* **2013**, *51*, 747–749. [CrossRef] [PubMed]
13. George, S.; Geldhof, P.; Albonico, M.; Ame, S.M.; Bethony, J.M.; Engels, D.; Mekonnen, Z.; Montresor, A.; Hem, S.; Tchuem-Tchuente, L.A.; et al. The molecular speciation of soil-transmitted helminth eggs collected from school children across six endemic countries. *Trans. R. Soc. Trop. Med. Hyg.* **2017**. [CrossRef] [PubMed]
14. Bahgat, M.A.; El Gindy, A.E.; Mahmoud, L.A.; Hegab, M.H.; Shahin, A.M. Evaluation of the role of *Ancylostoma caninum* in humans as a cause of acute and recurrent abdominal pain. *J. Egypt. Soc. Parasitol.* **1999**, *29*, 873–882. [PubMed]
15. Leles, D.; Gardner, S.L.; Reinhard, K.; Iniguez, A.; Araujo, A. Are *Ascaris lumbricoides* and *Ascaris suum* a single species? *Parasit. Vectors* **2012**, *5*, 42. [CrossRef] [PubMed]
16. Siddiqui, A.A.; Berk, S.L. Diagnosis of *Strongyloides stercoralis* infection. *Clin. Infect. Dis.* **2001**, *33*, 1040–1047. [CrossRef] [PubMed]
17. Genta, R.M. Global prevalence of strongyloidiasis: Critical review with epidemiologic insights into the prevention of disseminated disease. *Rev. Infect. Dis.* **1989**, *11*, 755–767. [CrossRef] [PubMed]
18. Magnaval, J.-F.; Glickman, L.T.; Dorchies, P.; Morassin, B. Highlights of human toxocariasis. *Korean J. Parasitol.* **2001**, *39*, 1–11. [CrossRef] [PubMed]
19. WHO. Metrics: Disability-Adjusted Life Year (DALY). Available online: http://www.who.int/healthinfo/global_burden_disease/metrics_daly/en/ (accessed on 6 July 2017).
20. Pullan, R.L.; Smith, J.L.; Jasrasaria, R.; Brooker, S.J. Global numbers of infection and disease burden of soil transmitted helminth infections in 2010. *Parasit. Vectors* **2014**, *7*, 37. [CrossRef] [PubMed]
21. Murray, C.J.; Vos, T.; Lozano, R.; Naghavi, M.; Flaxman, A.D.; Michaud, C.; Ezzati, M.; Shibuya, K.; Salomon, J.A.; Abdalla, S.; et al. Disability-adjusted life years (DALYs) for 291 diseases and injuries in 21

regions, 1990–2010: A systematic analysis for the Global Burden of Disease Study 2010. *Lancet* **2012**, *380*, 2197–2223. [CrossRef]

22. Murray, C.J.; Barber, R.M.; Foreman, K.J.; Ozgoren, A.A.; Abd-Allah, F.; Abera, S.F.; Aboyans, V.; Abraham, J.P.; Abubakar, I.; Abu-Raddad, L.J.; et al. Global, regional, and national disability-adjusted life years (DALYs) for 306 diseases and injuries and healthy life expectancy (HALE) for 188 countries, 1990–2013: Quantifying the epidemiological transition. *Lancet* **2015**. [CrossRef]
23. Osiro, S.; Hamula, C.; Glaser, A.; Rana, M.; Dunn, D. A case of *Strongyloides* hyperinfection syndrome in the setting of persistent eosinophilia but negative serology. *Diagn. Microbiol. Infect. Dis.* **2017**, *88*, 168–170. [CrossRef] [PubMed]
24. Ramamoorthy, K.G. Anaesthesia and *Ascaris* pneumonia (Loeffler's syndrome). *Indian J. Anaesth.* **2015**, *59*, 125–126. [CrossRef] [PubMed]
25. Cataño, J.C.; Pinzón, M.A. *Strongyloides* Pneumonia. *Am. J. Trop. Med. Hyg.* **2012**, *87*, 195. [CrossRef] [PubMed]
26. Cheepsattayakorn, A.; Cheepsattayakorn, R. Parasitic pneumonia and lung involvement. *BioMed Res. Int.* **2014**, *2014*, 18. [CrossRef] [PubMed]
27. Fan, C.K.; Holland, C.V.; Loxton, K.; Barghouth, U. Cerebral toxocariasis: Silent progression to neurodegenerative disorders? *Clin. Microbiol. Rev.* **2015**, *28*, 663–686. [CrossRef] [PubMed]
28. Keiser, P.B.; Nutman, T.B. *Strongyloides stercoralis* in the immunocompromised population. *Clin. Microbiol. Rev.* **2004**, *17*, 208–217. [CrossRef] [PubMed]
29. Einsiedel, L.; Fernandes, L. *Strongyloides stercoralis*: A cause of morbidity and mortality for indigenous people in Central Australia. *Intern. Med. J.* **2008**, *38*, 697–703. [CrossRef] [PubMed]
30. Jaleta, T.G.; Zhou, S.; Bemm, F.M.; Schar, F.; Khieu, V.; Muth, S.; Odermatt, P.; Lok, J.B.; Streit, A. Different but overlapping populations of *Strongyloides stercoralis* in dogs and humans - dogs as a possible source for zoonotic strongyloidiasis. *PLoS Negl. Trop. Dis.* **2017**, *11*, e0005752. [CrossRef] [PubMed]
31. Kouassi, R.Y.; McGraw, S.W.; Yao, P.K.; Abou-Bacar, A.; Brunet, J.; Pesson, B.; Bonfoh, B.; N'Goran, E.K.; Candolfi, E. Diversity and prevalence of gastrointestinal parasites in seven non-human primates of the Tai National Park, Cote d'Ivoire. *Parasite* **2015**, *22*, 1. [CrossRef] [PubMed]
32. Thanchomnang, T.; Intapan, P.M.; Sanpool, O.; Rodpai, R.; Tourtip, S.; Yahom, S.; Kullawat, J.; Radomyos, P.; Thammasiri, C.; Maleewong, W. First molecular identification and genetic diversity of *Strongyloides stercoralis* and *Strongyloides fuelleborni* in human communities having contact with long-tailed macaques in Thailand. *Parasitol. Res.* **2017**, *116*, 1917–1923. [CrossRef] [PubMed]
33. Bergquist, R.; Yang, G.J.; Knopp, S.; Utzinger, J.; Tanner, M. Surveillance and response: Tools and approaches for the elimination stage of neglected tropical diseases. *Acta Trop.* **2015**, *141*, 229–234. [CrossRef] [PubMed]
34. Nagayasu, E.; Aung, M.; Hortiwakul, T.; Hino, A.; Tanaka, T.; Higashiarakawa, M.; Olia, A.; Taniguchi, T.; Win, S.M.T.; Ohashi, I.; et al. A possible origin population of pathogenic intestinal nematodes, *Strongyloides stercoralis,* unveiled by molecular phylogeny. *Sci. Rep.* **2017**, *7*, 4844. [CrossRef] [PubMed]
35. *Pet Ownership Statistics*; Animal Medicines Australia: Barton ACT, Australia, 2016.
36. Caruana, S.R.; Kelly, H.A.; Ngeow, J.Y.; Ryan, N.J.; Bennett, C.M.; Chea, L.; Nuon, S.; Bak, N.; Skull, S.A.; Biggs, B.A. Undiagnosed and potentially lethal parasite infections among immigrants and refugees in Australia. *J. Travel Med.* **2006**, *13*, 233–239. [CrossRef] [PubMed]
37. De Silva, S.; Saykao, P.; Kelly, H.; MacIntyre, C.R.; Ryan, N.; Leydon, J.; Biggs, B.A. Chronic *Strongyloides stercoralis* infection in Laotian immigrants and refugees 7–20 years after resettlement in Australia. *Epidemiol. Infect.* **2002**, *128*, 439–444. [CrossRef] [PubMed]
38. Einsiedel, L.; Spelman, D. *Strongyloides stercoralis*: Risks posed to immigrant patients in an Australian tertiary referral centre. *Intern. Med. J.* **2006**, *36*, 632–637. [CrossRef] [PubMed]
39. Speare, R.; Bradbury, R.S.; Croese, J. A case of *Ancylostoma ceylanicum* infection occurring in an Australian soldier returned from Solomon Islands. *Korean J. Parasitol.* **2016**, *54*, 533–536. [CrossRef] [PubMed]
40. Rahmanian, H.; MacFarlane, A.C.; Rowland, K.E.; Einsiedel, L.J.; Neuhaus, S.J. Seroprevalence of *Strongyloides stercoralis* in a South Australian Vietnam veteran cohort. *Aust. N. Z. J. Public Health* **2015**, *39*, 331–335. [CrossRef] [PubMed]
41. Pattison, D.A.; Speare, R. Strongyloidiasis in personnel of the Regional Assistance Mission to Solomon Islands (RAMSI). *Med. J. Aust.* **2008**, *189*, 203–206. [PubMed]

42. Crowe, A.L.; Smith, P.; Ward, L.; Currie, B.J.; Baird, R. Decreasing prevalence of *Trichuris trichiura* (whipworm) in the Northern Territory from 2002 to 2012. *Med. J. Aust.* **2014**, *200*, 286–289. [CrossRef] [PubMed]
43. Davies, J.; Majumdar, S.S.; Forbes, R.T.; Smith, P.; Currie, B.J.; Baird, R.W. Hookworm in the Northern Territory: Down but not out. *Med. J. Aust.* **2013**, *198*, 278–281. [CrossRef] [PubMed]
44. Chaves, N.J.; Gibney, K.B.; Leder, K.; O'Brien, D.P.; Marshall, C.; Biggs, B.-A. Screening practices for infectious diseases among Burmese refugees in Australia. *Emerg. Infect. Dis.* **2009**, *15*, 1769–1772. [CrossRef] [PubMed]
45. Biggs, B.A.; Caruana, S.; Mihrshahi, S.; Jolley, D.; Leydon, J.; Chea, L.; Nuon, S. Management of chronic strongyloidiasis in immigrants and refugees: Is serologic testing useful? *Am. J. Trop. Med. Hyg.* **2009**, *80*, 788–791. [PubMed]
46. Mounsey, K.; Kearns, T.; Rampton, M.; Llewellyn, S.; King, M.; Holt, D.; Currie, B.J.; Andrews, R.; Nutman, T.; McCarthy, J. Use of dried blood spots to define antibody response to the *Strongyloides stercoralis* recombinant antigen NIE. *Acta Trop.* **2014**, *138*, 78–82. [CrossRef] [PubMed]
47. Shield, J.; Aland, K.; Kearns, T.; Gongdjalk, G.; Holt, D.; Currie, B.; Prociv, P. Intestinal parasites of children and adults in a remote Aboriginal community of the Northern Territory, Australia, 1994. *West. Pac. Surveill. Response J.* **2015**, *6*, 44–51. [CrossRef]
48. Lim, L.; Biggs, B.A. Fatal disseminated strongyloidiasis in a previously-treated patient. *Med. J. Aust.* **2001**, *174*, 355–356. [PubMed]
49. Koehler, A.V.; Bradbury, R.S.; Stevens, M.A.; Haydon, S.R.; Jex, A.R.; Gasser, R.B. Genetic characterization of selected parasites from people with histories of gastrointestinal disorders using a mutation scanning-coupled approach. *Electrophoresis* **2013**, *34*, 1720–1728. [CrossRef] [PubMed]
50. Traub, R.J. *Ancylostoma ceylanicum*, a re-emerging but neglected parasitic zoonosis. *Int. J. Parasitol.* **2013**, *43*, 1009–1015. [CrossRef] [PubMed]
51. Traub, R.J.; Inpankaew, T.; Sutthikornchai, C.; Sukthana, Y.; Thompson, R.C.A. PCR-based coprodiagnostic tools reveal dogs as reservoirs of zoonotic ancylostomiasis caused by *Ancylostoma ceylanicum* in temple communities in Bangkok. *Vet. Parasitol.* **2008**, *155*, 67–73. [CrossRef] [PubMed]
52. Schär, F.; Inpankaew, T.; Traub, R.J.; Khieu, V.; Dalsgaard, A.; Chimnoi, W.; Chhoun, C.; Sok, D.; Marti, H.; Muth, S.; et al. The prevalence and diversity of intestinal parasitic infections in humans and domestic animals in a rural Cambodian village. *Parasitol. Int.* **2014**, *63*, 597–603. [CrossRef] [PubMed]
53. Bradbury, R.; Traub, R.J. Hookworm Infection in Oceania. In *Neglected Tropical Diseases—Oceania*; Loukas, A., Ed.; Springer International Publishing: Cham, Switzerland, 2016; pp. 33–68.
54. Ngui, R.; Mahdy, M.A.; Chua, K.H.; Traub, R.; Lim, Y.A. Genetic characterization of the partial mitochondrial cytochrome oxidase c subunit I (*cox 1*) gene of the zoonotic parasitic nematode, *Ancylostoma ceylanicum* from humans, dogs and cats. *Acta Trop.* **2013**, *128*, 154–157. [CrossRef] [PubMed]
55. Hookworm biology. Available online: https://www.cdc.gov/parasites/hookworm/biology.html (accessed on 18 August 2017).
56. Whipworm biology. Available online: https://www.cdc.gov/parasites/whipworm/biology.html (accessed on 18 August 2017).
57. Ascariasis biology. Available online: https://www.cdc.gov/parasites/ascariasis/biology.html (accessed on 18 August 2017).
58. Strongyloidiasis biology. Available online: https://www.cdc.gov/dpdx/strongyloidiasis/index.html (accessed on 18 August 2017).
59. Yamada, M.; Matsuda, S.; Nakazawa, M.; Arizono, N. Species-specific differences in heterogonic development of serially transferred free-living generations of *Strongyloides planiceps* and *Strongyloides stercoralis*. *J. Parasitol.* **1991**, *77*, 592–594. [CrossRef] [PubMed]
60. Viney, M.E.; Lok, J.B. The biology of *Strongyloides spp.*. *WormBook Online Rev. C Elegans Biol.* **2015**, 1–17. [CrossRef] [PubMed]
61. Toxocariasis biology. Available online: https://www.cdc.gov/parasites/toxocariasis/biology.html (accessed on 18 August 2017).
62. Quattrocchi, G.; Nicoletti, A.; Marin, B.; Bruno, E.; Druet-Cabanac, M.; Preux, P.M. Toxocariasis and epilepsy: Systematic review and meta-analysis. *PLoS Negl. Trop. Dis.* **2012**, *6*, e1775. [CrossRef] [PubMed]
63. Jex, A.R.; Lim, Y.A.; Bethony, J.M.; Hotez, P.J.; Young, N.D.; Gasser, R.B. Soil-transmitted helminths of humans in Southeast Asia - towards integrated control. *Adv. Parasitol.* **2011**, *74*, 231–265. [PubMed]

64. Brooker, S.J.; Bundy, D.A.P. 55—Soil-transmitted Helminths (Geohelminths). In *Manson's Tropical Infectious Diseases (Twenty-Third Edition)*; Farrar, J., Hotez, P.J., Junghanss, T., Kang, G., Lalloo, D., White, N.J., Eds.; W.B. Saunders: London, UK, 2014.
65. De Silva, N.R.; Brooker, S.; Hotez, P.J.; Montresor, A.; Engels, D.; Savioli, L. Soil-transmitted helminth infections: Updating the global picture. *Trends Parasitol.* **2003**, *19*, 547–551. [CrossRef] [PubMed]
66. Gordon, C.A.; McManus, D.P.; Acosta, L.P.; Olveda, R.; Williams, M.; Ross, A.G.; Gray, D.J.; Gobert, G.N. Multiplex real-time PCR monitoring of intestinal helminths in humans reveals widespread polyparasitism in Northern Samar, the Philippines. *Int. J. Parasitol.* **2015**, *45*, 477–483. [CrossRef] [PubMed]
67. Laymanivong, S.; Hangvanthong, B.; Keokhamphavanh, B.; Phommasansak, M.; Phinmaland, B.; Sanpool, O.; Maleewong, W.; Intapan, P.M. Current status of human hookworm infections, ascariasis, trichuriasis, schistosomiasis mekongi and other trematodiases in Lao People's Democratic Republic. *Am. J. Trop. Med. Hyg.* **2014**, *90*, 667–669. [CrossRef] [PubMed]
68. Rim, H.-J.; Chai, J.-Y.; Min, D.-Y.; Cho, S.; Eom, K.S.; Hong, S.; Sohn, W.; Yong, T.; Deodato, G.; Standgaard, H.; et al. Prevalence of intestinal parasite infections on a national scale among primary schoolchildren in Laos. *Parasitol. Res.* **2003**, *91*, 267–272. [CrossRef] [PubMed]
69. Conlan, J.V.; Khamlome, B.; Vongxay, K.; Elliot, A.; Pallant, L.; Sripa, B.; Blacksell, S.D.; Fenwick, S.; Thompson, R.C. Soil-transmitted helminthiasis in Laos: A community-wide cross-sectional study of humans and dogs in a mass drug administration environment. *Am. J. Trop. Med. Hyg.* **2012**, *86*, 624–634. [CrossRef] [PubMed]
70. Meurs, L.; Polderman, A.M.; Vinkeles Melchers, N.V.; Brienen, E.A.; Verweij, J.J.; Groosjohan, B.; Mendes, F.; Mechendura, M.; Hepp, D.H.; Langenberg, M.C.; et al. Diagnosing polyparasitism in a high-prevalence setting in Beira, Mozambique: Detection of intestinal parasites in fecal samples by microscopy and real-time PCR. *PLoS Negl. Trop. Dis.* **2017**, *11*, e0005310. [CrossRef] [PubMed]
71. Elyana, F.N.; Al-Mekhlafi, H.M.; Ithoi, I.; Abdulsalam, A.M.; Dawaki, S.; Nasr, N.A.; Atroosh, W.M.; Abd-Basher, M.H.; Al-Areeqi, M.A.; Sady, H.; et al. A tale of two communities: Intestinal polyparasitism among Orang Asli and Malay communities in rural Terengganu, Malaysia. *Parasit. Vectors* **2016**, *9*, 398. [CrossRef] [PubMed]
72. Fleming, F.M.; Brooker, S.; Geiger, S.M.; Caldas, I.R.; Correa-Oliveira, R.; Hotez, P.J.; Bethony, J.M. Synergistic associations between hookworm and other helminth species in a rural community in Brazil. *Trop. Med. Int. Health* **2006**, *11*, 56–64. [CrossRef] [PubMed]
73. Mehta, R.S.; Rodriguez, A.; Chico, M.; Guadalupe, I.; Broncano, N.; Sandoval, C.; Tupiza, F.; Mitre, E.; Cooper, P.J. Maternal geohelminth infections are associated with an increased susceptibility to geohelminth infection in children: A case-control study. *PLoS Negl. Trop. Dis.* **2012**, *6*, e1753. [CrossRef] [PubMed]
74. Menzies, S.K.; Rodriguez, A.; Chico, M.; Sandoval, C.; Broncano, N.; Guadalupe, I.; Cooper, P.J. Risk Factors for soil-transmitted helminth infections during the first 3 years of life in the tropics; findings from a birth cohort. *PLoS Negl. Trop. Dis.* **2014**, *8*, e2718. [CrossRef] [PubMed]
75. Olsen, A.; van Lieshout, L.; Marti, H.; Polderman, T.; Polman, K.; Steinmann, P.; Stothard, R.; Thybo, S.; Verweij, J.J.; Magnussen, P. Strongyloidiasis–the most neglected of the neglected tropical diseases? *Trans. R. Soc. Trop. Med. Hyg.* **2009**, *103*, 967–972. [CrossRef] [PubMed]
76. Ngui, R.; Halim, N.A.; Rajoo, Y.; Lim, Y.A.; Ambu, S.; Rajoo, K.; Chang, T.S.; Woon, L.C.; Mahmud, R. Epidemiological characteristics of strongyloidiasis in inhabitants of indigenous communities in Borneo island, Malaysia. *Korean J. Parasitol.* **2016**, *54*, 673–678. [CrossRef] [PubMed]
77. Requena-Mendez, A.; Chiodini, P.; Bisoffi, Z.; Buonfrate, D.; Gotuzzo, E.; Munoz, J. The laboratory diagnosis and follow up of strongyloidiasis: A systematic review. *PLoS Negl. Trop. Dis.* **2013**, *7*, e2002. [CrossRef] [PubMed]
78. Verweij, J.J.; Canales, M.; Polman, K.; Ziem, J.; Brienen, E.A.T.; Polderman, A.M.; van Lieshout, L. Molecular diagnosis of *Strongyloides stercoralis* in faecal samples using real-time PCR. *Trans. R. Soc. Trop. Med. Hyg.* **2009**, *103*, 342–346. [CrossRef] [PubMed]
79. Intapan, P.M.; Maleewong, W.; Wongsaroj, T.; Singthong, S.; Morakote, N. Comparison of the quantitative formalin ethyl acetate concentration technique and agar plate culture for diagnosis of human strongyloidiasis. *J. Clin. Microbiol.* **2005**, *43*, 1932–1933. [CrossRef] [PubMed]

80. Boonjaraspinyo, S.; Boonmars, T.; Kaewsamut, B.; Ekobol, N.; Laummaunwai, P.; Aukkanimart, R.; Wonkchalee, N.; Juasook, A.; Sriraj, P. A cross-sectional study on intestinal parasitic infections in rural communities, northeast Thailand. *Korean J. Parasitol.* **2013**, *51*, 727–734. [CrossRef] [PubMed]
81. Kling, K.; Kuenzli, E.; Blum, J.; Neumayr, A. Acute strongyloidiasis in a traveller returning from South East Asia. *Travel Med. Infect. Dis.* **2016**, *14*, 535–536. [CrossRef] [PubMed]
82. Nguyen, T.; Cheong, F.W.; Liew, J.W.; Lau, Y.L. Seroprevalence of fascioliasis, toxocariasis, strongyloidiasis and cysticercosis in blood samples diagnosed in Medic Medical Center Laboratory, Ho Chi Minh City, Vietnam in 2012. *Parasit. Vectors* **2016**, *9*, 486. [CrossRef] [PubMed]
83. Nontasut, P.; Muennoo, C.; Sa-nguankiat, S.; Fongsri, S.; Vichit, A. Prevalence of *Strongyloides* in Northern Thailand and treatment with ivermectin vs albendazole. *Southeast Asian J. Trop. Med. Public Health* **2005**, *36*, 442–444. [PubMed]
84. Schär, F.; Trostdorf, U.; Giardina, F.; Khieu, V.; Muth, S.; Marti, H.; Vounatsou, P.; Odermatt, P. *Strongyloides stercoralis*: Global distribution and risk factors. *PLoS Negl. Trop. Dis.* **2013**, *7*, e2288. [CrossRef] [PubMed]
85. Smout, F.A.; Skerratt, L.F.; Butler, J.R.A.; Johnson, C.N.; Congdon, B.C.; Thompson, R.C.A. The hookworm *Ancylostoma ceylanicum*: An emerging public health risk in Australian tropical rainforests and Indigenous communities. *One Health (Amsterdam, Netherlands)* **2017**, *3*, 66–69. [CrossRef] [PubMed]
86. Smout, F.A.; Thompson, R.C.A.; Skerratt, L.F. First report of *Ancylostoma ceylanicum* in wild canids. *Int. J. Parasitol. Parasites Wildl.* **2013**, *2*, 173–177. [CrossRef] [PubMed]
87. Lee, A. Internal parasites of pigs. Available online: https://www.dpi.nsw.gov.au/__data/assets/pdf_file/0019/433018/internal-parasites-of-pigs.pdf (accessed on 4 July 2017).
88. Prociv, P.; Luke, R.A. The changing epidemiology of human hookworm infection in Australia. *Med. J. Aust.* **1995**, *162*, 150–154. [PubMed]
89. Health, V. Ascariasis (roundworm infection). Available online: https://www2.health.vic.gov.au/public-health/infectious-diseases/disease-information-advice/ascariasis-roundworm-infection (accessed on 27 July 2017).
90. Johnston, F.H.; Morris, P.S.; Speare, R.; McCarthy, J.; Currie, B.; Ewald, D.; Page, W.; Dempsey, K. Strongyloidiasis: A review of the evidence for Australian practitioners. *Aust. J. Rural Health* **2005**, *13*, 247–254. [CrossRef] [PubMed]
91. Jones, H.I. Intestinal parasite infections in Western Australian Aborigines. *Med. J. Aust.* **1980**, *2*, 375–380. [PubMed]
92. Prociv, P.; Luke, R. Observations on strongyloidiasis in Queensland aboriginal communities. *Med. J. Aust.* **1993**, *158*, 160–163. [PubMed]
93. Speare, R.; Miller, A.; Page, W.A. Strongyloidiasis: A case for notification in Australia? *Med. J. Aust.* **2015**, *202*, 523–524. [CrossRef] [PubMed]
94. Page, W.; Speare, R. Chronic strongyloidiasis—Don't look and you won't find. *Aust. Fam. Physician* **2016**, *45*, 40–44. [PubMed]
95. Hsu, Y.; Lin, J. Intestinal Infestation with *Ancylostoma ceylanicum*. *N. Engl. J. Med.* **2012**, *366*. [CrossRef] [PubMed]
96. Inpankaew, T.; Schar, F.; Dalsgaard, A.; Khieu, V.; Chimnoi, W.; Chhoun, C.; Sok, D.; Marti, H.; Muth, S.; Odermatt, P.; et al. High prevalence of *Ancylostoma ceylanicum* hookworm infections in humans, Cambodia, 2012. *Emerg. Infect. Dis.* **2014**, *20*, 976–982. [CrossRef] [PubMed]
97. Liu, Y.; Zheng, G.; Alsarakibi, M. The zoonotic risk of *Ancylostoma ceylanicum* isolated from stray dogs and cats in Guangzhou, South China. *BioMed Res. Int.* **2014**, *2014*, 208759. [CrossRef] [PubMed]
98. Mahdy, M.A.; Lim, Y.A.; Ngui, R.; Siti Fatimah, M.R.; Choy, S.H.; Yap, N.J.; Al-Mekhlafi, H.M.; Ibrahim, J.; Surin, J. Prevalence and zoonotic potential of canine hookworms in Malaysia. *Parasit. Vectors* **2012**, *5*, 88. [CrossRef] [PubMed]
99. Mohd Zain, S.N.; Sahimin, N.; Pal, P.; Lewis, J.W. Macroparasite communities in stray cat populations from urban cities in Peninsular Malaysia. *Vet. Parasitol.* **2013**, *196*, 469–477. [CrossRef] [PubMed]
100. Ngui, R.; Lim, Y.A.; Chua, K.H. Rapid detection and identification of human hookworm infections through high resolution melting (HRM) analysis. *PLoS ONE* **2012**, *7*, e41996. [CrossRef] [PubMed]
101. Ngui, R.; Lim, Y.A.; Ismail, W.H.; Lim, K.N.; Mahmud, R. Zoonotic *Ancylostoma ceylanicum* infection detected by endoscopy. *Am. J. Trop. Med. Hyg.* **2014**, *91*, 86–88. [CrossRef] [PubMed]

102. Pa Pa Aung, W.; Htoon, T.T.; Tin, H.H.; Sanpool, O.; Jongthawin, J.; Sadaow, L.; Phosuk, I.; Ropai, R.; Intapan, P.M.; Maleewong, W. First molecular identifications of *Necator americanus* and *Ancylostoma ceylanicum* infecting rural communities in lower Myanmar. *Am. J. Trop. Med. Hyg.* **2017**, *96*, 214–216. [CrossRef] [PubMed]
103. Palmer, C.S.; Traub, R.J.; Robertson, I.D.; Hobbs, R.P.; Elliot, A.; While, L.; Rees, R.; Thompson, R.C. The veterinary and public health significance of hookworm in dogs and cats in Australia and the status of *A. ceylanicum*. *Vet. Parasitol.* **2007**, *145*, 304–313. [CrossRef] [PubMed]
104. Traub, R.J.; Pednekar, R.P.; Cuttell, L.; Porter, R.B.; Abd Megat Rani, P.A.; Gatne, M.L. The prevalence and distribution of gastrointestinal parasites of stray and refuge dogs in four locations in India. *Vet. Parasitol.* **2014**, *205*, 233–238. [CrossRef] [PubMed]
105. Traub, R.J.; Robertson, I.D.; Irwin, P.; Mencke, N.; Thompson, R.C. Application of a species-specific PCR-RFLP to identify *Ancylostoma* eggs directly from canine faeces. *Vet. Parasitol.* **2004**, *123*, 245–255. [CrossRef] [PubMed]
106. Tun, S.; Ithoi, I.; Mahmud, R.; Samsudin, N.I.; Kek Heng, C.; Ling, L.Y. Detection of helminth eggs and identification of hookworm species in stray cats, dogs and soil from Klang Valley, Malaysia. *PLoS ONE* **2015**, *10*, e0142231. [CrossRef] [PubMed]
107. Kaya, D.; Yoshikawa, M.; Nakatani, T.; Tomo-Oka, F.; Fujimoto, Y.; Ishida, K.; Fujinaga, Y.; Aihara, Y.; Nagamatsu, S.; Matsuo, E.; et al. *Ancylostoma ceylanicum* hookworm infection in Japanese traveler who presented chronic diarrhea after return from Lao People's Democratic Republic. *Parasitol. Int.* **2016**, *65*, 737–740. [CrossRef] [PubMed]
108. George, S.; Levecke, B.; Kattula, D.; Velusamy, V.; Roy, S.; Geldhof, P.; Sarkar, R.; Kang, G. Molecular identification of hookworm isolates in humans, dogs and soil in a tribal area in Tamil Nadu, India. *PLoS Negl. Trop. Dis.* **2016**, *10*, e0004891. [CrossRef] [PubMed]
109. Pumidonming, W.; Salman, D.; Gronsang, D.; Abdelbaset, A.E.; Sangkaeo, K.; Kawazu, S.I.; Igarashi, M. Prevalence of gastrointestinal helminth parasites of zoonotic significance in dogs and cats in lower Northern Thailand. *J. Vet. Med. Sci.* **2017**, *78*, 1779–1784. [CrossRef] [PubMed]
110. Brunet, J.; Lemoine, J.P.; Lefebvre, N.; Denis, J.; Pfaff, A.W.; Abou-Bacar, A.; Traub, R.J.; Pesson, B.; Candolfi, E. Bloody diarrhea associated with hookworm infection in traveler returning to France from Myanmar. *Emerg. Infect. Dis.* **2015**, *21*, 1878–1879. [CrossRef] [PubMed]
111. Ng-Nguyen, D.; Hii, S.F.; Nguyen, V.A.; Van Nguyen, T.; Van Nguyen, D.; Traub, R.J. Re-evaluation of the species of hookworms infecting dogs in Central Vietnam. *Parasit. Vectors* **2015**, *8*, 401. [CrossRef] [PubMed]
112. Hu, W.; Yu, X.G.; Wu, S.; Tan, L.P.; Song, M.R.; Abdulahi, A.Y.; Wang, Z.; Jiang, B.; Li, G.Q. Levels of *Ancylostoma* infections and phylogenetic analysis of *cox 1* gene of *A. ceylanicum* in stray cat faecal samples from Guangzhou, China. *J. Helminthol.* **2016**, *90*, 392–397. [CrossRef] [PubMed]
113. George, S.; Kaliappan, S.P.; Kattula, D.; Roy, S.; Geldhof, P.; Kang, G.; Vercruysse, J.; Levecke, B. Identification of *Ancylostoma ceylanicum* in children from a tribal community in Tamil Nadu, India using a semi-nested PCR-RFLP tool. *Trans. R. Soc. Trop. Med. Hyg.* **2015**, *109*, 283–285. [CrossRef] [PubMed]
114. Jiraanankul, V.; Aphijirawat, W.; Mungthin, M.; Khositnithikul, R.; Rangsin, R.; Traub, R.J.; Piyaraj, P.; Naaglor, T.; Taamasri, P.; Leelayoova, S. Incidence and risk factors of hookworm infection in a rural community of central Thailand. *Am. J. Trop. Med. Hyg.* **2011**, *84*, 594–598. [CrossRef] [PubMed]
115. Sato, M.; Sanguankiat, S.; Yoonuan, T.; Pongvongsa, T.; Keomoungkhoun, M.; Phimmayoi, I.; Boupa, B.; Moji, K.; Waikagul, J. Copro-molecular identification of infections with hookworm eggs in rural Lao PDR. *Trans. R. Soc. Trop. Med. Hyg.* **2010**, *104*, 617–622. [CrossRef] [PubMed]
116. Scholz, T.; Uhlirova, M.; Ditrich, O. Helminth parasites of cats from the Vientiane province, Laos, as indicators of the occurrence of causative agents of human parasitoses. *Parasite* **2003**, *10*, 343–350. [CrossRef] [PubMed]
117. Chung, C.S.; Lin, C.K.; Su, K.E.; Liu, C.Y.; Lin, C.C.; Liang, C.C.; Lee, T.H. Diagnosis of *Ancylostoma ceylanicum* infestation by single-balloon enteroscopy (with video). *Gastrointest. Endosc.* **2012**, *76*, 671–672. [CrossRef] [PubMed]
118. Einsiedel, L.J.; Pham, H.; Woodman, R.J.; Pepperill, C.; Taylor, K.A. The prevalence and clinical associations of HTLV-1 infection in a remote Indigenous community. *Med. J. Aust.* **2016**, *205*, 305–309. [CrossRef] [PubMed]

119. Einsiedel, L.; Woodman, R.J.; Flynn, M.; Wilson, K.; Cassar, O.; Gessain, A. Human T-Lymphotropic Virus type 1 infection in an Indigenous Australian population: Epidemiological insights from a hospital-based cohort study. *BMC Public Health* **2016**, *16*, 787. [CrossRef] [PubMed]
120. Al Maslamani, M.A.; Al Soub, H.A.; Al Khal, A.L.M.; Al Bozom, I.A.; Abu Khattab, M.J.; Chacko, K.C. *Strongyloides stercoralis* hyperinfection after corticosteroid therapy: A report of two cases. *Ann. Saudi Med.* **2009**, *29*, 397–401. [PubMed]
121. Koticha, A.; Kuyare, S.; Nair, J.; Athvale, A.; Mehta, P. *Strongyloides stercoralis* hyperinfection syndrome in patients on prolonged steroid treatment: Two case reports. *J. Indian Med. Assoc.* **2013**, *111*, 272–274. [PubMed]
122. Aru, R.G.; Chilcutt, B.M.; Butt, S.; deShazo, R.D. Novel findings in HIV, immune reconstitution disease and *Strongyloides stercoralis* Infection. *Am. J. Med. Sci.* **2017**, *353*, 593–596. [CrossRef] [PubMed]
123. Llenas-Garcia, J.; Fiorante, S.; Salto, E.; Maseda, D.; Rodriguez, V.; Matarranz, M.; Hernando, A.; Rubio, R.; Pulido, F. Should we look for *Strongyloides stercoralis* in foreign-born HIV-infected persons? *J. Immigr. Minor. Health* **2013**, *15*, 796–802. [CrossRef] [PubMed]
124. Mobley, C.M.; Dhala, A.; Ghobrial, R.M. *Strongyloides stercoralis* in solid organ transplantation: Early diagnosis gets the worm. *Curr. Opin. Organ Transplant.* **2017**, *22*, 336–344. [CrossRef] [PubMed]
125. Medicinewise, N. Albendazole (Zentel) listing extended to treat hookworm and strongyloidiasis. Available online: https://www.nps.org.au/radar/articles/albendazole-zentel-listing-extended-to-treat-hookworm-and-strongyloidiasis (accessed on 4 July 2017).
126. Refugee health services. Available online: https://www.health.qld.gov.au/public-health/groups/multicultural/refugee-services (accessed on 27 September 2017).
127. Refugee and asylum seeker health and wellbeing. Available online: https://www2.health.vic.gov.au/about/populations/refugee-asylum-seeker-health (accessed on 27 September 2017).
128. NSW refugee health service. Available online: https://www.swslhd.health.nsw.gov.au/refugee/ (accessed on 27 September 2017).
129. Humanitarian entrant health service. Available online: http://ww2.health.wa.gov.au/Articles/F_I/Humanitarian-Entrant-Health-Service (accessed on 27 September 2017).
130. Refugee Health Program. Available online: https://www.ntphn.org.au/refugee-health (accessed on 27 September 2017).
131. Statistics, A.B.O. Migration, Australia, 2015–2016. Available online: http://www.abs.gov.au/ausstats/abs@.nsf/mf/3412.0 (accessed on 4 July 2017).
132. Bradbury, R.S.; Hii, S.F.; Harrington, H.; Speare, R.; Traub, R. *Ancylostoma ceylanicum* hookworm in the Solomon Islands. *Emerg. Infect. Dis.* **2017**, *23*, 252–257. [CrossRef] [PubMed]
133. Hanieh, S.; Ryan, N.; Biggs, B. Assessing enteric helminths in refugees, asylum seekers and new migrants. *Microbiol. Aust.* **2016**, 15–19. [CrossRef]
134. Mayer-Coverdale, J.K.; Crowe, A.; Smith, P.; Baird, R.W. Trends in *Strongyloides stercoralis* faecal larvae detections in the Northern Territory, Australia: 2002 to 2012. *Trop. Med. Infect. Dis.* **2017**, 2. [CrossRef]
135. Montes, M.; Sawhney, C.; Barros, N. *Strongyloides stercoralis*: There but not seen. *Curr. Opin. Infect. Dis.* **2010**, *23*, 500–504. [CrossRef] [PubMed]
136. Knopp, S.; Salim, N.; Schindler, T.; Voules, D.A.K.; Rothen, J.; Lweno, O.; Mohammed, A.S.; Singo, R.; Benninghoff, M.; Nsojo, A.A.; et al. Diagnostic accuracy of Kato-Katz, FLOTAC, Baermann, and PCR methods for the detection of light-intensity hookworm and *Strongyloides stercoralis* infections in Tanzania. *Am. J. Trop. Med. Hyg.* **2014**, *90*, 535–543. [CrossRef] [PubMed]
137. Knopp, S.; Speich, B.; Hattendorf, J.; Rinaldi, L.; Mohammed, K.A.; Khamis, I.S.; Mohammed, A.S.; Albonico, M.; Rollinson, D.; Marti, H.; et al. Diagnostic accuracy of Kato-Katz and FLOTAC for assessing anthelmintic drug efficacy. *PLoS Negl. Trop. Dis.* **2011**, *5*, e1036. [CrossRef] [PubMed]
138. Lin, D.-D.; Liu, J.-X.; Liu, Y.-M.; Hu, F.; Zhang, Y.-Y.; Xu, J.-M.; Li, J.-Y.; Ji, M.-J.; Bergquist, R.; Wu, G.-L.; et al. Routine Kato-Katz technique underestimates the prevalence of *Schistosoma japonicum*: A case study in an endemic area of the People's Republic of China. *Parasitol. Int.* **2008**, *57*, 281–286. [CrossRef] [PubMed]
139. McCarthy, J.S.; Lustigman, S.; Yang, G.-J.; Barakat, R.M.; García, H.H.; Sripa, B.; Willingham, A.L.; Prichard, R.K.; Basáñez, M.-G. A researcha genda for helminth diseases of humans: Diagnostics for control and elimination programmes. *PLoS Negl. Trop. Dis.* **2012**, *6*, e1601. [CrossRef] [PubMed]

140. Dacombe, R.J.; Crampin, A.C.; Floyd, S.; Randall, A.; Ndhlovu, R.; Bickle, Q.; Fine, P.E.M. Time delays between patient and laboratory selectively affect accuracy of helminth diagnosis. *Trans. R. Soc. Trop. Med. Hyg.* **2007**, *101*, 140–145. [CrossRef] [PubMed]
141. Cringoli, G. FLOTAC, a novel apparatus for a multivalent faecal egg count technique. *Parassitologica* **2006**, *48*, 381–384.
142. Glinz, D.; Silué, K.D.; Knopp, S.; Lohouringnon, L.K.; Yao, K.P.; Steinmann, P.; Rinaldi, L.; Cringoli, G.; N'Goran, E.K.; Utzinger, J. Comparing diagnostic accuraccy of Kato-Katz, koga agar plate, ether-concentration, and FLOTAC for *Schistosoma mansoni* and soli-transmitted helminths. *PLoS Negl. Trop. Dis.* **2010**, *4*, e754. [CrossRef] [PubMed]
143. Habtamu, K.; Degarege, A.; Ye-Ebiyo, Y.; Erko, B. Comparison of the Kato-Katz and FLOTAC techniques for the diagnosis of soil-transmitted helminth infections. *Parasitol. Int.* **2011**, *60*, 398–402. [CrossRef] [PubMed]
144. Knopp, S.; Rinaldi, R.; Khamis, I.S.; Stothard, J.R.; Rollinson, D.; Maurelli, M.P.; Steinmann, P.; Marti, H.; Cringoli, G.; Utzinger, J. A single FLOTAC is more sensitive than triplicate Kato-Katz for the diagnosis of low intensity soil-transmitted helminth infections. *Trans. R. Soc. Trop. Med. Hyg.* **2009**, *103*, 347–354. [CrossRef] [PubMed]
145. Speich, B.; Knopp, S.; Mohammed, A.K.; Khamis, I.S.; Rinaldi, L.; Cringoli, G.; Rollinson, D.; Utzinger, J. Comparative cost assessment of the Kato-Katz and FLOTAC techniques for soil-transmitted helminth diagnosis in epidemiological surveys. *Parasit. Vectors* **2010**, *3*. [CrossRef] [PubMed]
146. Buonfrate, D.; Formenti, F.; Perandin, F.; Bisoffi, Z. Novel approaches to the diagnosis of *Strongyloides stercoralis* infection. *Clin. Microbiol. Infect.* **2015**, *21*, 543–552. [CrossRef] [PubMed]
147. Buonfrate, D.; Perandin, F.; Formenti, F.; Bisoffi, Z. A retrospective study comparing agar plate culture, indirect immunofluorescence and real-time PCR for the diagnosis of *Strongyloides stercoralis* infection. *Parasitology* **2017**, 1–5. [CrossRef] [PubMed]
148. Van Doorn, H.R.; Koelewijn, R.; Hofwegen, H.; Gilis, H.; Wetsteyn, J.C.; Wismans, P.J.; Sarfati, C.; Vervoort, T.; van Gool, T. Use of enzyme-linked immunosorbent assay and dipstick assay for detection of *Strongyloides stercoralis* infection in humans. *J. Clin. Microbiol.* **2007**, *45*, 438–442. [CrossRef] [PubMed]
149. Anderson, N.W.; Klein, D.M.; Dornink, S.M.; Jespersen, D.J.; Kubofcik, J.; Nutman, T.B.; Merrigan, S.D.; Couturier, M.R.; Theel, E.S. Comparison of three immunoassays for detection of antibodies to *Strongyloides stercoralis*. *Clin. Vaccine Immunol. CVI* **2014**, *21*, 732–736. [CrossRef] [PubMed]
150. Gordon, C.A.; Gray, D.J.; Gobert, G.N.; McManus, D.P. DNA amplification approaches for the diagnosis of key parasitic helminth infections of humans. *Mol. Cell. Probes* **2011**, *25*, 143–152. [CrossRef] [PubMed]
151. Kumagai, T.; Furushima-Shimogawara, R.; Ohmae, H.; Wang, T.P.; Lu, S.; Chen, R.; Wen, L.; Ohta, N. Detection of early and single infections of *Schistosoma japonicum* in the intermediate host snail, *Oncomelania hupensis*, by PCR and loop-mediated isothermal amplification (LAMP) assay. *Am. J. Trop. Med. Hyg.* **2010**, *83*, 542–548. [CrossRef] [PubMed]
152. Mugambi, R.M.; Agola, E.L.; Mwangi, I.N.; Kinyua, J.; Shiraho, E.A.; Mkoji, G.M. Development and evaluation of a loop mediated isothermal amplification (LAMP) technique for the detection of hookworm (*Necator americanus*) infection in fecal samples. *Parasit. Vectors* **2015**, *8*, 574. [CrossRef] [PubMed]
153. Weerakoon, K.G.; Gordon, C.A.; Cai, P.; Gobert, G.N.; Duke, M.; Williams, G.M.; McManus, D.P. A novel duplex ddPCR assay for the diagnosis of schistosomiasis japonica: Proof of concept in an experimental mouse model. *Parasitology* **2017**, *144*, 1005–1015. [CrossRef] [PubMed]
154. Weerakoon, K.G.; Gordon, C.A.; Gobert, G.N.; Cai, P.; McManus, D.P. Optimisation of a droplet digital PCR assay for the diagnosis of *Schistosoma japonicum* infection: A duplex approach with DNA binding dye chemistry. *J. Microbiol. Methods* **2016**, *125*, 19–27. [CrossRef] [PubMed]
155. WHO. *KITS*; WHO: Geneva, Switzerland, 1998.
156. Pilotte, N.; Papaiakovou, M.; Grant, J.R.; Bierwert, L.A.; Llewellyn, S.; McCarthy, J.S.; Williams, S.A. Improved PCR-based detection of soil transmitted helminth infections using a next-generation sequencing approach to assay design. *PLoS Negl. Trop. Dis.* **2016**, *10*, e0004578. [CrossRef] [PubMed]
157. Belizario, V.Y.; Totanes, F.I.; de Leon, W.U.; Matias, K.M. School-based control of soil-transmitted helminthiasis in western Visayas, Philippines. *Southeast Asian J. Trop. Med. Public Health* **2014**, *45*, 556–567. [PubMed]

158. Insetta, E.R.; Soriano, A.J.; Totanes, F.I.; Macatangay, B.J.; Belizario, V.Y., Jr. Fear of birth defects is a major barrier to soil-transmitted helminth treatment (STH) for pregnant women in the Philippines. *PLoS ONE* **2014**, *9*, e85992. [CrossRef] [PubMed]
159. Ross, A.; Olveda, R.; Olveda, D.; Harn, D.; Gray, D.J.; McManus, D.P.; Tallo, V.; Chau, T.; Williams, G. Can mass drug administration lead to the sustainable control of schistosomiasis in the Philippines? *J. Infect. Dis.* **2015**, *211*, 283–289. [CrossRef] [PubMed]
160. Sanza, M.; Totanes, F.I.; Chua, P.L.; Belizario, V.Y., Jr. Monitoring the impact of a mebendazole mass drug administration initiative for soil-transmitted helminthiasis (STH) control in the Western Visayas Region of the Philippines from 2007 through 2011. *Acta Trop.* **2013**, *127*, 112–117. [CrossRef] [PubMed]
161. Geerts, S.; Gryseels, B. Drug resistance in human helminths: Current situation and lessons from livestock. *Clin. Microbiol. Rev.* **2000**, *13*, 207–222. [CrossRef] [PubMed]
162. WHO. *Monitoring Anthelmintic Efficacy for Soil Transmitted Helminths (STH)*; WHO: Geneva, Switzerland, 2008.
163. WHO. Soil-transmitted helminthiases: Number of children treated in 2014. *Wkly. Epidemiol. Rec.* **2015**, *90*, 701–712.
164. Gyorkos, T.W.; MacLean, J.D.; Viens, P.; Chheang, C.; Kokoskin-Nelson, E. Intestinal parasite infection in the Kampuchean refugee population 6 years after resettlement in Canada. *J. Infect. Dis.* **1992**, *166*, 413–417. [CrossRef] [PubMed]
165. Zaha, O.; Hirata, T.; Kinjo, F.; Saito, A.; Fukuhara, H. Efficacy of ivermectin for chronic strongyloidiasis: Two single doses given 2 weeks apart. *J. Infect. Chemother.* **2002**, *8*, 94–98. [CrossRef] [PubMed]
166. Hu, Y.; Miller, M.M.; Derman, A.I.; Ellis, B.L.; Monnerat, R.G.; Pogliano, J.; Aroian, R.V. *Bacillus subtilis* strain engineered for treatment of soil-transmitted helminth diseases. *Appl. Environ. Microbiol.* **2013**, *79*, 5527–5532. [CrossRef] [PubMed]
167. Osei-Atweneboana, M.Y.; Awadzi, K.; Attah, S.K.; Boakye, D.A.; Gyapong, J.O.; Prichard, R.K. Phenotypic evidence of emerging ivermectin resistance in *Onchocerca volvulus*. *PLoS Negl. Trop. Dis.* **2011**, *5*, e998. [CrossRef] [PubMed]
168. Diawara, A.; Schwenkenbecher, J.M.; Kaplan, R.M.; Prichard, R.K. Molecular and biological diagnostic tests for monitoring benzimidazole resistance in human soil-transmitted helminths. *Am. J. Trop. Med. Hyg.* **2013**, *88*, 1052–1061. [CrossRef] [PubMed]
169. Brockwell, Y.M.; Elliott, T.P.; Anderson, G.R.; Stanton, R.; Spithill, T.W.; Sangster, N.C. Confirmation of *Fasciola hepatica* resistant to triclabendazole in naturally infected Australian beef and dairy cattle. *Int. J. Parasitol. Drugs Drug Resist.* **2014**, *4*, 48–54. [CrossRef] [PubMed]
170. Wolstenholme, A.J.; Fairweather, I.; Prichard, R.; von Samson-Himmelstjerna, G.; Sangster, N.C. Drug resistance in veterinary helminths. *Trends Parasitol.* **2004**, *20*, 469–476. [CrossRef] [PubMed]
171. Vercruysse, J.; Albonico, M.; Behnke, J.M.; Kotze, A.C.; Prichard, R.K.; McCarthy, J.S.; Montresor, A.; Levecke, B. Is anthelmintic resistance a concern for the control of human soil-transmitted helminths? *Int. J. Parasitol. Drugs Drug Resist.* **2011**, *1*, 14–27. [CrossRef] [PubMed]
172. Bieri, F.A.M.; Gray, D.J.P.; Williams, G.M.P.; Raso, G.P.; Li, Y.-S.P.; Yuan, L.P.; He, Y.M.P.H.; Li, R.S.B.; Guo, F.-Y.B.A.; Li, S.-M.B.A.; et al. Health-education package to prevent worm infections in Chinese schoolchildren. *N. Engl. J. Med.* **2013**, *368*, 1603–1612. [CrossRef] [PubMed]
173. McManus, D.P.; Bieri, F.A.; Li, Y.S.; Williams, G.M.; Yuan, L.P.; Henglin, Y.; Du, Z.W.; Clements, A.C.; Steinmann, P.; Raso, G.; et al. Health education and the control of intestinal worm infections in China: A new vision. *Parasit. Vectors* **2014**, *7*, 344. [CrossRef] [PubMed]
174. Clarke, N.E.; Clements, A.C.; Bryan, S.; McGown, J.; Gray, D.; Nery, S.V. Investigating the differential impact of school and community-based integrated control programmes for soil-transmitted helminths in Timor-Leste: The (S)WASH-D for Worms pilot study protocol. *Pilot Feasibility Stud.* **2016**, *2*, 69. [CrossRef] [PubMed]
175. Nery, S.V.; McCarthy, J.S.; Traub, R.; Andrews, R.M.; Black, J.A.; Gray, D.J.; Weking, E.; Atkinson, J.A.; Campbell, S.; Francis, N.; et al. A cluster-randomised controlled trial integrating a community-based water, sanitation and hygiene programme, with mass distribution of albendazole to reduce intestinal parasites in Timor-Leste: The WASH for WORMS research protocol. *Br. Med. J.* **2015**, *5*. [CrossRef] [PubMed]

176. Yap, P.; Du, Z.W.; Wu, F.W.; Jiang, J.Y.; Chen, R.; Zhou, X.N.; Hattendorf, J.; Utzinger, J.; Steinmann, P. Rapid re-infection with soil-transmitted helminths after triple-dose albendazole treatment of school-aged children in Yunnan, People's Republic of China. *Am. J. Trop. Med. Hyg.* **2013**, *89*, 23–31. [CrossRef] [PubMed]
177. Mascarini-Serra, L. Prevention of soil-transmitted helminth infection. *J. Glob. Infect. Dis.* **2011**, *3*, 175–182. [CrossRef] [PubMed]
178. Hotez, P.J.; Bundy, D.A.P.; Beegle, K.; Brooker, S.; Drake, L.; de Silva, N.; Montresor, A.; Engels, D.; Jukes, M.; Chitsulo, L.; et al. Helminth infections: soil-transmitted helminth infections and schistosomiasis. In *Disease Control Priorities in Developing Countries*; Jamison, D.T., Breman, J.G., Measham, A.R., Alleyne, G., Claeson, M., Evans, D.B., Jha, P., Mills, A., Musgrove, P., Eds.; World Bank, The International Bank for Reconstruction and Development/The World Bank Group: Washington, DC, USA, 2006.
179. Conlan, J.V.; Sripa, B.; Attwood, S.; Newton, P.N. A review of parasitic zoonoses in a changing Southeast Asia. *Vet. Parasitol.* **2011**, *182*, 22–40. [CrossRef] [PubMed]
180. Overgaauw, P.A.M.; van Zutphen, L.; Hoek, D.; Yaya, F.O.; Roelfsema, J.; Pinelli, E.; van Knapen, F.; Kortbeek, L.M. Zoonotic parasites in fecal samples and fur from dogs and cats in The Netherlands. *Vet. Parasitol.* **2009**, *163*, 115–122. [CrossRef] [PubMed]
181. Overgaauw, P.A.M.; van Knapen, F. Veterinary and public health aspects of *Toxocara* spp. *Vet. Parasitol.* **2013**, *193*, 398–403. [CrossRef] [PubMed]
182. Simonato, G.; Frangipane di Regalbono, A.; Cassini, R.; Traversa, D.; Beraldo, P.; Tessarin, C.; Pietrobelli, M. Copromicroscopic and molecular investigations on intestinal parasites in kenneled dogs. *Parasitol. Res.* **2015**, *114*, 1963–1970. [CrossRef] [PubMed]
183. Paoletti, B.; Traversa, D.; Iorio, R.; De Berardinis, A.; Bartolini, R.; Salini, R.; Di Cesare, A. Zoonotic parasites in feces and fur of stray and private dogs from Italy. *Parasitol. Res.* **2015**. [CrossRef] [PubMed]
184. Roddie, G.; Stafford, P.; Holland, C.; Wolfe, A. Contamination of dog hair with eggs of *Toxocara canis*. *Vet. Parasitol.* **2008**, *152*, 85–93. [CrossRef] [PubMed]
185. Heyworth, J.S.; Cutt, H.; Glonek, G. Does dog or cat ownership lead to increased gastroenteritis in young children in South Australia? *Epidemiol. Infect.* **2006**, *134*, 926–934. [CrossRef] [PubMed]
186. Walker, N.I.; Croese, J.; Clouston, A.D.; Parry, M.; Loukas, A.; Prociv, P. Eosinophilic enteritis in northeastern Australia. Pathology, association with *Ancylostoma caninum*, and implications. *Am. J. Surg. Pathol.* **1995**, *19*, 328–337. [CrossRef] [PubMed]
187. Croese, J.; Loukas, A.; Opdebeeck, J.; Prociv, P. Occult enteric infection by *Ancylostoma caninum*: A previously unrecognized zoonosis. *Gastroenterology* **1994**, *106*, 3–12. [CrossRef]
188. Loukas, A.; Croese, J.; Opdebeeck, J.; Prociv, P. Detection of antibodies to secretions of *Ancylostoma caninum* in human eosinophilic enteritis. *Trans. R. Soc. Trop. Med. Hyg.* **1992**, *86*, 650–653. [CrossRef]
189. Loukas, A.; Opdebeeck, J.; Croese, J.; Prociv, P. Immunologic incrimination of *Ancylostoma caninum* as a human enteric pathogen. *Am. J. Trop. Med. Hyg.* **1994**, *50*, 69–77. [CrossRef] [PubMed]
190. Prociv, P.; Croese, J. Human enteric infection with *Ancylostoma caninum*: Hookworms reappraised in the light of a 'new' zoonosis. *Acta Trop.* **1996**, *62*, 23–44. [CrossRef]
191. Prociv, P.; Croese, J. Human eosinophilic enteritis caused by dog hookworm *Ancylostoma caninum*. *Lancet* **1990**, *335*, 1299–1302. [CrossRef]
192. Croese, J.; Fairley, S.; Loukas, A.; Hack, J.; Stronach, P. A distinctive aphthous ileitis linked to *Ancylostoma caninum*. *J. Gastroenterol. Hepatol.* **1996**, *11*, 524–531. [CrossRef] [PubMed]
193. McGuinness, S.L.; Leder, K. Global burden of toxocariasis: A common neglected infection of poverty. *Curr. Trop. Med. Rep.* **2014**, *1*, 52–61. [CrossRef]
194. Le, T.H.; Anh, N.T.; Nguyen, K.T.; Nguyen, N.T.; Thuy do, T.T.; Gasser, R.B. *Toxocara malaysiensis* infection in domestic cats in Vietnam—An emerging zoonotic issue? *Infect. Genet. Evol.* **2016**, *37*, 94–98. [CrossRef] [PubMed]
195. Li, M.W.; Lin, R.Q.; Song, H.Q.; Wu, X.Y.; Zhu, X.Q. The complete mitochondrial genomes for three *Toxocara* species of human and animal health significance. *BMC Genom.* **2008**, *9*, 224. [CrossRef] [PubMed]
196. Mohd Zain, S.N.; Rahman, R.; Lewis, J.W. Stray animal and human defecation as sources of soil-transmitted helminth eggs in playgrounds of Peninsular Malaysia. *J. Helminthol.* **2015**, *89*, 740–747. [CrossRef] [PubMed]
197. Arevalo, J.F.; Espinoza, J.V.; Arevalo, F.A. Ocular toxocariasis. *J. Pediatr. Ophthalmol. Strabismus* **2013**, *50*, 76–86. [CrossRef] [PubMed]

198. Blake, R.T.; Overend, D.J. The prevalence of *Dirofilaria immitis* and other parasites in urban pound dogs in north-eastern Victoria. *Aust. Vet. J.* **1982**, *58*, 111–114. [CrossRef] [PubMed]
199. Dunsmore, J.D.; Thompson, R.C.A.; Bates, I.A. Prevalence and survival of *Toxocara canis* eggs in the urban environment of Perth, Australia. *Vet. Parasitol.* **1984**, *16*, 303–311. [CrossRef]
200. Carden, S.M.; Meusemann, R.; Walker, J.; Stawell, R.J.; MacKinnon, J.R.; Smith, D.; Stawell, A.M.; Hall, A.J. *Toxocara canis*: Egg presence in Melbourne parks and disease incidence in Victoria. *Clin. Exp. Ophthalmol.* **2003**, *31*, 143–146. [CrossRef] [PubMed]
201. Nicholas, W.L.; Stewart, A.C.; Walker, J.C. Toxocariasis: A serological survey of blood donors in the Australian Capital Territory together with observations on the risks of infection. *Trans. R. Soc. Trop. Med. Hyg.* **1986**, *80*, 217–221. [CrossRef]
202. Nejsum, P.; Bertelsen, M.F.; Betson, M.; Stothard, J.R.; Murrell, K.D. Molecular evidence for sustained transmission of zoonotic *Ascaris suum* among zoo chimpanzees (*Pan Troglodytes*). *Vet. Parasitol.* **2010**, *171*, 273–276. [CrossRef] [PubMed]
203. Zhou, C.; Li, M.; Yuan, K.; Hu, N.; Peng, W. Phylogeography of *Ascaris lumbricoides* and *A. suum* from China. *Parasitol. Res.* **2011**, *109*, 329–338. [CrossRef] [PubMed]
204. Zhou, C.; Li, M.; Yuan, K.; Deng, S.; Peng, W. Pig *Ascaris*: An important source of human ascariasis in China. *Infect. Genet. Evol.* **2012**, *12*, 1172–1177. [CrossRef] [PubMed]
205. Traub, R.J.; Robertson, I.D.; Irwin, P.J.; Mencke, N.; Thompson, R.C.A.A. Canine gastrointestinal parasitic zoonoses in India. *Trends Parasitol.* **2005**, *21*, 42–48. [CrossRef] [PubMed]
206. Controlling worms in pigs. Available online: https://www.daf.qld.gov.au/animal-industries/pigs/pig-health-and-diseases/disease-prevention/controlling-worms-in-pigs (accessed on 11 October 2017).
207. Graves, S. Human infection with '*Ascaris suum*' in Tasmania? *Ann. ACTM* **2005**, *6*, 16.
208. Steinmann, P.; Yap, P.; Utzinger, J.; Du, Z.W.; Jiang, J.Y.; Chen, R.; Wu, F.W.; Chen, J.X.; Zhou, H.; Zhou, X.N. Control of soil-transmitted helminthiasis in Yunnan province, People's Republic of China: Experiences and lessons from a 5-year multi-intervention trial. *Acta Trop.* **2015**, *141*, 271–280. [CrossRef] [PubMed]
209. Tang, N.; Luo, N.J. A cross-sectional study of intestinal parasitic infections in a rural district of west China. *Can. J. Infect. Dis.* **2003**, *14*, 159–162. [CrossRef] [PubMed]
210. Yang, G.-J.; Liu, L.; Zhu, H.-R.; Griffiths, S.M.; Tanner, M.; Bergquist, R.; Utzinger, J.; Zhou, X.-N. China's sustained drive to eliminate neglected tropical diseases. *Lancet Infect. Dis.* **2014**, *14*, 881–892. [CrossRef]
211. Dunn, J.J.; Columbus, S.T.; Aldeen, W.E.; Davis, M.; Carroll, K.C. *Trichuris vulpis* recovered from a patient with chronic diarrhea and five dogs. *J. Clin. Microbiol.* **2002**, *40*, 2703–2704. [CrossRef] [PubMed]
212. Ravasi, D.F.; O'Riain, M.J.; Davids, F.; Illing, N. Phylogenetic evidence that two distinct *Trichuris* genotypes infect both humans and non-human primates. *PLoS ONE* **2012**, *7*, e44187. [CrossRef] [PubMed]
213. Hawash, M.B.F.; Andersen, L.O.; Gasser, R.B.; Stensvold, C.R.; Nejsum, P. Mitochondrial genome analyses suggest multiple *Trichuris* species in humans, baboons, and pigs from different geographical regions. *PLoS Negl. Trop. Dis.* **2015**, *9*, e0004059. [CrossRef] [PubMed]
214. Liu, G.H.; Zhou, W.; Nisbet, A.J.; Xu, M.J.; Zhou, D.H.; Zhao, G.H.; Wang, S.K.; Song, H.Q.; Lin, R.Q.; Zhu, X.Q. Characterization of *Trichuris trichiura* from humans and *T. suis* from pigs in China using internal transcribed spacers of nuclear ribosomal DNA. *J. Helminthol.* **2014**, *88*, 64–68. [CrossRef] [PubMed]
215. Liu, G.-H.; Gasser, R.B.; Su, A.; Nejsum, P.; Peng, L.; Lin, R.-Q.; Li, M.-W.; Xu, M.-J.; Zhu, X.-Q. Clear genetic distinctiveness between human- and pig-derived *Trichuris* based on analyses of mitochondrial datasets. *PLoS Negl. Trop. Dis.* **2012**, *6*, e1539. [CrossRef] [PubMed]
216. Bager, P.; Kapel, C.; Roepstorff, A.; Thamsborg, S.; Arnved, J.; Rønborg, S.; Kristensen, B.; Poulsen, L.K.; Wohlfahrt, J.; Melbye, M. Symptoms after ingestion of pig whipworm *Trichuris suis* eggs in a randomized placebo-controlled double-blind clinical trial. *PLoS ONE* **2011**, *6*, e22346. [CrossRef] [PubMed]
217. Helmby, H. Human helminth therapy to treat inflammatory disorders-where do we stand? *BMC Immunol.* **2015**, *16*, 12. [CrossRef] [PubMed]
218. Jackson, J.A.; Friberg, I.M.; Little, S.; Bradley, J.E. Review series on helminths, immune modulation and the hygiene hypothesis: Immunity against helminths and immunological phenomena in modern human populations: Coevolutionary legacies? *Immunology* **2009**, *126*, 18–27. [CrossRef] [PubMed]
219. Hewitson, J.P.; Grainger, J.R.; Maizels, R.M. Helminth immunoregulation: The role of parasite secreted proteins in modulating host immunity. *Mol. Biochem. Parasitol.* **2009**, *167*, 1–11. [CrossRef] [PubMed]

220. Feary, J.R.; Venn, A.J.; Mortimer, K.; Brown, A.P.; Hooi, D.; Falcone, F.H.; Pritchard, D.I.; Britton, J.R. Experimental hookworm infection: A randomized placebo-controlled trial in asthma. *Clin. Exp. Allergy* **2010**, *40*, 299–306. [CrossRef] [PubMed]
221. TOS. Available online: http://wormswell.com/science-research (accessed on 17 July 2017).
222. The helminthic therapy. Available online: https://tanawisa.com/ (accessed on 17 July 2017).
223. Turner, K.J.; Quinn, E.H.; Anderson, H.R. Regulation of asthma by intestinal parasites. Investigation of possible mechanisms. *Immunology* **1978**, *35*, 281–288. [PubMed]
224. Mpairwe, H.; Ndibazza, J.; Webb, E.L.; Nampijja, M.; Muhangi, L.; Apule, B.; Lule, S.; Akurut, H.; Kizito, D.; Kakande, M.; et al. Maternal hookworm modifies risk factors for childhood eczema: Results from a birth cohort in Uganda. *Pediatr. Allergy Immunol.* **2014**, *25*, 481–488. [CrossRef] [PubMed]
225. McSorley, H.J.; Gaze, S.; Daveson, J.; Jones, D.; Anderson, R.P.; Clouston, A.; Ruyssers, N.E.; Speare, R.; McCarthy, J.S.; Engwerda, C.R.; et al. Suppression of inflammatory immune responses in celiac disease by experimental hookworm infection. *PLoS ONE* **2011**, *6*, e24092. [CrossRef] [PubMed]
226. Daveson, A.J.; Jones, D.M.; Gaze, S.; McSorley, H.; Clouston, A.; Pascoe, A.; Cooke, S.; Speare, R.; Macdonald, G.A.; Anderson, R.; et al. Effect of hookworm infection on wheat challenge in celiac disease—A randomised double-blinded placebo controlled trial. *PLoS ONE* **2011**, *6*, e17366. [CrossRef] [PubMed]
227. Giacomin, P.; Zakrzewski, M.; Jenkins, T.P.; Su, X.; Al-Hallaf, R.; Croese, J.; de Vries, S.; Grant, A.; Mitreva, M.; Loukas, A.; et al. Changes in duodenal tissue-associated microbiota following hookworm infection and consecutive gluten challenges in humans with coeliac disease. *Sci. Rep.* **2016**, *6*, 36797. [CrossRef] [PubMed]
228. Cooper, P.; Walker, A.W.; Reyes, J.; Chico, M.; Salter, S.J.; Vaca, M.; Parkhill, J. Patent human infections with the whipworm, *Trichuris trichiura,* are not associated with alterations in the faecal microbiota. *PLoS ONE* **2013**, *8*, e76573. [CrossRef] [PubMed]
229. Williams, A.R.; Dige, A.; Rasmussen, T.K.; Hvas, C.L.; Dahlerup, J.F.; Iversen, L.; Stensvold, C.R.; Agnholt, J.; Nejsum, P. Immune responses and parasitological observations induced during probiotic treatment with medicinal *Trichuris suis* ova in a healthy volunteer. *Immunol. Lett.* **2017**, *188*, 32–37. [CrossRef] [PubMed]
230. Ruyssers, N.E.; De Winter, B.Y.; De Man, J.G.; Loukas, A.; Herman, A.G.; Pelckmans, P.A.; Moreels, T.G. Worms and the treatment of inflammatory bowel disease: Are molecules the answer? *Clin. Dev. Immunol.* **2008**, *2008*, 567314. [CrossRef] [PubMed]
231. Giacomin, P.; Croese, J.; Krause, L.; Loukas, A.; Cantacessi, C. Suppression of inflammation by helminths: A role for the gut microbiota? *Philos. Trans. R. Soc. Lond. B. Biol. Sci.* **2015**, *370*. [CrossRef] [PubMed]
232. Hays, R.; Esterman, A.; McDermott, R. Control of chronic *Strongyloides stercoralis* infection in an endemic community may be possible by pharmacological means alone: Results of a three-year cohort study. *PLoS Negl. Trop. Dis.* **2017**, *11*, e0005825. [CrossRef] [PubMed]
233. Flannery, G.; White, N. *Immunological Parameters in Northeast Arnhem Land Aboriginies: Consequences of Changing Settlement and Lifestyles;* Cambridge University Press: New York, NY, USA, 1993; pp. 202–220.

10

Potential Animal Reservoir of *Mycobacterium ulcerans*

Avishek Singh [1,*], William John Hannan McBride [1], Brenda Govan [2] and Mark Pearson [3]

1 Cairns Clinical School, College of Medicine and Dentistry, James Cook University, Cairns City, QLD 4870, Australia; john.mcbride@theiddoctor.com
2 College of Public Health, Medical & Vet Sciences, James Cook University, Townsville, QLD 4811, Australia; brenda.govan@jcu.edu.au
3 Australian Institute of Tropical Health & Medicine, James Cook University, Smithfield, QLD 4878, Australia; mark.pearson@jcu.edu.au
* Correspondence: avishek.singh@my.jcu.edu.au;

Abstract: *Mycobacterium ulcerans* is the causative agent of Buruli ulcer, also known in Australia as Daintree ulcer or Bairnsdale ulcer. This destructive skin disease is characterized by extensive and painless necrosis of the skin and soft tissue with the formation of large ulcers, commonly on the leg or arm. To date, 33 countries with tropical, subtropical and temperate climates in Africa, the Americas, Asia and the Western Pacific have reported cases of Buruli ulcer. The disease is rarely fatal, although it may lead to permanent disability and/or disfigurement if not treated appropriately or in time. It is the third most common mycobacterial infection in the world after tuberculosis and leprosy. The precise mode of transmission of *M. ulcerans* is yet to be elucidated. Nevertheless, it is possible that the mode of transmission varies with different geographical areas and epidemiological settings. The knowledge about the possible routes of transmission and potential animal reservoirs of *M. ulcerans* is poorly understood and still remains patchy. Infectious diseases arise from the interaction of agent, host and environment. The majority of emerging or remerging infectious disease in human populations is spread by animals: either wildlife, livestock or pets. Animals may act as hosts or reservoirs and subsequently spread the organism to the environment or directly to the human population. The reservoirs may or may not be the direct source of infection for the hosts; however, they play a major role in maintenance of the organism in the environment, and in the mode of transmission. This remains valid for *M. ulcerans*. Possums have been suggested as one of the reservoir of *M. ulcerans* in south-eastern Australia, where possums ingest *M. ulcerans* from the environment, amplify them and shed the organism through their faeces. We conducted a systematic review with selected key words on PubMed and INFORMIT databases to aggregate available published data on animal reservoirs of *M. ulcerans* around the world. After certain inclusion and exclusion criteria were implemented, a total of 17 studies was included in the review. A variety of animals around the world e.g., rodents, shrews, possums (ringtail and brushtail), horses, dogs, alpacas, koalas and Indian flap-shelled turtles have been recorded as being infected with *M. ulcerans*. The majority of studies included in this review identified animal reservoirs as predisposing to the emergence and reemergence of *M. ulcerans* infection. Taken together, from the selected studies in this systematic review, it is clear that exotic wildlife and native mammals play a significant role as reservoirs for *M. ulcerans*.

Keywords: *Mycobacterium ulcerans*; animal reservoir; transmission

1. Introduction

Sir Albert Cook, a British missionary doctor appointed at the Mengo Hospital in Kampala, Uganda, first noted the skin ulcer caused by *Mycobacterium ulcerans* in 1896. Later, in the late 1930s, two general practitioners, Drs. J. R. Searl and D. G. Alsop, working in rural Victoria, Australia, noticed a group of cases of mysterious skin ulcers around the town of Bairnsdale [1]. The cases were not published in the literature at the time and the causative organism was not identified or characterized. Professor Peter MacCallum and his colleagues first provided the detailed description of the disease in 1948, using presentation data of six patients in the Bairnsdale district, near Melbourne. They were the first to isolate *M. ulcerans* as the causative organism of the mysterious skin ulcer [2]. The first large cluster of *M. ulcerans* infection was identified in the Buruli County of Uganda (now called Nakasongola District) in the 1960s and the disease was termed 'Buruli ulcer' (BU) thereafter [3].

There have been several known outbreaks of Buruli ulcer around the world and each outbreak has its own unique characteristics in terms of epidemiology and the animals reported to be involved in transmission [4,5]. The World Health Organization (WHO) has classified BU as a neglected tropical disease [6]. Presently, BU has been reported (but not always microbiologically confirmed) in more than 30 countries spread over Africa, the Americas, Asia, and Oceania [7]. Australia is the only developed country with significant local transmission of BU, with foci of infection in tropical Far North Queensland [8,9], the Capricorn Coast region of central Queensland [10], the Northern Territory [11] and temperate coastal Victoria [10]. Non-human cases of *M. ulcerans* are prevalent in Australia only, where several cases of BU have been described in both native wildlife and domestic mammal species such as koalas (*Phascolarctos cinereus*) [12,13], common ringtail possums (*Pseudocheirus peregrinus*) [14,15], a mountain brushtail possum (*Trichosurus cunninghami*) [5,14,15], two horses [16], an alpaca [17], four dogs [18] and a cat [19]. Recent research in Victoria, Australia, has suggested the transmission of infection by mosquitoes, and possums with chronic BU as an important environmental reservoir of *M. ulcerans* in Victoria [14].

2. Materials and Methods

The PRISMA guidelines developed by the Centre for Review Dissemination (CRD) were used as the methodology for the systematic review [20]. A review protocol was registered with PROSPERO international prospective register of systematic reviews, which can be viewed online [21]. The systematic literature review was conducted using online databases MEDLINE and INFORMIT to aggregate all the published literature. Initially, MEDLINE was used to retrieve all the scientific information concerning the research topic. INFORMIT was searched with same search strategies adopted for MEDLINE. The following key words were chosen after a series of trial searches in order to ensure an adequate number of relevant articles were reviewed: (Buruli OR '*Mycobacterium ulcerans*') AND (Host OR Vector OR Reservoir OR Animal), accessed on 6 May 2018. The title and abstract of each of the articles were initially scanned to ensure that the included articles met the aim and scope of the systematic review. Articles that were deemed irrelevant to the aim of this systematic review or out of the research scope were excluded. For those articles that were not clear by the title and abstract, the full text was retrieved and further analyzed in order to determine if they met the inclusion and exclusion criteria below. The studies that reported only experimental or laboratory exposure of *M. ulcerans* in animals were excluded. The search strategy exclusively focused on potential animal reservoirs, not the vectors. The detection of the causative agent had to be confirmed by culture of bacteria and/or PCR. To be considered positive a sample needed to be confirmed either by culture of bacteria or positive for IS 2404 and reconfirmed by KR and IS 2606. Undoubtedly, PCR targeting IS 2404 is highly specific for detecting *M. ulcerans* in clinical specimen [22]. However, for detecting *M. ulcerans* from environmental samples, confirmatory PCR targeting two additional insertion sequences, IS 2606 and the ketoreductase B domain (KR), is essential to differentiate *M. ulcerans* from other environmental mycobacteria that may carry IS 2404 and other non-mycolactone-producing mycobacteria [22]. Thus, IS 2404-PCR used in conjunction with IS 2606 and KR-PCR confirms that the detected organism is *M.*

ulcerans. There were no language restrictions. Risk of bias was assessed by one reviewer on the basis of independent factors such as sample size, location and nature of infection.

3. Results

3.1. Results of the Literature Search and Method of Inclusion

The total number of discovered articles in MEDLINE database was 351. Three hundred and fourteen articles were excluded after reading the title and abstracts as they were not relevant to the research question. Full texts of thirty-seven studies were retrieved in portable document format (PDF) for further analysis. Of these remaining 37 studies, 19 were excluded as they clearly did not meet inclusion criteria (i.e., they were review articles, focused on vectors rather than on animal reservoirs, or pertained to laboratory or experimental exposure). One additional duplicate article was excluded as well. The remaining 17 studies from the PubMed database were included for systematic review. There were no additional articles in INFORMIT that did not appear in the initial MEDLINE search results. The flow chart for study selection process is shown in Figure 1.

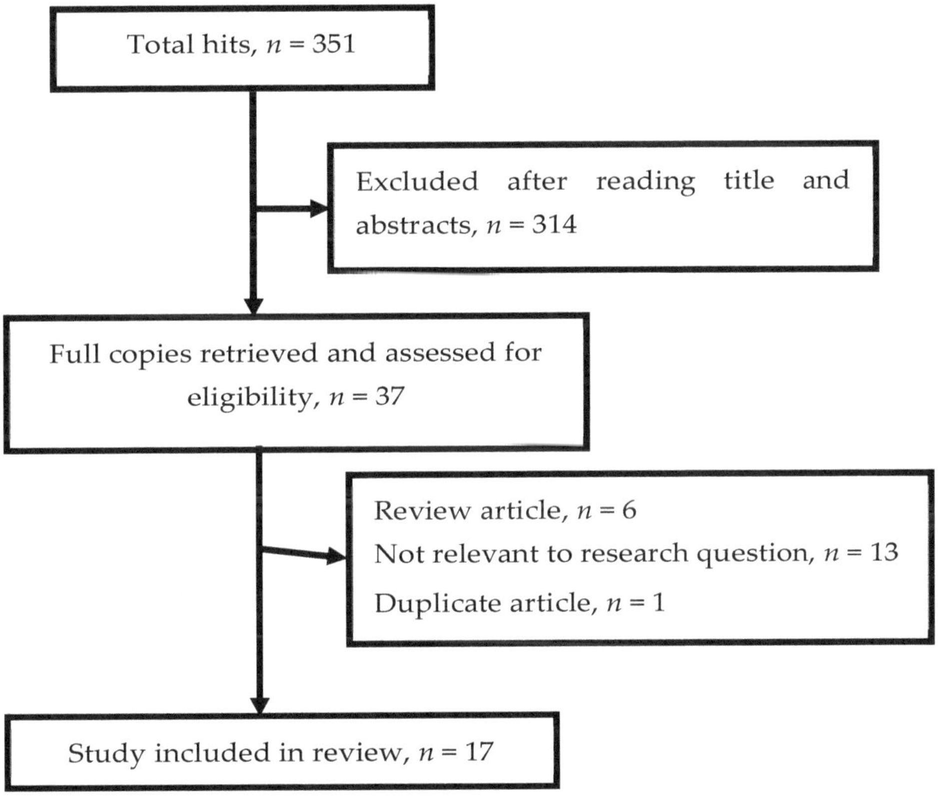

Figure 1. Flow chart of study selection process.

3.2. Basic Characteristics of Selected Studies

Out of the 17 included studies, ten were conducted in Australia, two in Ghana and one was conducted in each of Ivory Coast, North America, United States, Benin and Japan. The basic characteristics of selected studies for review are shown in Table 1 below.

Table 1. Basic characteristics of selected studies on occurrence of *Mycobacterium ulcerans*.

Author and Year	Sample and Sample Size	Collection Year, Location and Setting	Detection Method, Result or *M. ulcerans* Positive Signal
Roltgen, Pluschke, Johnson, & Fyfe, 2017 [9]	102 environmental samples: 55 from soil/vegetation; 35 from insects or small insects pool and 12 from animal excreta	September 2013 Northern Queensland, Australia	RT-PCR IS 2404 positive: 1 soil specimen: 2 bandicoot faeces, one individual mosquito and 1 pool of 2 mosquitoes IS 2606 and KR (ketoreductase) positive: 2 bandicoot faeces and pool of two mosquitoes
Tobias et al., 2016 [23]	180 faecal specimens from dominant domestic animals (ovine, porcine, avian, reptiles, canine)	September 2013 4 BU-endemic and one non-endemic villages of Ghana, West Africa	RT-PCR IS 2404 positive: 2/86 ovine; 1/69 avian: 1/16 reptiles IS 2606 and KR: all negative
Tian, Niamke, Tissot-Dupont, &Drancourt, 2016 [24]	496 environmental samples: 100 from soil (endemic n = 50 and non-endemic n = 50); 200 from stagnant water (endemic n = 100 and non-endemic n = 100); 100 from plants (endemic n = 50 and non-endemic n = 50) and 96 animal faeces (*Thryonomys swinderianus* (agouti) stools) (endemic n = 48 and non-endemic n = 48)	June–October 2014 Ivory Coast, West Africa	RT-PCR 43 samples with at least one positive IS 2404 and KR Out of 43, only 10 positive for both IS2404 and KR, IS 2606 not performed: 7 water specimen; 2 *T. swinderianus* (agouti) faeces and one soil specimen
Carson et al., 2014 [5]	Fecal sample: 216 common ringtail possums and 6 common brushtail possums	Southeast Australia, State Victoria	RT-PCR targeting IS 2404, IS 2606 and KR 20 common ringtail possums and 4 common brushtail possums
O'Brien et al., 2014 [15]	69 possums (ringtail and brushtail) trapped at Point Lonsdale: Faecal samples: 57; blood samples: 63; buccal swab: 67; urine sample: 16; pouch swab: 15; cloacal swab: 20 69 fecal samples from 15 mountain brushtail possums	1998–2011 Victoria, Australia	RT-PCR targeting IS 2404, IS 2606 and KR Point Lonsdale: Positive: faecal sample: 12 (25%); blood sample: 0; buccal swab: 7 (16%); urine sample: 0; pouch swab: 3 (20%) Bellbird Creek: Positive: 4 mountain brushtail possums (27%)
C. O'Brien et al., 2013 [17]	Case report: two alpacas (*Vicugna pacos*) ulcerated tissue	Case 1: September 1997 Case 2: May 2011 Victoria, Australia	RT-PCR targeting IS 2404, IS 2606 and KR positive
Willson et al., 2013 [25]	587 fish representing 13 genera and 17 species and 351 amphibians representing 10 genera: external swab	2008–2009 Ghana, West Africa	RT-PCR targeting IS 2606 and KR not performed. Not confirmed
C. R. O'Brien et al., 2011 [18]	Case report: Case 1: 14 months old female kelpie Case 2: 3 years old female kelpie Case 3: 6 years old male whippet Case 4: 3 years old male koolie	2011 Victoria, Australia	RT-PCR targeting IS 2404, IS 2606 and KR All 4 dogs positive for *M. ulcerans*
Sakaguchi et al., 2011 [26]	Case report; Indian flap-shelled turtle, *Lissemys punctata punctata*	Imported from India to aquarium in Japan	PCR assays targeting the *rpoβ* gene: unable to differentiate *M. ulcerans* from mycolactone-producing *M. marinum* (MPMM)

Table 1. *Cont.*

Author and Year	Sample and Sample Size	Collection Year, Location and Setting	Detection Method, Result or *M. ulcerans* Positive Signal
Fyfe et al., 2010 [14]	589 fecal samples from ringtail possums and 250 samples from brushtail possums. Live trapping: 42 ringtail possums and 21 brushtail possums	2007–2009 Victoria, Australia	RT-PCR targeting IS 2404, IS 2606 and KR *M. ulcerans* DNA detected in 43% of ringtail possum and 29% of brushtail possum faecal samples. 38% ringtail possum have *M. ulcerans* lesion and/or positive faeces Lower in brushtail possums: 1 with *M. ulcerans* lesion and/or positive faeces and 4 with no lesions and low *M. ulcerans* DNA in faeces.
Durnez et al., 2010 [27]	565 small mammals: 326 rodents and 222 shrews	2006 Benin, West Africa	RT-PCR: No *M. ulcerans* specific DNA detected
Van Zyl et al., 2010 [16]	2 horses: Case report Case 1: 21-year-old quarterhorse-cross Case 2: 32-year-old standard bredgelding	Case 1: May 2006 Case 2: October 2006 Southeastern Australia	RT-PCR *M. ulcerans* specific DNA detected from both horses
Elsner et al., 2008 [19]	Cat: Case report 10-year-old castrated male domestic cat	2006 Victoria, Australia	RT-PCR *M. ulcerans* specific DNA detected
Appleyard & Clark, 2002 [28]	Case report: three cats Case 1: An 8-year-old spayed female shorthair Case 2: 6-year-old spayed female shorthair Case 3: 11-year-old domestic longhair cat	2002 North America	PCR Could not differentiate *M. ulcerans* from other *Mycobacterium* spp. (a new *Mycobacterial* spp. namely '*Mycobacterium visibilis*' suggested)
Heckert, Elankumaran, Milani, &Baya, 2001 [29]	60 wild striped bass: Swab from external ulcerative dermatitis and granulomatous-like lesions in the internal organs	1997 Chesapeake Bay, USA	PCR No *M. ulcerans* specific DNA detected (a new mycobacterial spp. suggested)
Mitchell, McOrist, &Bilney, 1987 [13]	36 male and 51 female adult koalas captured	1980–1985 Raymond Island, southeastern Australia	Pathological and bacteriological examination 18 out of 87 captured koalas had skin wound 11 koalas were found positive for *M. ulcerans*
McOrist, Jerrett, Anderson, & Hayman, 1985 [12]	Case study: 2 koalas: one male and one female Ulcerated tissue	1982 Raymond Island, southeastern Australia	Pathological and bacteriological examination Both koalas suggested positive for *M. ulcerans*

4. Discussion on Possible Reservoirs and Vectors of *Mycobacterium ulcerans* by Country

This systematic review assessed the potential animal reservoir of *M. ulcerans* around the world recorded to date. This is essential for understanding the epidemiology and mode of transmission of the disease, which subsequently aids in prevention, control and elimination strategies.

4.1. Australia

Out of 17 studies included in this review, 10 were conducted in Australia. In Australia, the disease is more prevalent in the southeastern state of Victoria and in Far North Queensland. After the detection of *M. ulcerans* infection in four koalas in 1980 at Raymond Island, Australia [13], the entire island was searched for koalas in the following year. Thirty-six male and 51 female koalas were captured and examined. Of these, 18 out of 87 animals had skin wounds and 11 were found positive for *M. ulcerans*. Diagnosis was made on pathological and bacteriological examination; the PCR-based method used for the identification of *M. ulcerans* from clinical and environmental samples was only implemented in 1996 [30]. Non-human cases of *M. ulcerans* in Australia have been reported in marsupial species such as koalas [13], ringtail and brushtail possums [14,15,31], horses [16], alpacas [17], dogs [18] and cats [19]. A study conducted by Fyfe and colleagues between 2007–2009, at Point Lonsdale, a small coastal town south east of Melbourne, Australia, which is also endemic for BU, found that 43% of ringtail possum and 29% of brushtail possum faecal samples were positive for *M. ulcerans* DNA [14]. Only 1% of faecal samples from non-endemic area possums were positive for *M. ulcerans* DNA in this study, suggesting terrestrial mammals such as possums are potential reservoirs of *M. ulcerans* in southeast Australia. Several studies have identified possums (both ringtail and brushtail) as potential reservoirs since then [5,15]. In Australia, other than the southeastern state of Victoria, BU is also prevalent in Far North Queensland [8]. Inspired by the evidence of possums as potential reservoirs of *M. ulcerans* in Victoria, a study conducted by Roltgen and colleagues (2013) in northern Queensland, Australia, detected *M. ulcerans* DNA from two bandicoot faecal samples, suggesting the possibility that bandicoots are a potential reservoir of *M. ulcerans* in Far North Queensland [9].

4.2. Africa

Out of the 17 studies included in this review, four were conducted in West African countries: two in Ghana [23,25], one in the Ivory Coast [24] and one in Benin [27]. Durnez and colleagues (2006) caught 326 rodents and 222 shrews from endemic and non-endemic villages of Benin and tested for *M. ulcerans,* but no specific DNA was detected from any of their samples [27]. Despite their results, they suggested the necessity of more intensive research focusing on small mammals in Africa. Willson reported positive PCR with IS 2404 only from tadpoles and fishes from Ghana [25]. Similarly, two faecal specimens from *Thryonomys swinderianus* (agouti) were reported positive for *M. ulcerans* in a study conducted by Bi Diangoné Tian and colleagues (2014) from the Ivory Coast [24]. They suggested agouti, which are closely related to Australian possums, could be a potential reservoir of *M. ulcerans* in Africa. However, RT-PCR targeting IS 2606 was not conducted to confirm *M. ulcerans*. A faecal survey of domestic animals in rural Ghana for *M. ulcerans* conducted by Tobias and associates suggested no evidence of association between domestic animals and *M. ulcerans* in endemic and non-endemic villages in Ghana [23]. Unlike Australia, not a single study in Africa has reported the presence of *M. ulcerans*-positive DNA or cases in non-human species, suggesting that transmission dynamics may be different in Africa and Australia or, alternatively, a host animal is yet to be identified in Africa.

4.3. Other Countries

No study has reported *M. ulcerans* DNA or cases in non-human species in any country other than Australia. A study conducted by Heckert in 1997 at Chesapeake Bay, USA detected a new *Mycobacterium* species from wild striped bass [29]. This new isolate was closely related to *M. marinum, M. ulcerans,* and *M. tuberculosis*. Similarly, Sakaguchi and associates reported an atypical mycobacterial infection in an Indian flap-shelled turtle (*Lissemys punctata punctata)*, imported from India to Japan in an aquarium [26]. A PCR assay targeting the *rpoβ* gene revealed the isolate had 89–100% homology to *M. ulcerans* and *M. marinum*. Again, this study could not differentiate *M. ulcerans* from mycolactone-producing *M. marinum* (MPMM). Appleyard and Clark (2002) reported a new *Mycobacterial* species, namely '*Mycobacterium visibilis*' from three cats initially suspected of having *M. ulcerans* infection [28].

5. Conclusions

Human cases of BU have been reported in more than 30 countries from Africa, America, Asia and Oceania. Since the implementation of PCR-based methods for the detection and identification of *M. ulcerans* from clinical and environmental samples, there has been a significant increase in overall knowledge of BU. There is no record of direct human-to-human transmission of *M. ulcerans*, unlike tuberculosis and leprosy. Australia is the only country where non-human cases of BU have been identified, with small mammals, especially possums and, to some extent, bandicoots, being implicated as potential reservoirs of *M. ulcerans*. Despite there having been several outbreaks in African countries, no non-human cases have been recorded so far and there is no evidence of any animal acting as a potential reservoir for this organism. None of the studies included in this review discussed strain variation of *M. ulcerans* in different geographical regions leading to an increase or decrease in susceptibility among animal or human population. Compared to other mycobacteria, such as *M. tuberculosis*, there is very little genetic diversity among isolates of *M. ulcerans*. Some variation among the strains of *M. ulcerans* from Africa, the Americas, Asia and the Western Pacific has been recorded; however, the linkage between these various strains and virulence in human or animal population has not been recognized so far. Remarkable differences in the type of mycolactone produced by *M. ulcerans* in different geographical location has been recorded. African strains produce more mycolactone variant A and B, whereas strains from Australia produce more mycolactone variant C. However, this variation has nothing to do with host susceptibility to *M. ulcerans*; rather, it determines cytopathogenecity and thus clinical presentation of disease.

This systematic review suggests the need for extensive laboratory and field research focusing on domestic animals and wildlife to elucidate their roles in BU-endemic countries.

Author Contributions: A.S. and W.J.H.M. designed the study. A.S. collected and analyzed the data. A.S. wrote the paper with input from all authors. All authors reviewed the final manuscript.

Acknowledgments: The authors would like to acknowledge Janet A. Fyfe, Victorian Infectious Diseases Reference Laboratory, Melbourne, VIC 3000, Australia, for her continuous support and feedback. We would like to thank Far North Queensland Hospital Foundation and James Cook University for funding this research.

References

1. Alsop, D.G. The Bairnsdale ulcer. *Aust. N. Z. J. Surg.* **1972**, *41*, 317–319. [CrossRef] [PubMed]
2. MacCallum, P.T.J.C.; Tolhurst, J.C.; Buckle, G.; Sissons, H.A. A new mycobacterial infection in man. *J. Pathol. Bacteriol.* **1948**, *60*, 93–122. [CrossRef] [PubMed]
3. Clancey, J.; Dodge, R.; Lunn, H.F. Study of a *Mycobacterium* causing skin ulceration in Uganda. *Ann. Soc. Belg. Med. Trop.* **1920**, *42*, 585–590.
4. Johnson, P.D.; Azuolas, J.; Lavender, C.J.; Wishart, E.; Stinear, T.P.; Hayman, J.A.; Brown, L.; Jenkin, G.A.; Fyfe, J.A. *Mycobacterium ulcerans* in mosquitoes captured during outbreak of Buruli ulcer, southeastern Australia. *Emerg. Infect. Dis.* **2007**, *13*, 1653–1660. [CrossRef] [PubMed]
5. Carson, C.; Lavender, C.J.; Handasyde, K.A.; O'Brien, C.R.; Hewitt, N.; Johnson, P.D.; Fyfe, J.A. Potential wildlife sentinels for monitoring the endemic spread of human Buruli ulcer in south-east Australia. *PLoS Negl. Trop. Dis.* **2014**, *8*, e2668. [CrossRef] [PubMed]

6. World Health Organization. Neglected Tropical Diseases. 2018. Available online: http://www.who.int/neglected_diseases/diseases/en/ (accessed on 4 October 2017).
7. World Health Organization. *Distribution of Buruli Ulcer, Worldwide 2014*; WHO: Geneva, Switzerland, 2014.
8. Steffen, C.M.; Smith, M.; McBride, W.J. *Mycobacterium ulcerans* infection in North Queensland: The 'Daintree ulcer'. *ANZ J. Surg.* **2010**, *80*, 732–736. [CrossRef] [PubMed]
9. Röltgen, K.; Pluschke, G.; Johnson, P.D.; Fyfe, J. *Mycobacterium ulcerans* DNA in bandicoot excreta in Buruli ulcer-endemic area, northern Queensland, Australia. *Emerg. Infect. Dis.* **2017**, *23*, 2042–2045. [CrossRef] [PubMed]
10. Francis, G.; Whitby, M.; Woods, M. *Mycobacterium ulcerans* infection: A rediscovered focus in the Capricorn Coast region of central Queensland. *Med. J. Aust.* **2006**, *185*, 179–180. [PubMed]
11. Radford, A.J. *Mycobacterium ulcerans* in Australia. *Aust. N. Z. J. Med.* **1975**, *5*, 162–169. [CrossRef] [PubMed]
12. McOrist, S.; Jerrett, I.V.; Anderson, M.; Hayman, J. Cutaneous and respiratory tract infection with *Mycobacterium ulcerans* in two koalas (*Phascolarctos cinereus*). *J. Wildl. Dis.* **1985**, *21*, 171–173. [CrossRef] [PubMed]
13. Mitchell, P.J.; McOrist, S.; Bilney, R. Epidemiology of *Mycobacterium ulcerans* infection in koalas (*Phascolarctos cinereus*) on Raymond Island, southeastern Australia. *J. Wildl. Dis.* **1987**, *23*, 386–390. [CrossRef] [PubMed]
14. Fyfe, J.A.; Lavender, C.J.; Handasyde, K.A.; Legione, A.R.; O'Brien, C.R.; Stinear, T.P.; Pidot, S.J.; Seemann, T.; Benbow, M.E.; Wallace, J.R.; et al. A major role for mammals in the ecology of *Mycobacterium ulcerans*. *PLoS Negl. Trop. Dis.* **2010**, *4*, e791. [CrossRef] [PubMed]
15. O'Brien, C.R.; Handasyde, K.A.; Hibble, J.; Lavender, C.J.; Legione, A.R.; McCowan, C.; Globan, M.; Mitchell, A.T.; McCracken, H.E.; Johnson, P.D.; et al. Clinical, microbiological and pathological findings of *Mycobacterium ulcerans* infection in three Australian possum species. *PLoS Negl. Trop. Dis.* **2014**, *8*, e2666. [CrossRef] [PubMed]
16. van Zyl, A.; Daniel, J.; Wayne, J.; McCowan, C.; Malik, R.; Jelfs, P.; Lavender, C.J.; Fyfe, J.A. *Mycobacterium ulcerans* infections in two horses in south-eastern Australia. *Aust. Vet. J.* **2010**, *88*, 101–106. [CrossRef] [PubMed]
17. O'Brien, C.; Kuseff, G.; McMillan, E.; McCowan, C.; Lavender, C.; Globan, M.; Jerrett, I.; Oppedisano, F.; Johnson, P.; Fyfe, J. *Mycobacterium ulcerans* infection in two alpacas. *Aust. Vet. J.* **2013**, *91*, 296–300. [CrossRef] [PubMed]
18. O'Brien, C.R.; McMillan, E.; Harris, O.; O'Brien, D.P.; Lavender, C.J.; Globan, M.; Legione, A.R.; Fyfe, J.A. Localised *Mycobacterium ulcerans* infection in four dogs. *Aust. Vet. J.* **2011**, *89*, 506–510. [CrossRef] [PubMed]
19. Elsner, L.; Wayne, J.; O'Brien, C.R.; McCowan, C.; Malik, R.; Hayman, J.A.; Globan, M.; Lavender, C.J.; Fyfe, J.A. Localised *Mycobacterium ulcerans* infection in a cat in Australia. *J. Feline Med. Surg.* **2008**, *10*, 407–412. [CrossRef] [PubMed]
20. Moher, D.; Liberati, A.; Tetzlaff, J.; Altman, D.G.; Prisma Group. Preferred reporting items for systematic reviews and meta-analyses: The PRISMA statement. *Int. J. Surg.* **2010**, *8*, 336–341.
21. PROSPERO Registered Study Protocol. Available online: https://www.crd.york.ac.uk/prospero/display_record.php?RecordID=85484 (accessed on 12 January 2018).
22. Fyfe, J.A.; Lavender, C.J.; Johnson, P.D.; Globan, M.; Sievers, A.; Azuolas, J.; Stinear, T.P. Development and application of two multiplex real-time PCR assays for the detection of *Mycobacterium ulcerans* in clinical and environmental samples. *Appl. Environ. Microbiol.* **2007**, *73*, 4733–4740. [CrossRef] [PubMed]
23. Tobias, N.J.; Ammisah, N.A.; Ahortor, E.K.; Wallace, J.R.; Ablordey, A.; Stinear, T.P. Snapshot faecal survey of domestic animals in rural Ghana for *Mycobacterium ulcerans*. *PeerJ* **2016**, *4*, e2065. [CrossRef] [PubMed]
24. Tian, R.B.; Niamké, S.; Tissot-Dupont, H.; Drancourt, M. Detection of *Mycobacterium ulcerans* DNA in the environment, Ivory Coast. *PLoS ONE* **2016**, *11*, e0151567. [CrossRef] [PubMed]
25. Willson, S.J.; Kaufman, M.G.; Merritt, R.W.; Williamson, H.R.; Malakauskas, D.M.; Benbow, M.E. Fish and amphibians as potential reservoirs of *Mycobacterium ulcerans*, the causative agent of Buruli ulcer disease. *Infect. Ecol. Epidemiol.* **2013**, *3*, 19946. [CrossRef] [PubMed]
26. Sakaguchi, K.; Iima, H.; Hirayama, K.; Okamoto, M.; Matsuda, K.; Miyasho, T.; Kasamatsu, M.; Hasegawa, K.; Taniyama, H. *Mycobacterium ulcerans* infection in an Indian flap-shelled turtle (*Lissemys punctata punctata*). *J. Vet. Med. Sci.* **2011**, *73*, 1217–1220. [CrossRef] [PubMed]

27. Durnez, L.; Suykerbuyk, P.; Nicolas, V.; Barriere, P.; Verheyen, E.; Johnson, C.R.; Leirs, H.; Portaels, F. Terrestrial small mammals as reservoirs of *Mycobacterium ulcerans* in Benin. *Appl. Environ. Microbiol.* **2010**, *76*, 4574–4577. [CrossRef] [PubMed]
28. Appleyard, G.D.; Clark, E.G. Histologic and genotypic characterization of a novel *Mycobacterium* species found in three cats. *J. Clin. Microbiol.* **2002**, *40*, 2425–2430. [CrossRef] [PubMed]
29. Heckert, R.A.; Elankumaran, S.; Milani, A.; Baya, A. Detection of a new *Mycobacterium* species in wild striped bass in the Chesapeake Bay. *J. Clin. Microbiol.* **2001**, *39*, 710–715. [CrossRef] [PubMed]
30. Ross, B.C.; Marino, L.; Oppedisano, F.; Edwards, R.; Robins-Browne, R.M.; Johnson, P.D. Development of a PCR assay for rapid diagnosis of *Mycobacterium ulcerans* infection. *J. Clin. Microbiol.* **1997**, *35*, 1696–1700. [PubMed]
31. Portaels, F.; Hibble, J. *Mycobacterium ulcerans* in wild animals. *Rev. Sci. Technol.* **2001**, *20*, 252–264. [CrossRef]

11

Confronting the Emerging Threat to Public Health in Northern Australia of Neglected Indigenous Arboviruses

Narayan Gyawali [1,2] and Andrew W. Taylor-Robinson [3,*]

1 School of Health, Medical & Applied Sciences, Central Queensland University, Rockhampton, QLD 4702, Australia; n.gyawali@cqu.edu.au
2 Institute of Health & Biomedical Innovation, Queensland University of Technology, Brisbane, QLD 4059, Australia
3 School of Health, Medical & Applied Sciences, Central Queensland University, Brisbane, QLD 4000, Australia
* Correspondence: a.taylor-robinson@cqu.edu.au;

Abstract: In excess of 75 arboviruses have been identified in Australia, some of which are now well established as causative agents of debilitating diseases. These include Ross River virus, Barmah Forest virus, and Murray Valley encephalitis virus, each of which may be detected by both antibody-based recognition and molecular typing. However, for most of the remaining arboviruses that may be associated with pathology in humans, routine tests are not available to diagnose infection. A number of these so-called 'neglected' or 'orphan' arboviruses that are indigenous to Australia might have been infecting humans at a regular rate for decades. Some of them may be associated with undifferentiated febrile illness—fever, the cause of which is not obvious—for which around half of all cases each year remain undiagnosed. This is of particular relevance to Northern Australia, given the Commonwealth Government's transformative vision for the midterm future of massive infrastructure investment in this region. An expansion of the industrial and business development of this previously underpopulated region is predicted. This is set to bring into intimate proximity infection-naïve human hosts, native reservoir animals, and vector mosquitoes, thereby creating a perfect storm for increased prevalence of infection with neglected Australian arboviruses. Moreover, the escalating rate and effects of climate change that are increasingly observed in the tropical north of the country are likely to lead to elevated numbers of arbovirus-transmitting mosquitoes. As a commensurate response, continuing assiduous attention to vector monitoring and control is required. In this overall context, improved epidemiological surveillance and diagnostic screening, including establishing novel, rapid pan-viral tests to facilitate early diagnosis and appropriate treatment of febrile primary care patients, should be considered a public health priority. Investment in a rigorous identification program would reduce the possibility of significant outbreaks of these indigenous arboviruses at a time when population growth accelerates in Northern Australia.

Keywords: arbovirus; neglected; undifferentiated febrile illness; Northern Australia; diagnostics; control; prevention

---

1. Introduction

*Ar*thropod-*bo*rne*viruses* (arboviruses) are by definition transmitted between vertebrate hosts by biting arthropods (mosquitoes, ticks, sandflies, midges and gnats) [1], and the infections that they cause pose a significant public health risk worldwide. The International Catalogue of Arboviruses currently lists 537 registered viruses on the basis of their known transmission by arthropods, known for potential infectivity to humans or domestic animals, and antigenic or phylogenetic relationships to known arboviruses [2].

At present, more than 130 arboviruses are recognised as causing mild to fulminant disease in humans [3]. Symptoms of uncomplicated arboviral infection generally occur between 3 and 15 days after exposure to the virus and may persist for a week or so. The most common clinical features of infection are the indistinct influenza-like symptoms of fever, headache, and malaise, which, without recourse to further information regarding a patient's clinical and exposure history, often preclude a correct diagnosis [4].

Australia is home to over 75 arboviruses that have been isolated from its native arthropods [2]. While so far only 13 of these are found to be associated with human infection, just Barmah Forest virus (BFV) and Ross River virus (RRV) are tested for routinely. Moreover, laboratory tests are available for Murray Valley encephalitis virus (MVEV) and West Nile Kunjin virus (KUNV) but test requests are made on patients with highly suggestive signs and symptoms [5]. The ecology and role of other arboviruses in humans, whether they are associated with any serious infections or undiagnosed undifferentiated febrile illness (UFI), are unknown and their study is not prioritised. An analysis of the notifications of BFV, RRV, MVEV, and KUNV in the last two decades has clearly shown a higher distribution of these viruses in Northern Australia [6] (reviewed in [5]).

In this article, we describe briefly the neglected Australian arboviruses that are most likely to emerge as significant agents of human disease. The arboviruses that we discuss have been found to infect humans—serological evidence of host immune responses has been found. It is implicitly understood that a virus that is associated with human infection could potentially be a pathogen, i.e. it may have been causing a disease, the aetiology of which is so far unknown, or it could cause disease under certain circumstances, such as in immunocompromised persons, during pregnancy, or upon secondary infection. We also consider what action should be taken to confront the potential threat of such neglected indigenous arboviruses in the particular environment of Northern Australia. This is a largely tropical climatic region where both mosquito vectors and vertebrate reservoir hosts are abundant and in which a future major expansion of a human population primarily comprising relocating, previously non-exposed individuals, is predicted.

2. Arbovirus Ecology and Epidemiology

Most arboviruses studied thus far are transmitted in zoonotic cycles, i.e. the principal vertebrate host is an animal other than human [7]. The distribution of an arbovirus is restricted to areas inhabited by vertebrate hosts that serve as its reservoirs and vectors. Thus, many arboviruses have clearly defined ecological zones, while some, distributed globally, cause diseases of considerable public health and veterinary importance (reviewed in [8]). Examples of the latter include dengue (worldwide, approximately between the Tropics of Cancer and Capricorn), yellow fever (Africa and South America), Japanese encephalitis (eastern and southeast Asia and Australia), West Nile encephalitis (North America, Europe and the Middle East), chikungunya (Asia, Central and South America, parts of the Pacific), eastern and western equine encephalitis (North America), and Venezuelan equine encephalitis (South America). Due to focal, global, environmental, societal and/or demographic changes, many of these viruses have either emerged or re-emerged in the first years of this century [9–11].

Notably, the non-segmented, positive-strand RNA viruses belonging to the genus *Flavivirus*, family *Flaviviridae*, or genus *Alphavirus*, family *Togaviridae*, are the aetiological agents of several major global infectious diseases such as dengue, yellow fever, chikungunya and Zika. Other related pathogens belong to the segmented, negative strand RNA *Orthobunyavirus* genus. The vast majority of arbovirus-associated epidemics occur in the tropics and subtropics due to the prevailing hot and humid climate which is conducive to the habitation of vector mosquitoes, including members of *Aedes*, *Anopheles*, *Culex*, *Haemagogus*, and *Ochlerotatus* genera [12]. To this growing list of real or potential public health threats posed by arboviruses Mayarocan now be added, identified recently in the Amazon and other tropical regions of South America [13]. The issue of whether neglected

Australian arboviruses similarly present an emerging, hitherto unrecognised challenge to humans is a subject of discussion.

3. Arboviruses in Australia

Australia is the sixth largest country in the world by area, the largest country without land borders, and the largest country overall in the southern hemisphere. Early European settlement, urbanisation, increased sea and air travel and trade, globalisation, pathogen evolution, and elevated mean global temperature are some of the factors that may have influenced the introduction and expanded geographical reach of infectious diseases, including those caused by arboviruses, in Australia [14]. Furthermore, Australia spans tropical and subtropical latitudes, where arboviruses have access to an abundant source of both reservoir hosts and vectors.

While only 13 of the more than 75 identified arboviruses indigenous to Australia are currently known to cause disease in humans, information is scarce as to the potential human pathogenicity of most others [15]. Of those that are recognised to cause infection in humans in Australia (Figure 1), the alphaviruses RRV and BFV are the most well-known, infection with either of which triggers an incapacitating and occasionally chronic polyarthritis with accompanying myalgia and lethargy [16,17]. The flaviviruses MVEV and KUNV cause encephalitis, an acute inflammation of the brain [18].

Infection with the flavivirus dengue (DENV) is typically characterised by a febrile illness but a small proportion of cases manifest as a life-threatening haemorrhagic fever or shock syndrome (reviewed in [19]). DENV may be acquired outside Australia and brought back by returning travellers, a significant proportion of whom are hospitalised with unrecognised warning signs of severe disease. As intercontinental travel from Australia, particularly to Asia, continues to increase, in order to avert serious outcomes it is crucial that clinicians anticipate, and can recognise and manage, such tropical infectious diseases. While DENV has a transglobal distribution, local outbreaks are also reported regularly in far north Queensland, with foci in the vicinities of Cairns and Townsville [20], where it is well recognised by the resident population as a not insignificant threat to their health [21].

Several other arboviruses that are indigenous to Australia (Figure 1), such as the alphavirus Sindbis (SINV), the flaviviruses Alfuy (ALFV), Edge Hill (EHV), Kokobera (KOKV) and Stratford (STRV), and the orthobunyaviruses Gan Gan (GGV), Kowanyama (KOWV) and Trubanaman (TRUV), are recognised through eliciting mild symptoms of febrile illness, corroborated by detection of serum antibodies to viral antigens, as being able to infect humans [17,22,23] (reviewed in [5]). There are occasional reports of human disease caused by SINV, EHV and KOKV [24–26], but these are not currently included individually in the list of Australian national notifiable diseases by disease type [27]. The magnitude of each of these arboviral infections raises the question as to what is an appropriate threshold for recording cases for the purposes of annual notification at state/territory and national levels. SINV is reportedly the arbovirus most frequently isolated from mosquitoes in Australia [23], but as an alphavirus it does not come under the 'flavivirus infection (unspecified)' umbrella presently used for nationwide notification [27].

Other arboviruses have been isolated from arthropods in the Australia-Pacific region [15]. These include the newly identified Bamaga (BGV) and Fitzroy River (FRV) flaviviruses [28,29], which are closely related to the disease-causing yellow fever virus (YFV) and EHV, but for each of which there is scant information about its capacity to infect humans or to cause disease in humans.

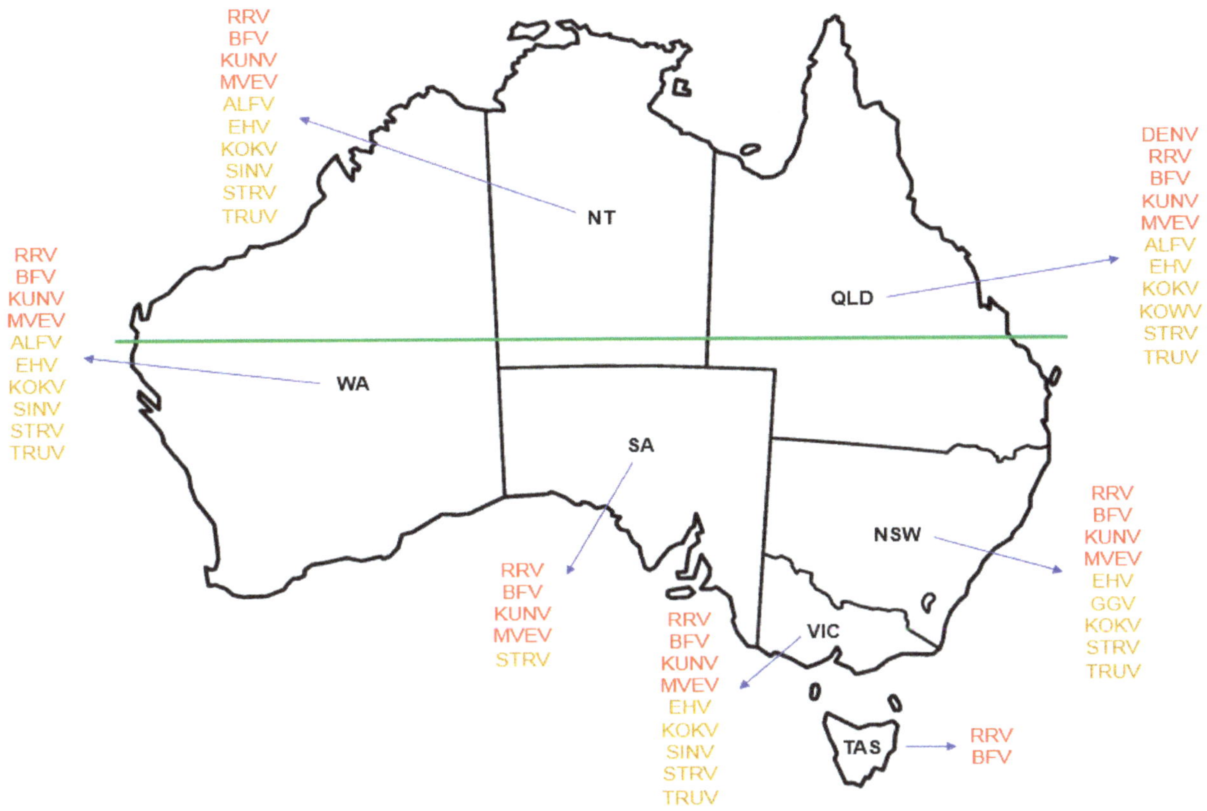

Figure 1. Geographical distribution of Australian indigenous arboviruses known to cause human infection. Use of red font for each named virus indicates the state or territory from which that virus is known to be recovered and the notifiable disease for which it is listed in the Australian National Notifiable Disease Surveillance System (ANNDSS). Use of amber font for each named virus indicates the reported recovery of that virus from mosquitoes during mosquito surveillance but that the corresponding virus-associated disease is not currently recorded in the ANNDSS. Named arboviruses: ALFV—Alfuy; BFV—Barmah Forest; DENV—Dengue; EHV—Edge Hill; GGV—Gan Gan; KOKV—Kokobera; KOWV—Kowanyama; KUNV—Kunjin; MVEV—Murray Valley encephalitis; RRV—Ross River; SINV—Sindbis; STRV—Stratford; Trubanaman—TRUV. The land mass above the horizontal green line, which marks the southern edge of the Pilbara Range (latitude 24° S, just south of the Tropic of Capricorn, 23.52° S), approximates to the region termed Northern Australia. States and territory: NSW—New South Wales; NT—Northern Territory; QLD—Queensland; SA—South Australia; TAS—Tasmania; VIC—Victoria; WA—Western Australia.

4. Undifferentiated Febrile Illness and Pyrexia of Unknown Origin

Fever, defined as an abnormally high body temperature (>100 °F, 37.8 °C), is a common symptom of patients seeking healthcare. Due to the non-specific clinical manifestations and a lack of positivity in initial laboratory testing, the cause of fever may not be identified. When the onset of fever is acute and no cause can be found after taking a full history and physical examination of the patient, it is called a UFI. If the UFI continues, it is classified as a pyrexia of unknown origin (PUO), defined in 1961 as an illness of more than three weeks' duration, with fever greater than 101 °F (38.3 °C) on several occasions, the cause of which is not identified after one week of in-hospital investigation [30]. Since this description does not include many self-limiting viral diseases, it was revised in 1991 [31]. The newer definition of PUO has four categories: classical; hospital-acquired; neutropenic (immune-deficient); and HIV-associated. Also, the revision proposed a minimum of three days of hospitalisation or at least three outpatient visits before this diagnosis may be made. Most commonly, PUO is the result of infection, malignancy, or non-malignant inflammatory diseases [32].

5. UFI/PUO as a Health Problem

Between 20% and 60% of UFI cases are attributed to infections [31,33–35]. The aetiological agents of UFI and PUO vary according to the geography and demography of the patients. For instance, in post-industrial countries, self-limited viral infections and infections with bacteria such as *Brucella* spp., *Leptospira* spp., and the atypical mycobacteria are major causes of UFI/PUO. In economically emerging nations, UFI/PUO include illnesses caused by a diverse range of human pathogens including *Mycobacterium tuberculosis*, *Neisseria meningitidis*, systemic *Salmonella enterica* infections, *Plasmodium* spp., DENV, Epstein-Barr virus, cytomegalovirus, and hantaviruses [36–38].

In a landmark prospective study in Belgium of patients hospitalised with febrile illness, depending on if and when a final diagnosis was in fact established, an estimated 12–35% were assessed to have died from PUO-associated complications [39]. The cause of the fever remained obscure in 48% of patients with episodic fever, compared to 26% of patients with continuous fever [39]. Prolonged febrile illnesses remain a diagnostic challenge; about one-third to half of PUO cases remain undiagnosed [40–42]. In developing countries, a diagnosis of UFI/PUO may result from a lack of laboratory resources but even in a high-income nation like Japan that has excellent diagnostic tools, 28.9% of PUO goes undiagnosed [43].

6. Diagnosis of Australian Arboviral Infection

For almost a decade after the identification of RRV in 1959 [44], only small numbers of patients were identified as having a clinical infection with this agent, because virological and serological diagnostic testing was available only within a research framework using an in-house test. Following the development of a commercial enzyme-linked immunosorbent assay (ELISA) to detect anti-RRV immunoglobulin (Ig)M antibody [45], the number of patients diagnosed annually rose to between 4000 and 6000 [46]. The number of localities from where RRV cases were reported increased almost two-fold from 1985 onwards [47].

Following its identification from northern Victoria in 1974 [48], a similar experience occurred with the diagnosis of BFV infection and its annual notification [49]. Epidemic polyarthritis, the now outmoded term that was then used to describe the autoimmune conditions associated with both RRV and BFV, became a nationally notifiable disease in 1990 [46]. While typically there are around 4500 notifications of epidemic polyarthritis per annum, 9554 cases were reported in 2015 [50].

Clinical infections with KUNV [51–54], EHV [25], GGV and KOKV [22,26] can now be confirmed in specialised laboratories, but only suspected KUNV infected cases undergo screening as standard.

7. A Causal Link between Neglected Arboviral Infections and UFI/PUO?

It has been proposed that arboviruses may be responsible for some cases of UFI observed in Australia [55]. While remarkably few systematic studies of UFI or PUO in an Australian setting have been undertaken, those that have been performed suggest that a large proportion of UFI/PUO cases remain undiagnosed (reviewed in [5]). This is despite the now-routine commercial testing for RRV and for BFV. A three-year retrospective study from 2008–2011 of a tertiary referral hospital in North Queensland found 58.8% of patients with UFI had no definitive diagnosis [56]. Neglected indigenous arboviruses may have infected humans regularly for decades, thereby being responsible for at least some of these UFI cases in this tropical north region. The possibility of arbovirus pathogens from Northern Australia causing more wide-scale outbreaks, such as the notified incidences of MVEV in 2001, 2008 and 2011, and the KUNV equine outbreak of 2011 in south-eastern Australia [57], should also be considered. While the horse-derived WNVNSW2011 strain of KUNV not only differed to, but was more virulent than, other KUNV strains that circulated previously in Australia [57], it may be argued that the ecology of this arbovirus changed alongside the emergence of virulence.

The introduction of commercial screening for RRV and BFV led to a highly significant rise in their respective reported rates of infection when compared to historical records [46,49]; these conspicuous examples of unforeseen prevalence may also apply to other arboviral infections. Hence, it is possible that further, neglected, arboviruses—for which diagnostic tests are not yet available outside research laboratories—are a major underlying cause of undiagnosed UFI/PUO cases in Australia.

8. Transmission Cycles of Australian Arboviruses

Over several decades, many arboviruses have been identified in Australian mosquitoes, ticks, and biting midges [5,15]. Little is known about their transmission cycles, their pathogenicity for humans, or their potential to cause epidemics. Although large marsupials such as kangaroos and wallabies are considered potential reservoirs for RRV [58,59] and BFV [59,60], and waterbirds such as herons and egrets are regarded as hosts for MVEV, ALFV and SINV [61,62], there are many other arboviruses whose relationship with reservoirs and vectors, and their role in human infections or diseases, are yet to be defined.

While the epidemiology of these arboviruses is poorly understood, it is likely that they are maintained in zoonotic cycles rather than by human-to-human transmission. It may be that these neglected viruses are harboured by apathogenic, persistent infections in native Australian reservoir mammals and birds, with occasional spillover into humans [5].

9. Northern Australia's Climate Favours Arboviruses

Many of Australia's indigenous arboviruses that are known to cause human disease have been recovered from Northern Australia (Figure 1). Since it had no previous political purpose, the term 'Northern Australia' was defined formally only very recently with the passing of the Northern Australia Infrastructure Facility Act 2016 [63]. Although there are several minor qualifications, broadly speaking it is considered to comprise the Northern Territory and the areas of Queensland and Western Australia that are north of the Tropic of Capricorn (latitude 23.5 degrees south of the Equator).

The northern coastal fringe of the country is made up of northern Queensland, the Northern Territory, and the remote Kimberley and Pilbara Ranges of Western Australia. Uniquely for Australia, the region experiences a tropical, often monsoonal, wet season during the southern hemisphere summer months of November to April each year [59,64]. Moreover, if the mean annual air temperature continues to rise as a consequence of global climate change, the spatial range of mosquito species able to transmit arboviruses is likely to broaden [65]. While the presence of vectors does not necessarily mean the emergence of human pathogens, these factors contribute to favourable breeding conditions for mosquito species that are especially well-suited to maintaining arboviruses of potential public health importance [66].

10. Potential Public Health Threat

The Australian Commonwealth Government is actively promoting increased settlement and economic activity in the currently less populated areas that lie to the north of the Tropic of Capricorn as an integral part of its 'Developing Northern Australia' white paper for massive infrastructure investment in this region over the coming decades [67]. Although it comprises nearly half of the total land mass of the country, Northern Australia includes only about one-quarter of the current Australian population. It is therefore considered to be a region of largely untapped potential that is ripe for 21st century population growth outside of the urban densification in the major metropolitan conurbations to the south [67]. An incentivised expansion of the industrial, business and agricultural development of this vast tract of land is predicted, with an increase in the residential population from the current 1.33 million to up to 2.9 million people by 2050 projected [68]. The anticipated increased human activity in many areas of the tropical north of Australia will lead to fast-growing urbanisation that places relocated immune-naïve people into closer proximity to native reservoir wildlife, as well as to vector mosquitoes, for Australian indigenous arboviruses.

The growth in agriculture and other economic developments proposed for these localities will inevitably alter the ecology of the native animals and birds that act as reservoir hosts for numerous neglected Australian arboviruses, as well as affecting the mosquito vectors [5]. Additionally, sudden climatic and environmental variations [69], including the high rainfall, more frequent cyclones and resultant increased intensity of flooding associated with outbreaks of MVEV [70] and RRV [71], have occurred with alarming regularity in recent years [72], potentially generating an ecological expansion of Australian arboviruses. These circumstances therefore create a perfect storm for greater prevalence of infection with neglected Australian arboviruses, particularly in the tropical north of the country. It is perhaps worth considering that notable close relatives of these many indigenous arboviruses have already caused global pandemics in recent decades [73].

11. A Call to Arms for Novel Diagnostic Tests and Therapy Targets

In this circumstance, therefore, there is a pressing obligation to determine the geographical range and true disease burden of neglected indigenous arboviruses in Northern Australia. This may be accomplished by implementing a scheme of systematic, continual surveillance of vectors, reservoirs and viruses in order to address where, when, and how virus transmission to humans occurs as well as building up a picture of its likely impact. This may also be progressed through performing routine testing by designated public health laboratories of a systematic sub-sample of UFI/PUO patients for evidence of recent infection with neglected arboviruses as well as other potential causative agents of UFI/PUO. Furthermore, to screen patients with UFI/PUO and other suspected cases of arboviral infection, in addition to serology testing, the development of novel diagnostic tools should be given high research priority. Already available methods of detection of pan-alphaviruses and pan-flaviviruses include IgM antibody-based ELISA, quantitative reverse transcription PCR (RT-qPCR), and microarray [74–76]. Other state-of-the-art methods, for example RNA-seq metagenomics, which reveal an individual's virome [77], could also be applied to this setting.

Notwithstanding the striking exceptions of YFV, Japanese encephalitis virus, and tick-borne encephalitis virus [78], an obstacle to the successful control of infections caused by arboviruses is the lack of effective, authority-registered vaccines [79]. Strenuous efforts to yield a commercially available vaccine against DENV are ongoing but these are exacerbated by media-fuelled concerns over suitability and side-effects in pilot immunisation programs [80,81]. Also, the phenomenon of antibody-dependent enhancement of infection of humans that has been shown for many flaviviruses and alphaviruses [82] is an impediment to any future potential consideration of therapeutic antibodies as an alternative treatment [83]. Given this scenario, there is a dire need to accelerate the quest for novel options for both diagnosis and therapy.

Therapy regimens that are syndrome-based are currently common practice, frequently informing the prescription of antibiotics in empirical treatment. Such antibacterial pharmaceutical agents are ineffective when the UFI/PUO is caused by arboviruses; indeed, their inappropriate use may contribute to the worsening problem of antimicrobial resistance. Early, on-site, and rapid screening for neglected Australian arboviruses could help to identify the cause of infection and thus reduce the often ill-informed perceived obligation to provide antibiotics. Adoption of this measure would also expedite early detection of outbreak foci, thereby facilitating a prompt, efficient and proportionate response. This would have the effect of limiting the spread of disease, as hindsight suggests public health policymakers could have achieved better during the recent epidemic in Latin America of the flavivirus Zika [84,85].

The existing funding model for diagnostic pathology services in Australia does not foster requests by a general practitioner or hospital clinician to test for infection with a little-known arbovirus, even if they are aware of its possible role in disease. Hence, many UFI/PUO cases are not diagnosed correctly as the treating clinicians may consider the cost of testing is not warranted or because samples for testing were collected at an inappropriate time or from an incorrect site. They also may go undiagnosed on account of the causative agent being novel, not known to cause human disease, or because there are no routine diagnostic tests available.

For cases of UFI/PUO, for reasons of both practical feasibility and cost, it is not a realistic proposition to recommend multiple, individual laboratory tests in order to detect most or all neglected arboviruses. In light of this, development of a generic assay that would provide for many pathogens and which may be applied in a broad range of settings should be prioritised. For example, routine testing by designated public health laboratories of a two-step protocol could be envisaged, starting with pan-flavivirus and pan-alphavirus IgM antibody rapid tests and, as required of a sub-sample of patients, followed by confirmatory detection of viral RNA by RT-qPCR [76]. Along with the ability to screen for multiple arboviruses in a short space of time there is a saving in resources for the testing laboratory by virtue of a quicker diagnosis. This means that any future decision not to request sample analysis may ultimately prove a false economy.

12. One Component of a 'One Health' Approach to Combating Arboviruses

The One Health approach is a currently promulgated systems-based movement in which biomedical researchers and professionals in public health, veterinary medicine, and ecology combine their expertise in order to monitor and control the threat of infectious diseases and determine how pathogens spread among people, animals, and the environment [86]. Involvement of biomedical researchers, pathologists, and clinicians in this transdisciplinary model may lead to more efficient diagnosis of, and improved outcomes for, patients with arboviral infections.

In order to achieve success in preventing outbreaks of neglected arboviruses within the context of Northern Australia, it will be necessary to engage all relevant stakeholders, from federal, state and local authorities, via tertiary care and general practice centres, to local neighbourhoods, schools, and households. Risk of outbreak is always amplified when people are unaware of a disease or its route of transmission. As with the ongoing threat posed by DENV in Queensland [21], raising awareness levels among residents of regional communities is an extremely important component of a future public health policy for Northern Australia. Well-targeted information campaigns would aim to increase individual knowledge of the symptoms and possible sequelae of UFI/PUO and, with regard to mosquito transmission of arboviral infections, personal preventive methods and vector control.

13. Conclusions and Future Directions

For the neglected arboviruses that are indigenous to Australia there is an inadequate understanding of their distribution, epidemiology, and transmission ecology. Information is also lacking with respect to theimmunopathology and true disease burden, including undiagnosed cases UFI/PUO, which they cause. This knowledge gap exists despite the potential for these neglected arboviruses to become significant human pathogens in the rapidly developing region of Northern Australia, thereby presenting a major challenge to the public health of the nation, and conceivably also globally [87]. Future research into the areas discussed herein, combined with production of diagnostic tools to include first-line screening of a suite of indigenous arboviruses, would help greatly to limit the impact of this emerging threat to human health and wellbeing in the tropical north of Australia. Preferably, this would form a key component of a holistic, transdisciplinary strategy to improve environmental health in order to prevent mosquito-borne diseases in Northern Australia [88].

Acknowledgments: We warmly thank Richard Bradbury (Central Queensland University, Rockhampton, Australia) and John Aaskov (Queensland University of Technology, Brisbane, Australia) for advice and insightful discussion throughout the conceptualisation of this study. Narayan Gyawali is in receipt of an International Postgraduate Research Scholarship and an Australian Postgraduate Award administered by Central Queensland University. Our research is supported in part through a Health Collaborative Research Network Merit Grant.

Author Contributions: Narayan Gyawali conceived the paper and Andrew Taylor-Robinson helped to refine ideas. Narayan Gyawali prepared the first draft and Andrew Taylor-Robinson critically reviewed and revised various versions. Both authors contributed to preparation of the final version and agreed to its submission.

References

1. World Health Organization. *Arboviruses and Human Disease: Report of a WHO Scientific Group*; Technical Report Series No. 369; WHO: Geneva, Switzerland, 1967.
2. Centers for Disease Control and Prevention. Arbovirus Catalog. Available online: https://wwwn.cdc.gov/arbocat/ (accessed on 11 September 2017).
3. Centers for Disease Control and Prevention. National Notifiable Diseases Surveillance System (NNDSS)—Arboviral Diseases, Neuroinvasive and Non-neuroinvasive 2015 Case Definition. Available online: https://wwwn.cdc.gov/nndss/conditions/arboviral-diseases-neuroinvasive-and-non-neuroinvasive/case-definition/2015/ (accessed on 11 September 2017).
4. Beckham, J.D.; Tyler, K.L. Arbovirus infections. *Continuum (Minneapolis, Minn)* **2015**, *21*, 1599–1611. [CrossRef] [PubMed]
5. Gyawali, N.; Bradbury, R.S.; Aaskov, J.G.; Taylor-Robinson, A.W. Neglected Australian arboviruses: Quam gravis? *Microbes Infect.* **2017**, *19*, 388–401. [CrossRef] [PubMed]
6. Australian Government Department of Health. National Notifiable Diseases Surveillance System. Notifications for All Diseases by State & Territory and Year. Available online: http://www9.health.gov.au/cda/source/rpt_2_sel.cfm (accessed on 11 September 2017).
7. Weaver, S.C.; Barrett, A.D. Transmission cycles, host range, evolution and emergence of arboviral disease. *Nat. Rev. Microbiol.* **2004**, *2*, 789–801. [CrossRef] [PubMed]
8. Young, P.R.; Ng, L.F.P.; Hall, R.A.; Smith, D.W.; Johansen, C.A. Arbovirus infection. In *Manson's Tropical Diseases*, 23rd ed.; Farrar, J., Hotez, P.J., Junghanss, T., Kang, G., Lalloo, D., White, N.J., Eds.; Elsevier: Amsterdam, The Netherlands, 2013; pp. 129–161.
9. Morens, D.M.; Fauci, A.S. Emerging infectious diseases: Threats to human health and global stability. *PLoS Pathog.* **2013**, *9*, e1003467. [CrossRef] [PubMed]
10. Cao-Lormeau, V.-M.; Musso, D. Emerging arboviruses in the Pacific. *Lancet* **2014**, *384*, 1571–1572. [CrossRef]
11. Gubler, D.J. Dengue viruses: Their evolution, history and emergence as a global public health problem. In *Dengue and Dengue Hemorrhagic Fever*; Gubler, D.J., Ooi, E., Vasudevan, S., Farrar, J., Eds.; CAB International: Wallingford, UK, 2014; pp. 1–29.
12. Mackenzie, J.S.; Gubler, D.J.; Peterson, L.R. Emerging flaviviruses: The spread and resurgence of Japanese encephalitis, West Nile and dengue viruses. *Nat. Med.* **2004**, *10*, S98–S109. [CrossRef] [PubMed]
13. Hotez, P.J.; Murray, K.O. Dengue, West Nile virus, chikungunya, Zika and now Mayaro? *PLoS Negl. Trop. Dis.* **2017**, *11*, e0005462. [CrossRef] [PubMed]
14. Sutherst, R.W. Global change and human vulnerability to vector-borne diseases. *Clin. Microbiol. Rev.* **2004**, *17*, 136–173. [CrossRef] [PubMed]
15. Russell, R.C. Mosquito-borne disease and climate change in Australia: Time for a reality check. *Aust. J. Entomol.* **2009**, *48*, 1–7. [CrossRef]
16. Fraser, J.R. Epidemic polyarthritis and Ross River virus disease. *Clin. Rheum. Dis.* **1986**, *12*, 369–388. [PubMed]
17. Vale, T.G.; Carter, I.W.; McPhie, K.A.; James, G.; Cloonan, M.J. Human arbovirus infections along the south coast of New South Wales. *Aust. J. Exp. Biol. Med. Sci.* **1986**, *64*, 307–309. [CrossRef] [PubMed]
18. Russell, R.C. Arboviruses and their vectors in Australia: An update on the ecology and epidemiology of some mosquito-borne arboviruses. *Rev. Med. Vet. Entomol.* **1995**, *83*, 141–158.
19. Gyawali, N.; Bradbury, R.S.; Taylor-Robinson, A.W. The epidemiology of dengue infection: Harnessing past experience and current knowledge to support implementation of future control strategies. *J. Vector Borne Dis.* **2016**, *53*, 293–304. [PubMed]
20. Naish, S.; Tong, S. Hot spot detection and spatio-temporal dynamics of dengue in Queensland, Australia. In Proceedings of the ISPRS Technical Commission VIII Symposium, Hyderabad, India, 9–12 December 2014; Dadhwal, V.K., Diwakar, P.G., Seshasai, M.V.R., Raju, P.L.N., Hakeem, A., Eds.; International Society of Photogrammetry and Remote Sensing. pp. 197–204.
21. Gyawali, N.; Bradbury, R.S.; Taylor-Robinson, A.W. Knowledge, attitude and recommendations for practice regarding dengue among the resident population of Queensland, Australia. *Asian Pac. J. Trop. Biomed.* **2016**, *6*, 360–366. [CrossRef]

22. Hawkes, R.A.; Boughton, C.R.; Naim, H.M.; Wild, J.; Chapman, B. Arbovirus infections of humans in New South Wales. Seroepidemiology of the flavivirus group of togaviruses. *Med. J. Aust.* **1985**, *143*, 555–561. [PubMed]
23. Mackenzie, J.; Lindsay, M.; Coelen, R.; Broom, A.; Hall, R.; Smith, D. Arboviruses causing human disease in the Australasian zoogeographic region. *Arch. Virol.* **1994**, *136*, 447–467. [CrossRef] [PubMed]
24. Guard, R.W.; McAuliffe, M.; Stallman, N.; Bramston, B. Haemorrhagic manifestations with Sindbis infection. Case report. *Pathology* **1982**, *14*, 89–90. [CrossRef] [PubMed]
25. Aaskov, J.G.; Phillips, D.A.; Wiemers, M.A. Possible clinical infection with Edge Hill virus. *Trans. R. Soc. Trop. Med. Hyg.* **1993**, *87*, 452–453. [CrossRef]
26. Boughton, C.R.; Hawkes, R.A.; Naim, H.M. Illness caused by a Kokobera-like virus in south-eastern Australia. *Med. J. Aust.* **1986**, *145*, 90–92. [PubMed]
27. Australian Government Department of Health. Australian National Notifiable Diseases by Disease Type. Available online: http://www.health.gov.au/internet/main/publishing.nsf/Content/cda-surveil-nndss-casedefs-distype.htm (accessed on 11 September 2017).
28. Colmant, A.M.; Bielefeldt-Ohmann, H.; Hobson-Peters, J.; Suen, W.W.; O'Brien, C.A.; van den Hurk, A.F.; Hall, R.A. A newly discovered flavivirus in the yellow fever virus group displays restricted replication in vertebrates. *J. Gen. Virol.* **2016**, *97*, 1087–1093. [CrossRef] [PubMed]
29. Johansen, C.A.; Williams, S.H.; Melville, L.F.; Nicholson, J.; Hall, R.A.; Bielefeldt-Ohmann, H.; Prow, N.A.; Chidlow, G.R.; Wong, S.; Sinha, R.; et al. Characterization of Fitzroy River virus and serologic evidence of human and animal infection. *Emerg. Infect. Dis.* **2017**, *23*, 1289–1299. [CrossRef] [PubMed]
30. Petersdorf, R.G.; Beeson, P.B. Fever of unexplained origin: Report on 100 cases. *Medicine* **1961**, *40*, 1–30. [CrossRef] [PubMed]
31. Durack, D.T.; Street, A.C. Fever of unknown origin—Reexamined and redefined. *Curr. Clin. Top. Infect. Dis.* **1991**, *11*, 35–51. [PubMed]
32. Mourad, O.; Palda, V.; Detsky, A.S. A comprehensive evidence-based approach to fever of unknown origin. *Arch. Intern. Med.* **2003**, *163*, 545–551. [CrossRef] [PubMed]
33. Jacoby, G.A.; Swartz, M.N. Fever of undetermined origin. *N. Engl. J. Med.* **1973**, *289*, 1407–1410. [CrossRef] [PubMed]
34. Larson, E.B.; Featherstone, H.J.; Petersdorf, R.G. Fever of undetermined origin: diagnosis and follow-up of 105 cases, 1970–1980. *Medicine* **1982**, *61*, 269–292. [CrossRef] [PubMed]
35. De Kleijn, E.M.; Vandenbroucke, J.P.; van der Meer, J.W.; Group, N.F.S. Fever of unknown origin (FUO): I. A prospective multicenter study of 167 patients with FUO, using fixed epidemiologic entry criteria. *Medicine* **1997**, *76*, 392–400. [CrossRef] [PubMed]
36. Boivin, G.; Hardy, I.; Tellier, G.; Maziade, J. Predicting influenza infections during epidemics with use of a clinical case definition. *Clin. Infect. Dis.* **2000**, *31*, 1166–1169. [CrossRef] [PubMed]
37. Rongrungruang, Y.; Leelarasamee, A. Characteristics and outcomes of adult patients with symptomatic dengue virus infections. *J. Infect. Dis. Antimicrob. Agents* **2001**, *18*, 19–23.
38. Efstathiou, S.P.; Pefanis, A.V.; Tsiakou, A.G.; Skeva, I.I.; Tsioulos, D.I.; Achimastos, A.D.; Mountokalakis, T.D. Fever of unknown origin: Discrimination between infectious and non-infectious causes. *Eur. J. Intern. Med.* **2010**, *21*, 137–143. [CrossRef] [PubMed]
39. Vanderschueren, S.; Knockaert, D.; Adriaenssens, T.; Demey, W.; Durnez, A.; Blockmans, D.; Bobbaers, H. From prolonged febrile illness to fever of unknown origin: The challenge continues. *Arch. Intern. Med.* **2003**, *163*, 1033–1041. [CrossRef] [PubMed]
40. Buysschaert, I.; Vanderschueren, S.; Blockmans, D.; Mortelmans, L.; Knockaert, D. Contribution of ^{18}fluoro-deoxyglucose positron emission tomography to the work-up of patients with fever of unknown origin. *Eur. J. Intern. Med.* **2004**, *15*, 151–156. [CrossRef] [PubMed]
41. Bleeker-Rovers, C.P.; Vos, F.J.; de Kleijn, E.M.; Mudde, A.H.; Dofferhoff, T.S.; Richter, C.; Smilde, T.J.; Krabbe, P.F.; Oyen, W.J.; van der Meer, J.W. A prospective multicenter study on fever of unknown origin: The yield of a structured diagnostic protocol. *Medicine* **2007**, *86*, 26–38. [CrossRef] [PubMed]
42. Robine, A.; Hot, A.; Maucort-Boulch, D.; Iwaz, J.; Broussolle, C.; Sève, P. Fever of unknown origin in the 2000s: Evaluation of 103 cases over eleven years. *Presse Méd.* **2014**, *43*, e233–e240. [CrossRef] [PubMed]

43. Yamanouchi, M.; Uehara, Y.; Yokokawa, H.; Hosoda, T.; Watanabe, Y.; Shiga, T.; Inui, A.; Otsuki, Y.; Fujibayashi, K.; Isonuma, H.; Naito, T. Analysis of 256 cases of classic fever of unknown origin. *Intern. Med.* **2013**, *53*, 2471–2475. [CrossRef]
44. Doherty, R.L.; Whitehead, R.H.; Gorman, B.M.; O'Gower, A.K. The isolation of a third group A arbovirus in Australia, with preliminary observations on its relationship to epidemic polyarthritis. *Aust. J. Sci.* **1963**, *26*, 183–184.
45. Oseni, R.A.; Donaldson, M.D.; Dalglish, D.A.; Aaskov, J.G. Detection by ELISA of IgM antibodies to Ross River virus in serum from patients with suspected epidemic polyarthritis. *Bull. World Health Organ.* **1983**, *61*, 703–708. [PubMed]
46. Hargreaves, J.; Longbottom, H.; Myint, H.; Herceg, A.; Oliver, G.; Curran, M.; Evans, D. Annual report of the National Notifiable Diseases Surveillance System, 1994. *Commun. Dis. Intell.* **1995**, *19*, 542–574.
47. Tong, S.; Bi, P.; Hayes, J.; Donald, K.; Mackenzie, J. Geographic variation of notified Ross River virus infections in Queensland, Australia, 1985–1996. *Am. J. Trop. Med. Hyg.* **2001**, *65*, 171–176. [CrossRef] [PubMed]
48. Marshall, I.D.; Woodroofe, G.M.; Hirsch, S. Viruses recovered from mosquitoes and wildlife serum collected in the Murray Valley of south-eastern Australia, February 1974, during an epidemic of encephalitis. *Aust. J. Exp. Biol. Med. Sci.* **1982**, *60*, 457–470. [CrossRef] [PubMed]
49. Jacups, S.P.; Whelan, P.I.; Currie, B.J. Ross River virus and Barmah Forest virus infections: A review of history, ecology, and predictive models, with implications for tropical northern Australia. *Vector Borne Zoonotic Dis.* **2008**, *8*, 283–298. [CrossRef] [PubMed]
50. Australian Government Department of Health. National Notifiable Diseases: Australia's Notifiable Diseases Status. Annual Reports of the National Notifiable Diseases Surveillance System, 1994–2014. Available online: http://www.health.gov.au/internet/main/publishing.nsf/Content/cda-pubs-annlrpt-nndssar.htm (accessed on 11 September 2017).
51. Doherty, R.L.; Carley, J.G.; Filippich, C.; White, J.; Gust, I.D. Murray Valley encephalitis in Australia, 1974: Antibody response in cases and community. *Aust. N.Z. J. Med.* **1976**, *6*, 446–453. [CrossRef] [PubMed]
52. Phillips, D.A.; Aaskov, J.G.; Atkin, C.; Wiemers, M.A. Isolation of Kunjin virus from a patient with a naturally acquired infection. *Med. J. Aust.* **1992**, *157*, 190–191. [PubMed]
53. Mackenzie, J.; Smith, D.; Broom, A.; Bucens, M. Australian encephalitis in Western Australia, 1978–1991. *Med. J. Aust.* **1993**, *158*, 591–595. [PubMed]
54. Broom, A.; Whelan, P.; Smith, D.; Lindsay, M.; Melville, L.; Bolisetty, S.; Wheaton, G.; Brown, A.; Higgins, G. An outbreak of Australian encephalitis in Western Australia and Central Australia (Northern Territory and South Australia) during the 2000 wet season. *Arbovirus Res. Aust.* **2001**, *8*, 37–42.
55. Doherty, R.L. Arthropod-borne viruses in Australia and their relation to infection and disease. *Prog. Med. Virol.* **1974**, *17*, 136–192. [PubMed]
56. Susilawati, T.N.; McBride, W.J.H. Undiagnosed undifferentiated fever in far north Queensland, Australia: A retrospective study. *Int. J. Infect. Dis.* **2014**, *27*, 59–64. [CrossRef] [PubMed]
57. Frost, M.J.; Zhang, J.; Edmonds, J.H.; Prow, N.A.; Gu, X.; Davis, R.; Hornitzky, C.; Arzey, K.E.; Finlaison, D.; Hick, P.; et al. Characterization of virulent West Nile virus Kunjin strain, Australia, 2011. *Emerg. Infect. Dis.* **2012**, *18*, 792–800. [CrossRef] [PubMed]
58. Doherty, R.L.; Gorman, B.M.; Whitehead, R.H.; Carley, J.G. Studies of arthropod-borne virus infections in Queensland. V. Survey of antibodies to group A arboviruses in man and other animals. *Aust. J. Exp. Biol. Med. Sci.* **1966**, *44*, 365–377. [CrossRef] [PubMed]
59. Inglis, T.J.; Bradbury, R.S.; McInnes, R.L.; Frances, S.P.; Merritt, A.J.; Levy, A.; Nicholson, J.; Neville, P.J.; Lindsay, M.; Smith, D.W. Deployable molecular detection of arboviruses in the Australian Outback. *Am. J. Trop. Med. Hyg.* **2016**, *95*, 633–638. [CrossRef] [PubMed]
60. Vale, T.G.; Spratt, D.M.; Cloonan, M.J. Serological evidence of arbovirus infection in native and domesticated mammals on the south coast of New South Wales. *Aust. J. Zool.* **1991**, *39*, 1–7. [CrossRef]
61. Anderson, S.G. Murray Valley encephalitis and Australian X disease. *Epidemiol. Infect.* **1954**, *52*, 447–468. [CrossRef]
62. Doherty, R. Arboviruses of Australia. *Aust. Vet. J.* **1972**, *48*, 172–180. [CrossRef] [PubMed]
63. Australian Government. Northern Australia Infrastructure Facility Act 2016. Available online: https://www.legislation.gov.au/Details/C2016A00041 (accessed on 11 September 2017).

64. Australian Government. Australian Weather and Seasons—A Variety of Climates. Available online: http://www.australia.gov.au/about-australia/australian-story/austn-weather-and-the-seasons (accessed on 11 September 2017).
65. Parham, P.E.; Waldock, J.; Christophides, G.K.; Hemming, D.; Agusto, F.; Evans, K.J.; Fefferman, N.; Gaff, H.; Gumel, A.; LaDeau, S.; et al. Climate, environmental and socio-economic change: Weighing up the balance in vector-borne disease transmission. *Philos. Trans. R. Soc. Lond. B Biol. Sci.* **2015**, *370*, 20130551. [CrossRef] [PubMed]
66. Van den Hurk, A.F.; Craig, S.B.; Tulsiani, S.M.; Jansen, C.C. Emerging tropical diseases in Australia. Part 4. Mosquito-borne diseases. *Ann. Trop. Med. Parasitol.* **2010**, *104*, 623–640. [CrossRef] [PubMed]
67. Australian Government. Our North, Our Future: White Paper on Developing Northern Australia. Available online: http://northernaustralia.gov.au/sites/prod.office-northern-australia.gov.au/files/files/NAWP-FullReport.pdf (accessed on 11 September 2017).
68. Cummings Economics, March 2015. Long-Term Population Growth in Northern Australia. Available online: http://www.cummings.net.au/pdf/recent/J2806NthnAusLongTermPopulationGrowth.pdf (accessed on 11 September 2017).
69. Inglis, T.J. Climate change and infectious diseases in Australia. *Aust. Prescr.* **2009**, *32*, 58–59. [CrossRef]
70. Selvey, L.A.; Johansen, C.A.; Broom, A.K.; Antão, C.; Lindsay, M.D.; Mackenzie, J.S.; Smith, D.W. Rainfall and sentinel chicken seroconversions predict human cases of Murray Valley encephalitis in the north of Western Australia. *BMC Infect. Dis.* **2014**, *14*, 672. [CrossRef] [PubMed]
71. Tall, J.A.; Gatton, M.L.; Tong, S. Ross River virus disease activity associated with naturally occurring nontidal flood events in Australia: A systematic review. *J. Med. Entomol.* **2014**, *51*, 1097–1108. [CrossRef] [PubMed]
72. Knutson, T.R.; McBride, J.L.; Chan, J.; Emanuel, K.; Holland, G.; Landsea, C.; Held, I.; Kossin, J.P.; Srivastava, A.K.; Sugi, M. Tropical cyclones and climate change. *Nat. Geosci.* **2010**, *3*, 157–163. [CrossRef]
73. Mayer, S.V.; Tesh, R.B.; Vasilakis, N. The emergence of arthropod-borne viral diseases: A global prospective on dengue, chikungunya and Zika fevers. *Acta Trop.* **2017**, *166*, 155–163. [CrossRef] [PubMed]
74. Palacios, G.; Quan, P.L.; Jabado, O.J.; Conlan, S.; Hirschberg, D.L.; Liu, Y.; Zhai, J.; Renwick, N.; Hui, J.; Hegyi, H.; et al. Panmicrobial oligonucleotide array for diagnosis of infectious diseases. *Emerg. Infect. Dis.* **2007**, *13*, 73–81. [CrossRef] [PubMed]
75. Giry, C.; Roquebert, B.; Li-Pat-Yuen, G.; Gasque, P.; Jaffar-Bandjee, M.C. Improved detection of genus-specific *Alphavirus* using a generic TaqMan®assay. *BMC Microbiol.* **2017**, *17*, 164. [CrossRef] [PubMed]
76. Vina-Rodriguez, A.; Sachse, K.; Ziegler, U.; Chaintoutis, S.C.; Keller, M.; Groschup, M.H.; Eiden, M. A novel pan-*Flavivirus* detection and identification assay based on RT-qPCR and microarray. *Biomed. Res. Int.* **2017**, 4248756. [CrossRef] [PubMed]
77. Rosani, U.; Gerdol, M. A bioinformatics approach reveals seven nearly-complete RNA-virus genomes in bivalve RNA-seq data. *Virus Res.* **2017**, *239*, 33–42. [CrossRef] [PubMed]
78. Khou, C.; Pardigon, N. Identifying attenuating mutations: Tools for a new vaccine design against flaviviruses. *Intervirology* **2017**, *60*, 8–18. [CrossRef] [PubMed]
79. Gautam, R.; Mishra, S.; Milhotra, A.; Nagpal, R.; Mohan, M.; Singhal, A.; Kumari, P. Challenges with mosquito-borne viral diseases: Outbreak of the monsters. *Curr. Top. Med. Chem.* **2017**, *17*, 2199–2214. [CrossRef] [PubMed]
80. Sun Star Manila, 25 April 2016. DOH Records 362 Adverse Reactions of Dengue Vaccine. Available online: http://www.sunstar.com.ph/manila/local-news/2016/04/25/doh-records-362-adverse-effects-dengue-vaccine-469921 (accessed on 11 September 2017).
81. Malay Mail Online, 7 April 2017. Controversial Dengue Vaccine Approved for Further Trials in Malaysia. Available online: http://www.themalaymailonline.com/malaysia/article/controversial-dengue-vaccine-approved-for-further-trials-in-malaysia#sErjCc1APGerWKmy.99 (accessed on 11 September 2017).
82. Pierson, T.C.; Fremont, D.H.; Kuhn, R.J.; Diamond, M.S. Structural insights into the mechanisms of antibody-mediated neutralization of flavivirus infection: Implications for vaccine development. *Cell Host Microbe* **2008**, *4*, 229–238. [CrossRef] [PubMed]
83. Gautam, S.; Subedi, D.; Taylor-Robinson, A.W. Anti-idiotype antibody against pre-membrane-specific antibody as an adjunct to current dengue vaccination strategy. *Immun. Dis.* **2015**, *3*, 1–7.
84. Fauci, A.S.; Morens, D.M. Zika virus in the Americas—Yet another arbovirus threat. *N. Engl. J. Med.* **2016**, *374*, 601–604. [CrossRef] [PubMed]

85. Lazear, H.M.; Stringer, E.M.; de Silva, A.M. The emerging Zika virus epidemic in the Americas: Research priorities. *JAMA* **2016**, *315*, 1945–1946. [CrossRef] [PubMed]
86. Rüegg, S.R.; McMahon, B.J.; Häsler, B.; Esposito, R.; Nielsen, L.R.; Ifejika Speranza, C.; Ehlinger, T.; Peyre, M.; Aragrande, M.; Zinsstag, J.; et al. A blueprint to evaluate One Health. *Front. Public Health* **2017**, *5*, 20.
87. Gyawali, N.; Bradbury, R.S.; Taylor-Robinson, A.W. Do neglected Australian arboviruses pose a global epidemic threat? *Aust. N. Z. J. Public Health* **2016**, *40*, 596. [CrossRef] [PubMed]
88. Hardy, M.C.; Barrington, D.J. A transdisciplinary approach to managing emerging and resurging mosquito-borne diseases in the Western Pacific Region. *Trop. Med. Infect. Dis.* **2017**, *2*, 1. [CrossRef]

12

Long-Range Diagnosis of and Support for Skin Conditions in Field Settings

Victoria Williams * and Carrie Kovarik

Department of Dermatology, Perelman School of Medicine, University of Pennsylvania, Philadelphia, PA 19104, USA; carrie.kovarik@uphs.upenn.edu

* Correspondence: tori22@gmail.com;

Abstract: Skin diseases are a significant cause of morbidity and mortality worldwide; however, access to dermatology services are critically limited, particularly in low- to middle-income countries (LMIC), where there is an overall shortage of physicians. Implementation of long-range technological support tools has been growing in an effort to provide quality dermatology care to even the most remote settings globally. eHealth strategies can provide realistic healthcare solutions if implemented in a feasible and sensitive way, customizing tools to address the unique needs and resource limitations of the local setting. This article summarizes the various types of telemedicine and mobile health (mHealth) tools and their practical applications and benefits for patient care. The challenges and barriers of teledermatology are discussed, as well as steps to consider when implementing a new teledermatology initiative. eHealth arguably offers one of the most flexible and realistic tools for providing critically needed access to dermatology skills in underserved LMICs.

Keywords: teledermatology; eHealth; mHealth; long range diagnosis; dermatology; telepathology; technology; skin disease

---

1. Introduction

Skin diseases are a significant cause of morbidity and mortality worldwide; however, access to dermatology services are critically limited, particularly in low- to middle-income countries (LMICs), where there is an overall shortage of physicians [1]. The World Health Organization (WHO) has estimated that there is a worldwide shortage of 4.3 million physicians and nurses, and countries with the lowest density of healthcare workers such as sub-Saharan Africa, have the highest level of disease burden [2–4]. When an estimated 1 billion people across the world do not have access to a trained healthcare worker, access to specialty services like dermatology care is very rare [3,4]. Many regions completely lack a dermatology specialist or have dermatologists that live only in urban areas, leaving remote populations without access to care [5,6]. Skin diseases are reported to be the 4th leading cause of disability worldwide, but with the limited number and distribution of dermatologists, it is nearly impossible to provide adequate care to everyone in need using traditional methods [7]. Thus, the implementation of long-range technological support tools has been growing in an effort to provide quality dermatology care to even the most remote settings globally. eHealth strategies can provide realistic healthcare solutions if implemented in a feasible and sensitive way, customizing tools to address the unique needs and resource limitations of the local setting.

The WHO defines eHealth as the overall use of information and communication technology for health, which can broadly apply to all parts of the healthcare system from electronic medical record systems, education, research, clinical care, and hospital information systems [8]. There are numerous subsets of eHealth that can augment the delivery of healthcare; however, when looking to improve the diagnosis and management of skin diseases in remote field settings, mobile health (mHealth) and more specifically mobile telemedicine tools can provide flexible and innovative solutions.

Telemedicine is a subset of eHealth that encompasses the use of electronic communications technology to exchange medical information for the purposes of health and education. Dermatology is uniquely suited for telemedicine because of the largely visual component involved in diagnosis. Teledermatology can be delivered using either store and forward or live methods. Store and forward (SAF) methods, which are the most commonly utilized, involve gathering data that is then sent to a distant provider to be reviewed at a later time. Live telemedicine utilizes videoconference technology to connect a patient or provider in real time with a distant provider for consultation. Live telemedicine is infrequently used in the developing world due to the difficulty in sustaining a live connection.

Mobile health encompasses the use of mobile devices to support healthcare practices via various applications. The estimated penetration of unique mobile subscribers worldwide reached 66% (5.0 billion) in 2017, and is expected to be 71% (5.9 billion) by 2025 [9]. The majority of the world's cell phone subscriptions are now in the developing world, and mobile phones offer an accessible healthcare tool that can be utilized even in the most remote settings. The type of healthcare that can be delivered through mHealth depends on the device and network connectivity. In 2017, smartphones as a percentage of mobile phone penetration were 34% in sub-Saharan Africa, and are projected to be 68% in 2025. Including 3G, mobile broadband network coverage reached 83% globally in 2016 [9]. As the connectivity advances in LMIC, the opportunities for mHealth expand.

2. Types of Mobile Health (mHealth) and Telemedicine Tools

eHealth tools come in a variety of formats that may be customized depending on the needs of the users. Table 1 outlines the various platforms that can be leveraged to practice teledermatology and summarizes their associated advantages and disadvantages. Formal telemedicine platforms utilize programs that have been specially designed to transmit secure healthcare information between providers. Traditionally, SAF teledermatology platforms were created solely for desktop use and required uploading photographs to a web-based program, which could prove challenging for providers with low computer literacy, limited internet access, and poor computer resources. In recent years, most web-based teledermatology platforms have also developed an associated mobile application that functions in parallel to the web-based program and allows for easier data collection and flexible connectivity over mobile networks or wifi. Providers can work directly from their mobile smartphones to transmit photos and patient information to remote consultants.

Formal SAF teledermatology platforms require each user to be registered in the program and are tailored to collect a predetermined set of information. A customized dermatology template can be provided for patient data collection, which allows providers with limited dermatology knowledge to perform a thorough skin history without significant prior dermatology experience. Photos of the patient can then be attached to the consultation (Figure 1). Benefits of this type of service include secure data transmission and higher likelihood of pertinent patient information being included in consultations. Limitations include the need to individually register users and train them to use the application. Most programs will work over a mobile connection but require a strong network signal for ideal performance. Examples of successful long-term teledermatology programs using formal SAF platforms to support developing countries include the Africa Teledermatology Project [10], the Swinfen Charitable Trust [11,12], the Médecins Sans Frontières Telemedicine Network [13] and Réseau Afrique Francophone de Télémédecine (RAFT) project [14].

Informal telemedicine platforms include any method that allows the electronic SAF transmission of patient data. These tools allow for the quick and easy exchange of data without the need to individually identify, register and train all users. However, they have the drawback of not providing any formal framework for the collection or organization of data. The consultation information provided may be missing key elements and the security of transmitted information cannot be guaranteed.

Table 1. Description of teledermatology and telepathology platform types, advantages, disadvantages and examples.

Platform Type	Advantages	Disadvantages	Examples
Formal Teledermatology Platforms			
Web and/or Mobile Teledermatology Applications	secure, guides referring providers through a dermatology consult, stores a record of all consults, most applications can be used on desktop or mobile device	must identify and register all users, must train all users, cost associated with creation of application or subscription to use, most time intensive for providers to utilize, difficult for providers to ask follow up questions, usually no mechanism for long term follow-up of cases, requires wifi or strong network signal	Africa Teledermatology Project [10], Swinfen Charitable Trust [11,12], MSF [13], ClickMedix [15], Azova [16]
Informal Teledermatology Platforms			
Secure Email	can be used on desktop or mobile device, minimal training needed for users, minimally time intensive, fits into most providers daily routine, options for free access	security depends on email server, requires wifi or moderate network signal, no structure to guide consults, email accounts may have limited storage capacity, provider must identify and obtain emails of consultants to connect	free encrypted email services: Proton mail [17], Tutanota [18]
Secure Cloud Based File Sharing	can be used on desktop or mobile device, options for free access, provides a mechanism for organized storage of patient information, minimally time intensive	limited storage on free versions, requires some training for users, users must register, requires wifi or strong network signal, moderately secure, no structure to guide consults	Dropbox [19], Google Drive [20], OneDrive [21], Box [22]
Secure Direct Messaging Applications	fits into providers daily routine, least time intensive, minimal training needed, allows real time communication during patient visits, options for text/photos/videos/audio messaging, allows open communication for follow up questions and patient follow up, options for free access, secure end to end encryption, allows one-on-one or group chats, works well with low signal or wifi	provider must identify a consultant and obtain a phone number to connect, no structure to guide consults, no organized record of consults or communications	Free: WhatsApp [23,24], MedTunnel [25],Bloomtext [26] Paid: Imprivata [27], TigerConnect [28], Voalte [29], QliqSoft [30], Spok Mobile [31]
Social Networking Sites	free, low time commitment, minimal training needed, allows connection to a single provider or a global network, any provider can register and connect, works well with low signal or wifi	cannot guarantee security, difficult to guarantee credentials and expertise of consultants providing advice, no structure to guide consults, no organized record of consults or communications	Telederm.org [32], Sermo [33], Facebook [34]
Telepathology Platforms			
Virtual Slide Microscopy (VSM)	secure, highest quality images, can view any part of the slide at any magnification, creates an organized library of cases for teaching or research, least time intensive for reviewer when slides are pre-scanned	high cost to purchase, ongoing costs to maintain equipment and software, requires significant training, needs high storage capacity for images, needs consistent and high bandwidth to function, slide scanning can be time intensive for sender	Olympus VS 120 [35], Zeiss Axio Scan.Z1 [36], Leica Aperio AT2 [37]

Table 1. *Cont.*

Platform Type	Advantages	Disadvantages	Examples
Dynamic Slide Microscopy (DSM)	secure, can view any part of the slide at any magnification, potentially lower cost to implement compared to VSM	highest bandwidth requirements which may limit image quality, requires strict program compatibility for viewing, requires significant training, ongoing costs to maintain equipment and software, most time intensive to use for sender and reviewer	Leica Aperio LV1 [38], 3dHistech Panoramic DESK II DW [39]
Static Imaging	lowest cost, works with any microscope, no software requirements, does not require consistent wifi	risk of sampling error, quality of images varies based on skills of photographer, can only view areas of tissue and magnification chosen by photographer, time intensive for sender and reviewer	smartphone to eyepiece attachments: LabCam [40], Magnifi [41], Snapzoom [42]; any smartphone camera through eyepiece; any digital microscope camera

Abbreviations: MSF = Médecins Sans Frontières.

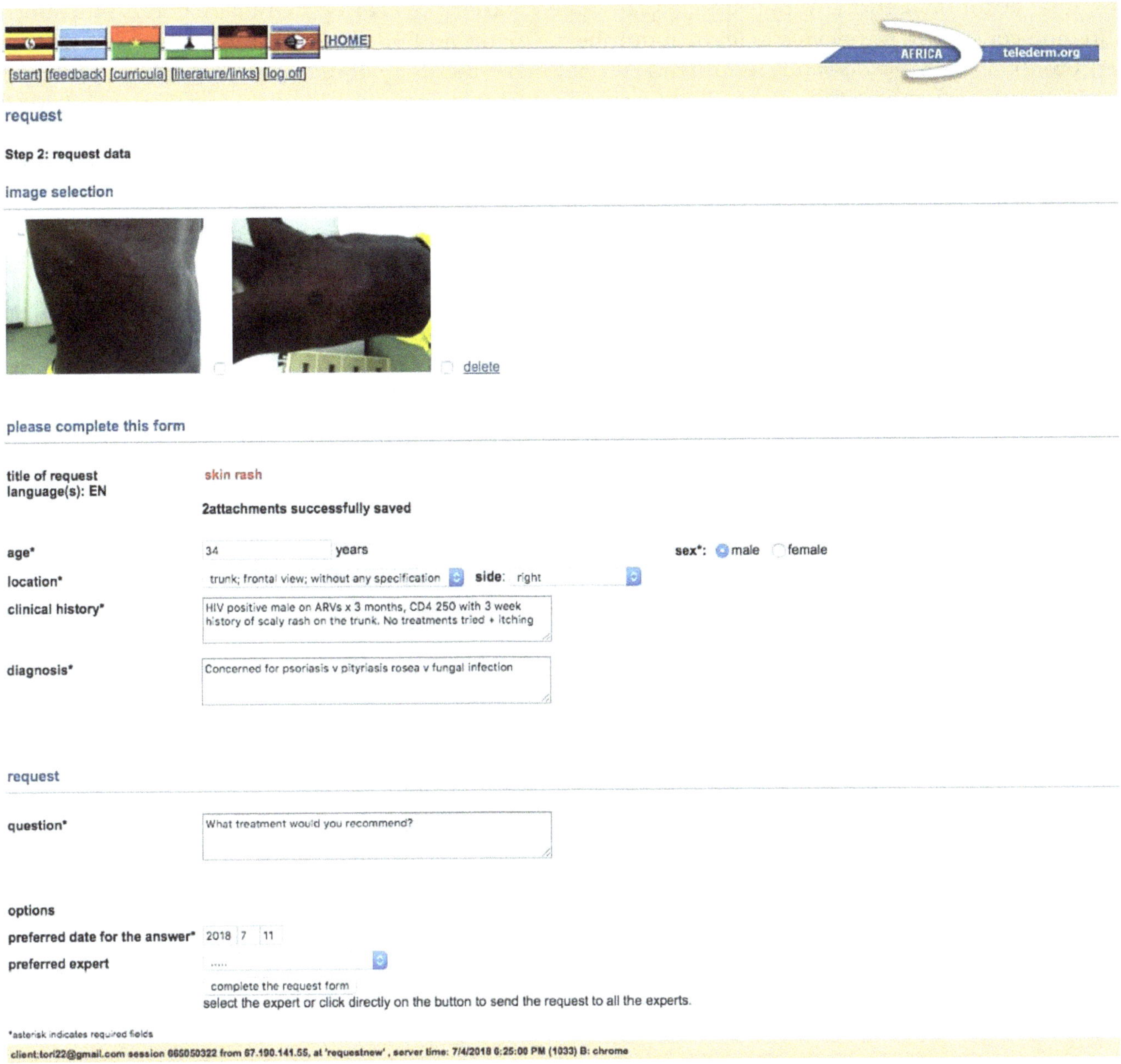

Figure 1. An example of a formal web-based teledermatology platform, the Africa Teledermatology Project, which uses a simple template to collect patient data for consultations.

Email is one of the more commonly utilized informal teledermatology platforms. Photos and pertinent patient information are included in an email message which can be sent to one provider or a group of providers for consultation. For the patient data to be secure, the sender and each recipient included must utilize a secure email service. Academic institutions with teledermatology links to developing countries via email platforms include Emory University to a teaching hospital in Kabul, Afghanistan [43]; the Medical College of Wisconsin to Hillside Healthcare International in Belize [44]; and the University of Basel, which is linked to several remote clinical sites globally [45].

Secure mobile messaging services allow the exchange of text, photos, audio, video and document files using mobile data or wifi. A widely used free mobile instant messaging application, Whatsapp, has been reported as a particularly powerful tool for teledermatology in several resource limited settings [23,24]. Because Whatsapp is already in use by more than 1 billion people in over 180 countries worldwide [46], the application can integrate seamlessly into the daily clinic routine of providers with minimal additional effort. Whatsapp can facilitate a variety of rapid patient care communications, allowing consulting physicians to learn about their patients and provide appropriate care in real time (Figure 2). Whatsapp does not require additional investments in equipment or dedicated internet access for users because it can be utilized on a provider's own smartphone with either mobile data or wifi. Most importantly, Whatsapp maintains high functionality even in areas of poor connectivity. There are several other secure mobile messaging systems that have been designed for healthcare; however, most require paid subscriptions which limit their usage in LMICs [25–31,47].

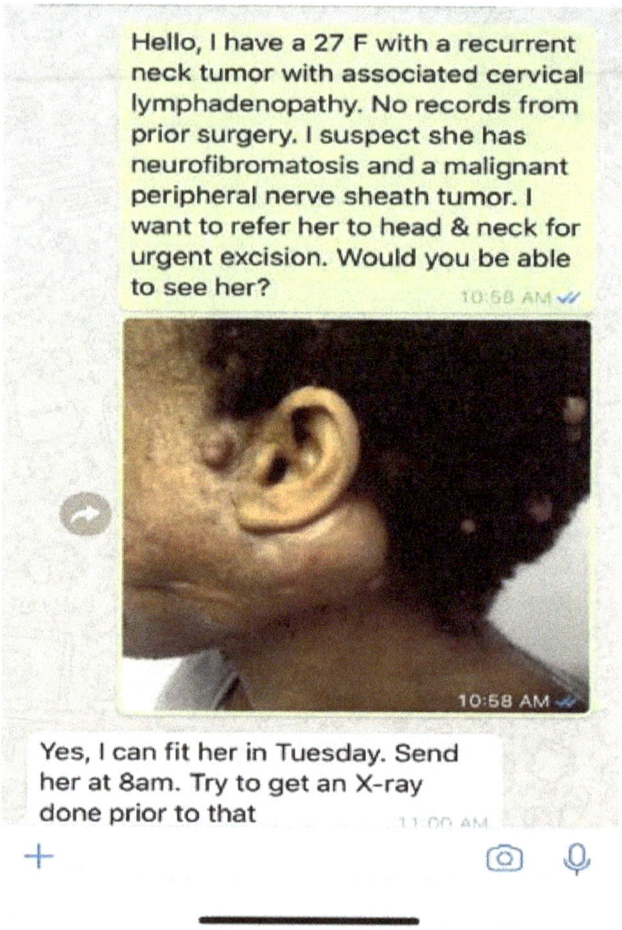

Figure 2. An example of secure direct messaging being used as a platform for teledermatology. Whatsapp is being utilized to tele-triage and coordinate care for a dermatology patient to sub-specialty care in Botswana.

Teledermatology can also be leveraged using cloud based file-hosting services that can provide a secure method for online file storage and sharing. Dropbox and Google drive are two popular cloud platforms that can facilitate Health Insurance Portability and Accountability Act (HIPAA) compliant sharing of protected patient information if utilized appropriately [19,20,48]. A recent study in Egypt, which used Dropbox for teledermatology consultation, found it to be a reliable diagnostic method with high rates of patient satisfaction [49]. Although cloud-based applications can function over mobile networks, they typically require a strong signal or wifi for optimal performance.

There has been a steady rise in the use of social networking among physicians who are starting to utilize crowdsourcing as a tool for patient care. Telederm.org is a free web-based dermatology networking platform that was started in 2002 and now has more than 2000 users [32]. After registering and creating an online profile, users can submit questions or cases to discussion forums that are divided by topic. Sermo is a similar website that connects more than 800,000 physicians of different specialties across the world via anonymous user profiles to allow the discussion of cases and other healthcare related topics [33]. Facebook, which connects users via a public profile, now has the ability to host private groups that are reportedly secure and only accessible by invitation [34]. Providers from any setting can come together to form collaborative groups in order to share challenging cases and request input from other members. Facebook groups can be tailored to specific topics of interest such as dermatopathology, tropical medicine or skin of color. Garcia-Romero et al. reported on the use of Facebook to create a teledermatology link between a rural clinic and a dermatology department at an urban general hospital in Mexico, which achieved clinical improvement in 75% of patients who received remote consultation [50]. Social media platforms have the benefit of a simple interface that requires negligible training for users and, most importantly, allows remote providers to connect with potentially thousands of dermatologists and other physicians across the world. Bandwidth requirements are low for these applications so they can be easily utilized on mobile devices in low-connectivity areas. However, there has been significant controversy about the use of social media platforms for healthcare, mainly due to the difficulty in guaranteeing patient privacy, confidentiality and security of the exchanged data. These methods should be used with caution.

Telepathology is a powerful component of teledermatology because histological analysis is vital for diagnostic confirmation in many dermatologic conditions, particularly in areas with high HIV burdens where clinical presentations are often atypical. Reliable pathology consultation services are critically needed in developing countries. Half of all fellowship trained pathologists work in the US, serving less than 5% of the global population [51]. Access to pathologists with dermatopathology experience or dermatopathology specialization is even more difficult to find in the global setting, creating an additional layer of challenges for physicians caring for skin diseases in remote settings.

Telepathology methods can also be tailored to the needs of the local community and available resources. The three methods of telepathology currently described are static imaging, dynamic imaging, and virtual slide systems (Table 1).

Static imaging is arguably the simplest telepathology method with the lowest budget requirements. The process involves taking photographs of slides at different magnifications and transmitting them to a remote dermatopathologist via any secure messaging, email or file-sharing platform. The most basic static technique utilizes a camera or smartphone to photograph a slide directly through a microscope eyepiece. Specialized adaptors and eyepiece attachments (Figure 3) have also been developed for use in combination with a smartphone to simplify the process of image capturing and improve the quality of images [52]. However, Bellina and Missoni demonstrated that quality images can be produced using any type of camera-equipped smartphone without the need for adaptors or additional technology [53], making this method ideal for low-resource settings. Digital camera attachments for microscopes are widely available and offer another simple mechanism for photographing slides. Multiple remote settings have achieved successful implementation of static telepathology programs with reported diagnostic concordance rates of up to 90.2% [45,54,55]. Major advantages of static image telepathology include minimal investment needed in equipment, training and maintenance, as well as the ability to function with unstable internet access. Static methods have the disadvantage of lower image quality, risk of sampling error and higher time requirements due to the need to select representative fields of view and take numerous pictures at different magnifications [56].

In dynamic imaging systems, slide images are examined in real time using a live microcopy viewing platform. Control of the live streaming images is either done directly by on site personnel or by the remote pathologist via robotic control of the microscope.

Live viewing systems have the advantage of allowing the pathologist to view the entire slide including different focus planes. Live view also allows cases to be discussed in real time which can increase the educational quality of consultations [57,58]. The feasibility of implementing a dynamic system has been demonstrated by the long-term use of a robotic telepathology system in a resource-limited government hospital in Botswana [59].

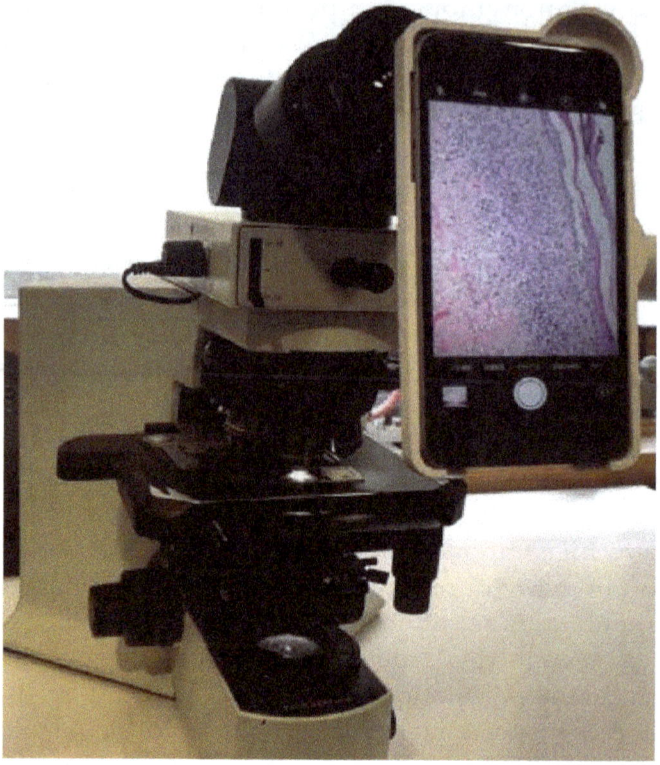

Figure 3. An example of a low-cost method for telepathology, the LabCam smartphone attachment, which allows photography of slides through the eyepiece of any microscope using an iPhone.

Virtual slide microscopy, also known as whole slide imaging systems, creates high-resolution scanned images of histology slides that can be digitally stored and then reviewed by a remote pathologist using specialized virtual slide viewing software [60]. This is also referred to as a hybrid method because it allows a pathologist to analyze the entire histology slide image dynamically by viewing selected areas digitally at higher magnification [61]. Major advantages include the ability to automate slide scanning; reduce interpretation time compared to robotic or static methods; the ability to manipulate, annotate and analyze slide images with viewing software; and the numerous educational applications that can be generated by creating a virtual 'teaching set' [61,62].

Virtual and dynamic slide telepathology systems can offer visual quality that is comparable to viewing slides in person under light microscopy, and several studies support good diagnostic concordance compared to a traditional glass slide review [63–70].

However, commercial slide-imaging systems are difficult to implement in low-resource settings due to the high cost of hardware and software, the need for skilled technicians to operate and maintain the systems locally, and the need for consistent high-bandwidth connectivity to transmit quality images [56,60,71].

In an effort to overcome the cost barriers of commercial slide-imaging systems, several low-cost interventions have been piloted utilizing innovative telepathology methods. Dudas et al. tested three low-cost telecytology systems including a Raspberry Pi attached to a webcam, an iPhone 4S with FaceTime, and an iPhone 4S with a live-streaming application [72]. All systems were able to stream live video of cytology slides to remote locations at a resolution that was suitable for a pathologist's review [72]. Meléndez-Álvarez et al. designed a telepathology prototype manufactured with plastic materials made using an open design 3D printer, a conventional optical microscope, a Celestron camera attachment, open-sourced software and electronic components that are readily available in most electronic shops [73]. The prototype had a total cost of less than $910 and the resulting images were judged to be of diagnostic quality by a pathologist [73]. Utilization of free web-based teleconferencing software such as Skype, Google Hangouts, GoToMeetings, Windows Live Messenger, Fuze, and Webex, can provide a low-cost alternative to commercial live view microscopy systems [60,74–76]. Yu et al. described the newly realized capacity of smartphones to power whole-slide imaging systems via software which splits the image digitalization process between smartphone applications and remote cloud servers [77]. An android or iOS smartphone mounted on the eyepiece of a standard optical microscope has the ability to scan whole-slide images into a virtual slide with a resulting image quality comparable to high end commercial slide-scanning systems [77,78]. This innovative smartphone technology offers the potential to bring slide scanning technology to more widespread settings in LMICs.

Implementation of any telepathology system requires careful planning and a strong partnership between local and remote providers. Additionally, it is important to note that none of these telepathology tools can overcome the need for local training and resources to perform quality skin biopsies and histopathological processing at the local site which is often the limiting factor in resource-limited settings [56]. Table 2 summarizes the advantages and disadvantages of each type of telepathology tool.

Table 2. Summary of the methods in which teledermatology can be utilized in practice, associated benefits and recommended platforms for remote providers in field settings.

Applications of Teledermatology	Benefits	Recommended Platforms for Remote Providers
Tele-Triage	appropriate and timely scheduling of patients into dermatology clinic, timely referral of dermatology patients to other specialists	secure direct messaging
Primary Care to Dermatology Consultation	diagnostic and management support, building dermatology skills over time	secure direct messaging
Specialist to Dermatology Consultation	diagnostic and management support, care coordination, building dermatology skills over time	secure direct messaging
Dermatologist to Dermatologist Consultation	second opinion, subspecialty dermatologist consultation, super specialist consultation for rare diseases, decreases isolation and burnout	formal teledermatology application, secure email, secure direct messaging, cloud based file sharing
Telepathology	expert analysis of skin biopsy specimens, improved diagnostic accuracy of skin disease, training of local pathologists	static images via smartphone or digital microscope camera
Long Term Management	allows for provider to dermatologist follow up, allows patient to dermatologist follow up, improves patient compliance and patient outcomes	secure direct messaging, secure email, cloud based file sharing
Care Coordination	allows for group chats between various providers to save time and resources	secure direct messaging, secure email, cloud based file sharing
Dermatology Education	remote access to dermatology education in any setting, builds local capacity	web based learning modules, video lectures, virtual patient encounters, email or web based access to lectures/handouts/guidelines, clinical decision support tools

In addition to supporting teledermatology functions, eHealth tools can provide access to education in many forms. The RAFT network is an example of a robust telemedicine network spanning four continents that focuses on providing medical education through a variety of low-bandwidth technologies such as interactive video lectures, virtual patient encounters, continuing medical education curriculums, tele-consults, clinical decision support tools, and web-casting of scientific conferences [14,79]. The emphasis on local involvement in coordinating and creating educational content that is most relevant to local providers has helped to make this project sustainable and successful [79].

mHealth applications are powerful educational tools because they can provide vital information to clinicians at the point of care. In recent years the number of mHealth applications has rapidly expanded to include programs to assist with disease diagnosis, management guidelines, drug reference, evidence-based medicine search tools, medical calculators, medical training tools, and clinical decision support pathways for navigating difficult clinical scenarios [80]. DynaMed, Epocrates, Medscape, Visual Dx, and UpToDate are some of the more commonly used mHealth tools, which allow clinicians to have rapid access to reference material with only a smartphone and/or mobile connection [81–85]. However, some of these applications require subscription costs, which can limit widespread usage in LMICs.

3. Benefits and Practical Applications of eHealth Tools

eHealth tools can be harnessed in a variety of different formats and combinations to benefit all levels of providers. Table 2 summarizes various methods in which teledermatology can provide solutions for the challenges of dermatology care in remote settings.

Teledermatology methods have been utilized to extend dermatologic care to developing countries since the early 1990s. The benefits of utilizing eHealth technologies are many and reports of successful programs have been published from numerous centers in Africa, Asia, and Latin America [5,10,11,44,86–89]. The growing transition to mobile teledermatology applications is supported by reports of successful implementation including satisfactory diagnosis and management of skin disease, diagnostic concordance with traditional face to face visits, patient satisfaction and provider satisfaction [23,89–96]. Utilization of tele-triage has the potential to significantly decrease the time to first evaluation of a patient by a dermatology specialist, which can in turn decrease morbidity from skin disease and increase patient satisfaction [23,97]. mHealth tools can improve the dermatology skills of front line providers who are more likely to retain knowledge because they are discussing and learning from their own patients [94]. Resident trainees in Botswana who were provided with smartphones pre-loaded with clinical decision support applications and training on how to best utilize the applications, reported multiple benefits including increased collaboration between primary care physicians and trainees, as well as increased clinician empowerment [77]. Teledermatology opens new communication and collaboration possibilities for providers and patients in isolated rural settings which can increase job satisfaction and improve care for patients with skin disease. Teledermatology can reduce healthcare costs by reducing the travel burden for patients, improving long-term follow-up and increasing successful care collaboration to improve patient outcomes [98,99]. Importantly, several studies have shown there is diagnostic concordance between teledermatology consultation and face-to-face visits, ensuring that patients are benefitting from use of the telemedicine without sacrificing quality of care [88,89,91].

4. Challenges and Barriers to Use of Teledermatology

Teledermatology is not without its challenges. Principally, sustainability becomes a key concern when setting up a program. Formal teledermatology platforms in particular require a significant amount of funding to implement, including but not limited to creation of the application, providing the necessary equipment, and training local providers. If the resources are not in place to continue the program long term, it becomes difficult to rationalize the initiation. The computer literacy of the providers being supported, local power supply, internet access, local mobile network connectivity, and availability of local technological resources all need to be carefully considered [14]. A major key to sustainability is ensuring that local clinicians are supportive of the program. Effective training on the tools being implemented can be challenging due to the often rapid provider turnover in low-resource clinical settings. Programs have a better chance of long-term success if technologies that are already in place and regularly used by local providers can be harnessed for teledermatology. Integration of the teledermatology program into the local healthcare system is essential for sustainability. Ideally the dermatologists answering the consultations are located in the country of origin of the consultee, or at the minimum, they are highly familiar with the diseases, work flow, and resources of the local healthcare system. Treatment plans being recommended must be realistic within the local socio-cultural and healthcare environment. Ideally, consultants should be available for continued collaboration and follow-up to address the common challenges that come with dermatology care in resource-limited settings. However, many teledermatology applications lack a method for long-term follow-up. Additionally, in certain cultures, teledermatology may not be an acceptable form of healthcare because patients expect face to face care or are resistant to having their skin condition photographed. Although teledermatology and mHealth applications give providers access to dermatology expertise, they do not solve the inherent challenges of local resource limitations such as medication stock outs, lack of available specialists for referral and limited diagnostic testing services.

The use of teledermatology requires a critical sensitivity to patient privacy and data security. It can be challenging to ensure that all providers participating in teledermatology are obtaining patient consent to share their information, sharing it over a secure platform, and using de-identified information to maintain patient confidentiality. Social media-based platforms must be used with caution because security settings and data-sharing policies can change rapidly and affect the ethical use of the program for patient data.

5. Practical Tips for Implementation of a New Teledermatology Initiative

The most important part of developing a new teledermatology initiative is a thorough local needs assessment of the area to be supported [12,44]. The first step in this process is evaluating the local healthcare environment. Most importantly, do local providers want to engage in teledermatology? Is there a need for or an interest in improving dermatology skills? Who would need to approve the program? Until clear need and firm local support can be secured, it is not advisable to initiate a teledermatology collaboration.

Review the current methods and workflow being used for dermatology patients. Where is the closest dermatology provider? Who cares for dermatology patients in rural areas versus urban areas? How far do most patients have to travel to see a dermatologist? How does the local healthcare system work? What is the cost of care for patients?

Then, review the locally available technological resources. Do most providers and patients use mobile phones? How prevalent are smartphones? How widespread are cellphone networks and how strong/reliable is the signal in the areas being supported? Are computers and/or wifi available in the local clinics or hospitals being supported? How technologically literate are the providers and patients being supported?

Next, identify partners that will participate in the initiative. Clearly outline the requirements and duties of all parties to be involved from the beginning to prevent problems developing later on. Have a discussion with local providers to get a firsthand understanding of their biggest concerns and the major challenges they face in caring for dermatology patients. Present your ideas for teledermatology solutions and get local feedback on the feasibility and interest in the proposed platforms. Ensure the platform can maintain patient privacy and provide a secure exchange of information.

Then, utilize the information gathered to narrow down the best options for a teledermatology platform. Identify the costs required to initiate and sustain the proposed platforms. Identify funding sources that can meet the needs of your proposal. Organize an implementation team to train all providers involved on both sides. Most importantly, identify a local means of providing ongoing training and support for the program to ensure sustainability.

If funding and resources appear to be major limitations, but local providers and leadership are supportive of developing a collaboration, consider starting with a free secure messaging application like Whatsapp. It can be integrated into even the most limited resource settings with little need for training and a low burden of time and effort for local providers to implement. If there is a robust interest in teledermatology at the local level, a strong health infrastructure that includes a dermatologist, and funding available for supplying and maintaining technological tools, a more formal teledermatology program could be feasible.

For overall success, teledermatology partnerships need to benefit both sides and need to be set up with the clear involvement of local providers. Remote dermatologists need to be willing and able to offer realistic diagnosis and treatment advice by taking into consideration local cultural norms and resource limitations. This is made possible by creating an open dialogue with local providers for exchange of information to allow both sides to learn from the interaction and improve care over time.

6. Conclusions

eHealth arguably offers one of the most flexible and realistic tools for providing critically needed access to dermatology skills in underserved LMICs. eHealth resources are ideal because they offer a wide range of customizable tools to match the needs and available resources of local providers in any setting. As the cost of mobile technology continues to decrease, the opportunities for low-cost teledermatology applications will continue to increase, making it feasible for any provider in any setting to be connected to a global community of dermatologists.

Author Contributions: V.W.: Writing-original draft preparation, C.K.: Writing-review and editing.

References

1. Karimkhani, C.; Dellavalle, R.P.; Coffeng, L.E.; Flohr, C.; Hay, R.J.; Langan, S.M.; Nsoesie, E.O.; Ferrari, A.J.; Erskine, H.E.; Silverberg, J.I.; et al. Global skin disease morbidity and mortality: An update from the Global Burden of Disease Study 2013. *JAMA Dermatol.* **2017**, *153*, 406. [CrossRef] [PubMed]
2. Evans, T.; Chen, L.; Evans, D.; Sadana, R.; Stilwell, B.; Travis, O.; Van Lerberghe, W.; Zurn, P.; Aschwanden, C. *The World Health Report 2006 - Working Together for Health*; World Health Organization: Geneva, Switzerland, 2006; ISBN 978-92-4-156317-8.
3. Chen, L.; Evans, T.; Anand, S.; Boufford, J.I.; Brown, H.; Chowdhury, M.; Cueto, M.; Dare, L.; Dussault, G.; Elzinga, G.; et al. Human resources for health: Overcoming the crisis. *Lancet* **2004**, *364*, 1984–1990. [CrossRef]
4. Crisp, N.; Chen, L. Global supply of health professionals. *N. Engl. J. Med.* **2014**, *370*, 950–957. [CrossRef] [PubMed]
5. Desai, B.; McKoy, K.; Kovarik, C. Overview of international teledermatology. *Pan Afr. Med. J.* **2010**, *6*, 3. [CrossRef] [PubMed]
6. International Foundation for Dermatology International Foundation for Dermatology. Available online: http://www.ifd.org/about2.html (accessed on 20 June 2018).
7. Hay, R.J.; Johns, N.E.; Williams, H.C.; Bolliger, I.W.; Dellavalle, R.P.; Margolis, D.J.; Marks, R.; Naldi, L.; Weinstock, M.A.; Wulf, S.K.; et al. The global burden of skin disease in 2010: An analysis of the prevalence and impact of skin conditions. *J. Investig. Dermatol.* **2014**, *134*, 1527–1534. [CrossRef] [PubMed]
8. WHO Global Observatory for eHealth. *Global Diffusion of eHealth: Making Universal Health Coverage Achievable: Report of the Third Global Survey on eHealth*; World Health Organization: Geneva, Switzerland, 2016; ISBN 978-92-4-151178-0.
9. Groupe Speciale Mobile Association. *The Mobile Economy 2014*; GSMA & International Telecomm Union: London, UK, 2014.
10. Lipoff, J.B.; Cobos, G.; Kaddu, S.; Kovarik, C.L. The Africa Teledermatology Project: A retrospective case review of 1229 consultations from sub-saharan Africa. *J. Am. Acad. Dermatol.* **2015**, *72*, 1084–1085. [CrossRef] [PubMed]
11. Wootton, R.; Geissbuhler, A.; Jethwani, K.; Kovarik, C.; Person, D.A.; Vladzymyrskyy, A.; Zanaboni, P.; Zolfo, M. Long-running telemedicine networks delivering humanitarian services: Experience, performance and scientific output. *Bull. World Health Organ.* **2012**, *90*, 341D–347D. [CrossRef] [PubMed]
12. Kaddu, S.; Kovarik, C.; Gabler, G.; Soyer, H. Teledermatology in Developing Countries. In *Telehealth in the Developing World*; Royal Society of Medicine Press/IDRC: London, UK, 2009; ISBN 978-1-85315-784.

13. Delaigue, S.; Morand, J.J.; Olson, D.; Wootton, R.; Bonnardot, L. Teledermatology in low-resource settings: The MSF experience with a multilingual tele-expertise platform. *Front. Public Health* **2014**, *2*. [CrossRef] [PubMed]
14. Bagayoko, C.O.; Müller, H.; Geissbuhler, A. Assessment of internet-based tele-medicine in Africa (the RAFT project). *Comput. Med. Imaging Graph.* **2006**, *30*, 407–416. [CrossRef] [PubMed]
15. Clickmedix. Available online: https://clickmedix.com/ (accessed on 1 July 2018).
16. Azova. Available online: http://azovahealth.com/ (accessed on 1 July 2018).
17. Proton Mail. Available online: https://protonmail.com/ (accessed on 1 July 2018).
18. Tutanota. Available online: https://tutanota.com/ (accessed on 1 July 2018).
19. Dropbox Business and HIPAA/HITECH—An Overview. Available online: https://www.dropbox.com/help/security/hipaa-hitech-overview (accessed on 20 June 2018).
20. Google Drive. Available online: https://www.google.com/drive/ (accessed on 1 July 2018).
21. Microsoft OneDrive. Available online: https://onedrive.live.com/about/en-us/ (accessed on 1 July 2018).
22. Box. Available online: https://www.box.com/home (accessed on 1 July 2018).
23. Williams, V.; Kovarik, C. WhatsApp: An innovative tool for dermatology care in limited resource settings. *Telemed. e-Health* **2018**, *24*, 464–468. [CrossRef] [PubMed]
24. Mars, M.; Scott, R.E. WhatsApp in clinical practice: A literature review. *Stud. Health Technol. Inform.* **2016**, *231*, 82–90. [PubMed]
25. Medtunnel. Available online: http://www.medtunnel.com/ (accessed on 1 July 2018).
26. Bloomtext. Available online: https://www.bloomtext.com/#/ (accessed on 1 July 2018).
27. Imprivata. Available online: https://www.imprivata.com/secure-communications (accessed on 20 June 2018).
28. Tiger Connect. Available online: https://www.tigerconnect.com/ (accessed on 20 June 2018).
29. Voalte. Available online: http://www.voalte.com/healthcare-communication-platform-2 (accessed on 20 June 2018).
30. Qliqsoft. Available online: https://www.qliqsoft.com/ (accessed on 1 July 2018).
31. Spok Mobile. Available online: https://www.spok.com/spok-mobile (accessed on 1 July 2018).
32. Telederm.org. Available online: http://www.telederm.org/ (accessed on 20 June 2018).
33. Sermo. Available online: http://www.sermo.com/ (accessed on 20 June 2018).
34. Facebook. Available online: https://www.facebook.com/ (accessed on 20 June 2018).
35. Olympus VS120-S6-W Virtual Slide Microscope. Available online: www.olympuslifescience.com/Microscopes/VC120 (accessed on 1 July 2018).
36. ZEISS Axio Scan.Z1 Digital Slide Scanner. Available online: https://www.zeiss.com/microscopy/int/products/imaging-systems/axio-scan-z1.html (accessed on 1 July 2018).
37. Leica Biosystems Aperio AT2 Telepathology Platform. Available online: https://www.leicabiosystems.com/digital-pathology/scan/aperio-at2/ (accessed on 1 July 2018).
38. Leica Biosystems Aperio LV1 Telepathology Platform. Available online: www.leicabiosystems.com/Aperio/LV1 (accessed on 1 July 2018).
39. 3DHISTECH Pannoramic DESK II DW. Available online: https://www.3dhistech.com/pannoramic_desk_II_DW (accessed on 1 July 2018).
40. Lab Cam. Available online: https://www.ilabcam.com/ (accessed on 1 July 2018).
41. Magnifi. Available online: http://www.arcturuslabs.com (accessed on 1 July 2018).
42. Snapzoom. Available online: http://snapzooms.com (accessed on 1 July 2018).
43. Ismail, A.; McMichael, J.R.; Stoff, B.K. Utility of international store-and-forward teledermatopathology among a cohort of mostly female patients at a tertiary referral center in Afghanistan. *Int. J. Womens Dermatol.* **2018**, *4*, 83–86. [CrossRef] [PubMed]
44. Bobbs, M.; Bayer, M.; Frazer, T.; Humphrey, S.; Wilson, B.; Olasz, E.; Holland, K.; Kuzminski, J. Building a global teledermatology collaboration. *Int. J. Dermatol.* **2016**, *55*, 446–449. [CrossRef] [PubMed]
45. Brauchli, K.; Jagilly, R.; Oberli, H.; Kunze, K.D.; Phillips, G.; Hurwitz, N.; Oberholzer, M. Telepathology on the Solomon Islands—two years' experience with a hybrid web- and email-based telepathology System. *J. Telemed. Telecare* **2004**, *10*, 14–17. [CrossRef] [PubMed]
46. Yueng, K. Whatsapp Passes 1 Billion Monthly Active Users. Venture Beat 2016. Available online: https://venturebeat.com/2016/02/01/whatsapp-passes-1-billion-monthly-active-users/ (accessed on 20 June 2018).

47. Monegian, B. KLAS Names Top Secure Messaging Tools. Healthcare IT News 2015. Available online: https://www.healthcareitnews.com/news/tigertext-leads-messaging-market-now (accessed on 20 June 2018).
48. Kohgadai, A. Top 5 HIPAA-Compliant Cloud Storage Services. Cloud Security Blog. Available online: https://www.skyhighnetworks.com/cloud-security-blog/top-5-hipaa-compliant-cloud-storage-services/ (accessed on 20 June 2018).
49. Saleh, N.; Abdel Hay, R.; Hegazy, R.; Hussein, M.; Gomaa, D. Can teledermatology be a useful diagnostic tool in dermatology practice in remote areas? An Egyptian experience with 600 patients. *J. Telemed. Telecare* **2017**, *23*, 233–238. [CrossRef] [PubMed]
50. Garcia-Romero, M.T.; Prado, F.; Dominguez-Cherit, J.; Hojyo-Tomomka, M.T.; Arenas, R. Teledermatology via a social networking web site: A pilot study between a general hospital and a rural clinic. *Telemed. e-Health* **2011**, *17*, 652–655. [CrossRef] [PubMed]
51. Meyer, J.; Paré, G. Telepathology Impacts and Implementation Challenges: A Scoping Review. *Arch. Pathol. Lab. Med.* **2015**, *139*, 1550–1557. [CrossRef] [PubMed]
52. Roy, S.; Pantanowitz, L.; Amin, M.; Seethala, R.R.; Ishtiaque, A.; Yousem, S.A.; Parwani, A.V.; Cucoranu, I.; Hartman, D.J. Smartphone adapters for digital photomicrography. *J. Pathol. Inform.* **2014**, *5*, 24. [CrossRef] [PubMed]
53. Bellina, L.; Missoni, E. Mobile cell-phones (M-phones) in telemicroscopy: Increasing connectivity of isolated laboratories. *Diagn. Pathol.* **2009**, *4*, 19. [CrossRef] [PubMed]
54. Abdirad, A.; Sarrafpour, B.; Ghaderi-Sohi, S. Static telepathology in Cancer Institute of Tehran University: Report of the first academic experience in Iran. *Diagn. Pathol.* **2006**, *1*, 33. [CrossRef] [PubMed]
55. Desai, S.; Patil, R.; Chinoy, R.; Kothari, A.; Ghosh, T.K.; Chavan, M.; Mohan, A.; Nene, B.M.; Dinshaw, K.A. Experience with telepathology at a tertiary cancer centre and a rural cancer hospital. *Natl. Med. J. India* **2004**, *17*, 17–19. [PubMed]
56. Evans, A.; Garcia, B.; Godin, C.; Godlewski, M.; Jansen, G.; Kabani, A.; Louahlia, S.; Manning, L.; Maung, R.; Moore, L.; et al. Guidelines from the Canadian Association of Pathologists for establishing a telepathology service for anatomic pathology using whole-slide imaging. *J. Pathol. Inform.* **2014**, *5*, 15. [CrossRef] [PubMed]
57. Kayser, K. Introduction of virtual microscopy in routine surgical pathology–a hypothesis and personal view from Europe. *Diagn. Pathol.* **2012**, *7*, 48. [CrossRef] [PubMed]
58. Weinstein, R.S.; Graham, A.R.; Richter, L.C.; Barker, G.P.; Krupinski, E.A.; Lopez, A.M.; Erps, K.A.; Bhattacharyya, A.K.; Yagi, Y.; Gilbertson, J.R. Overview of telepathology, virtual microscopy, and whole slide imaging: Prospects for the future. *Hum. Pathol.* **2009**, *40*, 1057–1069. [CrossRef] [PubMed]
59. Fischer, M.K.; Kayembe, M.K.; Scheer, A.J.; Introcaso, C.E.; Binder, S.W.; Kovarik, C.L. Establishing telepathology in Africa: Lessons from Botswana. *J. Am. Acad. Dermatol.* **2011**, *64*, 986–987. [CrossRef] [PubMed]
60. Pantanowitz, L.; Farahani, N.; Parwani, A. Whole Slide Imaging in Pathology: Advantages, Limitations, and Emerging Perspectives. *Pathol. Lab. Med. Int.* **2015**, *23*. [CrossRef]
61. Pantanowitz, L. Digital images and the future of digital pathology. *J. Pathol. Inform.* **2010**, *1*, 15. [CrossRef] [PubMed]
62. Evans, A.J.; Chetty, R.; Clarke, B.A.; Croul, S.; Ghazarian, D.M.; Kiehl, T.R.; Perez Ordonez, B.; Ilaalagan, S.; Asa, S.L. Primary frozen section diagnosis by robotic microscopy and virtual slide telepathology: The University Health Network experience. *Hum. Pathol.* **2009**, *40*, 1070–1081. [CrossRef] [PubMed]
63. Al Habeeb, A.; Ghazarian, D.; Evans, A. Virtual microscopy using whole-slide imaging as an enabler for teledermatopathology: A paired consultant validation study. *J. Pathol. Inform.* **2012**, *3*, 2. [CrossRef] [PubMed]
64. Al-Janabi, S.; Huisman, A.; Vink, A.; Leguit, R.J.; Offerhaus, G.J.A.; ten Kate, F.J.W.; van Dijk, M.R.; van Diest, P.J. Whole slide images for primary diagnostics in dermatopathology: A feasibility study. *J. Clin. Pathol.* **2012**, *65*, 152–158. [CrossRef] [PubMed]
65. Kent, M.N.; Olsen, T.G.; Feeser, T.A.; Tesno, K.C.; Moad, J.C.; Conroy, M.P.; Kendrick, M.J.; Stephenson, S.R.; Murchland, M.R.; Khan, A.U.; et al. Diagnostic accuracy of virtual pathology vs. traditional microscopy in a large dermatopathology study. *JAMA Dermatol.* **2017**, *153*, 1285. [CrossRef] [PubMed]
66. Koch, L.H.; Lampros, J.N.; Delong, L.K.; Chen, S.C.; Woosley, J.T.; Hood, A.F. Randomized comparison of virtual microscopy and traditional glass microscopy in diagnostic accuracy among dermatology and pathology residents. *Hum. Pathol.* **2009**, *40*, 662–667. [CrossRef] [PubMed]

67. Molin, J.; Thorstenson, S.; Lundström, C. Implementation of large-scale routine diagnostics using whole slide imaging in Sweden: Digital pathology experiences 2006–2013. *J. Pathol. Inform.* **2014**, *5*, 14. [CrossRef] [PubMed]
68. Nielsen, P.S.; Lindebjerg, J.; Rasmussen, J.; Starklint, H.; Waldstrøm, M.; Nielsen, B. Virtual Microscopy: An Evaluation of its Validity and Diagnostic Performance in Routine Histologic Diagnosis of Skin Tumors. *Hum. Pathol.* **2010**, *41*, 1770–1776. [CrossRef] [PubMed]
69. Shah, K.K.; Lehman, J.S.; Gibson, L.E.; Lohse, C.M.; Comfere, N.I.; Wieland, C.N. Validation of diagnostic accuracy with whole-slide imaging compared with glass slide review in dermatopathology. *J. Am. Acad. Dermatol.* **2016**, *75*, 1229–1237. [CrossRef] [PubMed]
70. Wamala, D.; Katamba, A.; Dworak, O. Feasibility and diagnostic accuracy of internet-based dynamic telepathology between Uganda and Germany. *J. Telemed. Telecare* **2011**, *17*, 222–225. [CrossRef] [PubMed]
71. Della Mea, V.; Cortolezzis, D.; Beltrami, C.A. The economics of telepathology-a case study. *J. Telemed. Telecare* **2000**, *6* (Suppl. 1), S168–S169. [PubMed]
72. Dudas, R.; VandenBussche, C.; Baras, A.; Ali, S.Z.; Olson, M.T. Inexpensive Telecytology solutions that use the Raspberry Pi and the iPhone. *J. Am. Soc. Cytopathol.* **2014**, *3*, 49–55. [CrossRef]
73. Meléndez-Álvarez, B.; Robayo, O.; Gil-Guillén, V.; Carratalá-Munuera, M. Design and validation of a low-cost telepathology system. *Telemedicine e-Health* **2017**, *23*, 976–982. [CrossRef] [PubMed]
74. Klock, C.; Gomes, R. Web conferencing systems: Skype and MSN in telepathology. *Diagn. Pathol.* **2008**, *3*, S13. [CrossRef] [PubMed]
75. Sirintrapun, S.; Cimic, A. Dynamic nonrobotic telemicroscopy via Skype: A cost effective solution to teleconsultation. *J. Pathol. Inform.* **2012**, *3*, 28. [CrossRef] [PubMed]
76. Speiser, J.J.; Hughes, I.; Mehta, V.; Wojcik, E.M.; Hutchens, K.A. Mobile teledermatopathology: Using a tablet PC as a novel and cost-efficient method to remotely diagnose dermatopathology cases. *Am. J. Dermatopathol.* **2014**, *36*, 54–57. [CrossRef] [PubMed]
77. Yu, H.; Gao, F.; Jiang, L.; Ma, S. Development of a whole slide imaging system on smartphones and evaluation with frozen section samples. *JMIR mHealth uHealth* **2017**, *5*, e132. [CrossRef] [PubMed]
78. Huang, Y.N.; Peng, X.C.; Ma, S.; Yu, H.; Jin, Y.B.; Zheng, J.; Fu, G.H. Development of whole slide imaging on smartphones and evaluation with ThinPrep cytology test samples: Follow-up study. *JMIR mHealth uHealth* **2018**, *6*, e82. [CrossRef] [PubMed]
79. Randriambelonoro, M.; Bagayoko, C.O.; Geissbuhler, A. Telemedicine as a tool for digital medical education: A 15-year journey inside the RAFT network. Digital medical education using the RAFT network. *Ann. N. Y. Acad. Sci.* **2018**. [CrossRef] [PubMed]
80. Mosa, A.S.M.; Yoo, I.; Sheets, L. A systematic review of healthcare applications for smartphones. *BMC Med. Inform. Decis. Mak.* **2012**, *12*. [CrossRef] [PubMed]
81. Dynamed. Available online: https://dynamed.com/home/ (accessed on 20 June 2018).
82. Epocrates. Available online: http://www.epocrates.com/ (accessed on 20 June 2018).
83. Medscape. Available online: www.medscape.com (accessed on 20 June 2018).
84. Visual Dx. Available online: https://www.visualdx.com/ (accessed on 20 June 2018).
85. UpToDate. Available online: https://www.uptodate.com/home (accessed on 20 June 2018).
86. Colven, R.; Shim, M.H.M.; Brock, D.; Todd, G. dermatological diagnostic acumen improves with use of a simple telemedicine system for underserved areas of South Africa. *Telemed. e-Health* **2011**, *17*, 363–369. [CrossRef] [PubMed]
87. Osei-tutu, A.; Shih, T.; Rosen, A.; Amanquah, N.; Chowdhury, M.; Nijhawan, R.I.; Siegel, D.; Kovarik, C. Mobile teledermatology in Ghana: Sending and answering consults via mobile platform. *J. Am. Acad. Dermatol.* **2013**, *69*, e90–e91. [CrossRef] [PubMed]
88. Patro, B.; Tripathy, J.; Sinha, S.; Singh, A.; De, D.; Kanwar, A. Diagnostic agreement between a primary care physician and a teledermatologist for common dermatological conditions in North India. *Indian Dermatol. Online J.* **2015**, *6*, 21. [CrossRef] [PubMed]
89. Tran, K.; Ayad, M.; Weinberg, J.; Cherng, A.; Chowdhury, M.; Monir, S.; El Hariri, M.; Kovarik, C. Mobile teledermatology in the developing world: Implications of a feasibility study on 30 Egyptian patients with common skin diseases. *J. Am. Acad. Dermatol.* **2011**, *64*, 302–309. [CrossRef] [PubMed]

90. Azfar, R.S.; Weinberg, J.L.; Cavric, G.; Lee-Keltner, I.A.; Bilker, W.B.; Gelfand, J.M.; Kovarik, C.L. HIV-positive patients in Botswana state that mobile teledermatology is an acceptable method for receiving dermatology care. *J. Telemed. Telecare* **2011**, *17*, 338–340. [CrossRef] [PubMed]
91. Azfar, R.S.; Lee, R.A.; Castelo-Soccio, L.; Greenberg, M.S.; Bilker, W.B.; Gelfand, J.M.; Kovarik, C.L. Reliability and validity of mobile teledermatology in human immunodeficiency virus–positive patients in Botswana: A pilot study. *JAMA Dermatol.* **2014**, *150*, 601. [CrossRef] [PubMed]
92. Frühauf, J.; Hofman-Wellenhof, R.; Kovarik, C.; Mulyowa, G.; Alitwala, C.; Soyer, H.; Kaddu, S. Mobile teledermatology in sub-Saharan Africa: A useful tool in supporting health workers in low-resource centres. *Acta Derm. Venereol.* **2013**, *93*, 122–123. [CrossRef] [PubMed]
93. Greisman, L.; Nguyen, T.M.; Mann, R.E.; Baganizi, M.; Jacobson, M.; Paccione, G.A.; Friedman, A.J.; Lipoff, J.B. Feasibility and cost of a medical student proxy-based mobile teledermatology consult service with Kisoro, Uganda, and Lake Atitlán, Guatemala. *Int. J. Dermatol.* **2015**, *54*, 685–692. [CrossRef] [PubMed]
94. Littman-Quinn, R.; Mibenge, C.; Antwi, C.; Chandra, A.; Kovarik, C.L. Implementation of m-Health applications in Botswana: Telemedicine and education on mobile devices in a low resource setting. *J. Telemed. Telecare* **2013**, *19*, 120–125. [CrossRef] [PubMed]
95. Mars, M.; Scott, R.E. Being spontaneous: The future of telehealth implementation? *Telemed. e-Health* **2017**. [CrossRef] [PubMed]
96. Sáenz, J.P.; Novoa, M.P.; Correal, D.; Eapen, B.R. On using a mobile application to support teledermatology: A case study in an underprivileged area in Colombia. *Int. J. Telemed. Appl.* **2018**, *2018*, 1–8. [CrossRef] [PubMed]
97. Chansky, P.B.; Simpson, C.L.; Lipoff, J.B. Implementation of a dermatology teletriage system to improve access in an underserved clinic: A retrospective study. *J. Am. Acad. Dermatol.* **2017**, *77*, 975–977. [CrossRef] [PubMed]
98. Ferrándiz, L.; Moreno-Ramírez, D.; Ruiz-de-Casas, A.; Nieto-García, A.; Moreno-Alvarez, P.; Galdeano, R.; Camacho, F.M. An economic analysis of presurgical teledermatology in patients with nonmelanoma skin cancer. *Actas Dermo-Sifiliogr.* **2008**, *99*, 795–802. [CrossRef]
99. Moreno-Ramirez, D.; Ferrandiz, L.; Ruiz-de-Casas, A.; Nieto-Garcia, A.; Moreno-Alvarez, P.; Galdeano, R.; Camacho, F.M. Economic evaluation of a store-and-forward teledermatology system for skin cancer patients. *J. Telemed. Telecare* **2009**, *15*, 40–45. [CrossRef] [PubMed]

13

Soil-Transmitted Helminths in Children in a Remote Aboriginal Community in the Northern Territory: Hookworm is Rare but *Strongyloides stercoralis* and *Trichuris trichiura* Persist

Deborah C. Holt [1], Jennifer Shield [1,2], Tegan M. Harris [1], Kate E. Mounsey [3], Kieran Aland [4], James S. McCarthy [5,6], Bart J. Currie [1] and Therese M. Kearns [1,*]

1 Menzies School of Health Research, Charles Darwin University, Darwin NT 0811, Australia; deborah.holt@menzies.edu.au (D.C.H.); j.shield@latrobe.edu.au (J.S.); tegan.harris@menzies.edu.au (T.M.H.); bart.currie@menzies.edu.au (B.J.C.)
2 Department of Pharmacy and Applied Science, La Trobe University, Bendigo VIC 3550, Australia
3 School of Health and Sports Science, University of the Sunshine Coast, Maroochydore QLD 4558, Australia; kmounsey@usc.edu.au
4 Queensland Museum, South Brisbane QLD 4101, Australia; bioscreenoz@gmail.com
5 QIMR Berghofer Medical Research Institute, Herston QLD 4006, Australia; j.mcarthy@uq.edu.au
6 School of Medicine, University of Queensland, Brisbane QLD 4072, Australia
* Correspondence: therese.kearns@menzies.edu.au;

Abstract: (1) Background: soil-transmitted helminths are a problem worldwide, largely affecting disadvantaged populations. The little data available indicates high rates of infection in some remote Aboriginal communities in Australia. Studies of helminths were carried out in the same remote community in the Northern Territory in 1994–1996 and 2010–2011; (2) Methods: fecal samples were collected from children aged <10 years and examined for helminths by direct smear microscopy. In the 2010–2011 study, some fecal samples were also analyzed by agar plate culture and PCR for *Strongyloides stercoralis* DNA. Serological analysis of fingerprick dried blood spots using a *S. stercoralis* NIE antigen was also conducted; (3) Results and Conclusions: a reduction in fecal samples positive for *S. stercoralis*, hookworm and *Trichuris trichiura* was seen between the studies in 1994–1996 and 2010–2011, likely reflecting public health measures undertaken in the region to reduce intestinal helminths. Comparison of methods to detect *S. stercoralis* showed that PCR of fecal samples and serological testing of dried blood spots was at least as sensitive as direct smear microscopy and agar plate culture. These methods have advantages for use in remote field studies.

Keywords: *Strongyloides stercoralis*; strongyloidiasis; *Trichuris trichiura*; *Rodentolepis nana*; Northern Territory; Aboriginal

---

1. Introduction

Soil-transmitted helminths are a worldwide problem generally affecting poor and vulnerable populations [1]. In Australia, there is a paucity of studies documenting the prevalence of soil-transmitted helminths due to the difficulties in diagnosing infection in communities, and timely transport to the nearest diagnostic laboratory. A cross-sectional survey in a remote Aboriginal community in the north of Western Australia in 1992 found hookworm infection in 77% of participants with the highest prevalence in children aged 5–14 years (93%) [2]. In a remote community in the Northern Territory (NT), a study in the mid-1990s of children and adults documented high rates of infection with hookworm, *Strongyloides stercoralis*, *Trichuris trichiura* and *Rodentolepis* (*Hymenolepis*) *nana* [3]. More recent surveys of *S. stercoralis* prevalence indicate that it is endemic in many northern Australian Aboriginal communities [4–6].

Currently, there is no gold standard test for diagnosing *S. stercoralis* [7,8]. Stool examination underestimates the prevalence of the parasite in population-based studies, while serological testing gives a higher prevalence [9]. When examining stools, the larval density is often low and output sporadic, resulting in variation in detection between samples in the same individuals [10]. Routine direct smear microscopy of single stool specimens has a low sensitivity in chronic cases and can fail to detect larvae in up to 70% of chronic infections [7,10]. The use of the agar culture plate technique has improved detection in chronic *S. stercoralis*, with a sensitivity of 96% when compared with direct fecal smear, formalin-ethyl acetate concentration and Harada-Mori filter paper culture [7]. A practical problem for the agar plate technique is that viable larvae are required for culture, which can be problematic for specimens that involve long delays (transport or otherwise) in reaching the laboratory. Serological examination for *S. stercoralis* antibodies improves detection in those with chronic infection. However, it may not readily detect those with acute infection as the prepatent period can be up to 28 days [8,11].

A study in a remote NT Aboriginal community in 1994–1996 revealed a high level of intestinal helminths by formol-ether concentration of fecal samples [3]. Concern of residents in this community about high rates of *S. stercoralis* infection resulted in a project in 2010–2011 to investigate the utility of mass drug administration to reduce the endemic prevalence of *S. stercoralis* and scabies [6,12]. The aim of this study was to compare the prevalence of intestinal parasites identified by direct smear microscopy between the 1994–1996 and 2010–2011 studies. In addition, due to the logistical challenges of handling and processing fecal samples during remote field studies, we also investigated the utility of alternative methods of *S. stercoralis* diagnosis during the 2010–2011 study. Serological testing of eluted dried blood spots and PCR were shown to be at least as sensitive as microscopy and culture, and have considerable advantages for use in remote community settings.

2. Materials and Methods

2.1. Sample Population

Samples were collected from consenting participants during two separate projects in a remote Aboriginal community with an estimated population of 2000, located 550 km east of Darwin, NT Australia. Ninety-four percent of the resident population are Australian Aboriginal with an average of 6.3 members per household, and 19.9% of the population are aged <10 years [13]. Each project received ethical approval from the Human Research Ethics Committee of the Northern Territory Department of Health and Menzies School of Health Research (EC00153; approvals 94/19 and 09/34).

2.2. Fecal Sample Collection and Processing

In the first study, surveys of intestinal parasites were conducted in the community from 1994–1996 [3]. Fecal samples were collected into disposable plastic containers by a parent or carer and collected by the researchers the following morning. Direct smears for the identification of intestinal parasites were undertaken in a field laboratory. Quantitative formol-ether counts conducted on fecal samples preserved in 4% formaldehyde were previously reported [3]. Treatment was administered by the local primary health care service and was not recorded as part of the study.

The 2010–2011 study consisted of two population censuses and mass drug administrations (MDAs) conducted 12 months apart in a staged roll-out. The full study design has been previously reported [6,12]. Fecal samples were collected from children by a parent or carer into disposable plastic containers and returned to the researchers. Direct smear microscopy on approximately 0.005 g of feces was performed on the majority of samples on site in a field laboratory within four hours of receipt. A small number of samples from 2011 were fixed in SAF (sodium acetate, acetic acid, formalin) and transported by aircraft to a commercial pathology laboratory for microscopic analysis the day after receipt. Only the results of the first fecal sample collected from each participant aged <10 years are reported here.

Fisher exact probability tests were performed at the VassarStats website [14].

2.3. Agar Plate Culture

For samples with sufficient fecal matter, agar plate culture was conducted, based on the method of Garcia [15], except that nutrient-deficient Mueller-Hinton agar plates were used, with the aim of reducing fungal growth. Specifically, a patch of ~2 cm diameter of feces was applied to the center of a nutrient-deficient Mueller-Hinton agar plate, sealed, and incubated at room temperature (~25 °C) overnight. The plates were then transported by aircraft to the research laboratory the following day in a foam container with a sweated ice brick to maintain a temperature of 17–25 °C. The plates were maintained in the research laboratory at 25 °C and examined macroscopically for larval tracks marked by bacterial colonies daily for up to five days after plating. Once tracks were observed, or after five days had elapsed, the plate was flooded with 10% formalin for five minutes, the liquid aspirated and centrifuged at $500\times g$, and the sediment examined microscopically for *S. stercoralis* and hookworm infective larvae.

2.4. Fecal DNA Extraction and PCR

Any remaining fecal material was transported to the research laboratory, where it was stored in ethanol at −20 °C. DNA extraction using up to 30 mg of stored fecal samples was performed using a PowerSoil® DNA isolation kit (MoBio Laboratories Inc, Carlsbad, CA, USA), according to the manufacturer's instructions. The PowerSoil kit is designed for use with complex samples and has been shown to be superior to four other DNA extraction methods in terms of sensitivity and ease of use, for extraction and detection of *Strongyloides ratti* DNA in spiked human stool samples [16]. DNA samples were tested using a published real-time PCR based method for the detection of *S. stercoralis* 18S rDNA [17]. Due to a high percentage of positive samples in 2010 that were detected using this method (34/39), the real-time PCR products were analyzed by agarose gel electrophoresis. Many samples did not have the correct 101 bp product, but had a smaller DNA fragment, possibly primer dimer, that presumably reacted with the probe to produce fluorescence in the real-time PCR. As a result, we designed an alternative forward primer (Stro18S-altF 5′ GGGCCGGACACTATAAGGAT 3′), which produced a 471 bp product with the published Stro18S-1630R primer (5′ TGCCTCTGGATATTGCTCAGTTC 3′) [17]. The original Stro18S-1530F and Stro18S-1630R primer set was shown to be highly specific for *S. stercoralis* [17]; however, the specificity when using the alternative forward primer designed here was not systematically tested. End-point PCR using this alternative primer combination was conducted using 2 μL of DNA extraction, 20 pmol each primer, 100 μM dNTPs, 1.5 mM Mg^{2+} and 1 U *Taq* polymerase in a total volume of 20 μL. Cycling conditions were 35 cycles of 95 °C for 30 s, 58 °C for 30 s, and 72 °C 30 s. A positive control plasmid was constructed by cloning a PCR product obtained from an agar plate culture-positive sample into pBlueScript II SK. The efficiency of the PCR was optimized using the plasmid control and a culture-positive fecal sample.

2.5. Blood Spot Collection and Serological Testing

Dried blood spots were collected by fingerprick onto filter paper cards, air dried and stored in zip-lock bags with silica desiccant at 4–8 °C. Serum was eluted from the dried blood spots and analyzed by ELISA using a recombinant *S. stercoralis* NIE antigen [18] as previously reported [19]. Briefly, dried blood spots were eluted in 150 μL phosphate buffered saline and 0.05% Tween 20 (PBS-T) overnight at room temperature. A 1:500 dilution of this eluate was used in the NIE ELISA. Plates were coated with 100 μL of 125 ng/mL NIE antigen, and blocked with 5% skim milk powder in PBS-T. Dried blood spot elutions were added and incubated at 37 °C for two hours. Alkaline phosphatase conjugated goat anti-human IgG was used as the secondary antibody at a dilution of 1:2500. Plates were developed with phosphatase substrate and optical density read at 405 nm. The assay was initially established and validated using a panel of sera from participants that were either positive or negative for *S. stercoralis* by fecal culture. Each ELISA assay included positive and negative control dried blood spots, which were used to validate the assay and normalize optical density (OD) results [19]. Normalized ODs were calculated by the ratio of test sample OD to positive control dried blood spot OD. The result of the first sample collected from each participant is reported here.

3. Results

3.1. Comparison of Intestinal Parasites Identified in Children <10 Years in 1994–1996 and 2010–2011

Fecal samples were collected from children aged <10 years and examined by direct smear. Samples were collected from 84 participants in 1994–1996 (mean age 5.6 years) and 85 children in 2010–2011 (mean age 3.7 years). The percentage of samples positive for hookworm and *T. trichiura* in 2010–2011 was significantly less than that reported in 1994–1996 ($p = 0.002$ and 0.012 respectively). The percentage of samples positive for *S. stercoralis* also reduced, however *R. nana* remained unchanged (Table 1). The mean number of intestinal parasites identified per fecal sample was 1.5 in 1994–1996 and 2 in 2010–2011 (data not shown).

Table 1. Intestinal parasites identified in fecal samples by direct smear microscopy.

n	1994–1996 84	2010–2011 85	Fisher Exact Probability Test *p* (Two-tail)
Average age (years)	5.6	3.7	
Strongyloides stercoralis	11 (13.1%)	4 (4.7%)	0.063
Hookworm	11 (13.1%)	1 (1.2%)	0.002 *
Rodentolepis nana	20 (23.8%)	19 (22.4%)	0.857
Trichuris trichiura	57 (67.9%)	41 (48.2%)	0.012 *

* $p < 0.05$.

3.2. Comparison of Diagnostic Methods for S. stercoralis

In addition to the direct smears, in the 2010–2011 study agar plate culture for helminth larvae, and PCR for *S. stercoralis* DNA was conducted on a subset of fecal samples, and serology was performed on sera eluted from dried blood spots (Table 2). *S. stercoralis* larvae were detected in five of 77 (6.5%) samples examined by agar plate culture and formalin sedimentation (Figure 1). Four of these samples were positive for *S. stercoralis* by direct smear, while one was negative. No hookworm larvae were detected. End point PCR for *S. stercoralis* 18S rDNA was positive for six (7.2%) of 83 samples tested, which included the five agar plate-positive samples. The percentage of samples considered positive by serology was higher than for the other methods with 25 (16.2%) of the dried blood spot samples considered positive.

Table 2. Comparison of *Strongyloides stercoralis* diagnostic methods in children aged <10 years in 2010–2011.

Method	+ve/n (%)
Direct smear	4/85 (4.7%)
Culture and formalin sedimentation	5/77 (6.5%)
S. stercoralis 18S rDNA PCR	6/83 (7.2%)
Serology on dried blood spots	25/154 (16.2%)

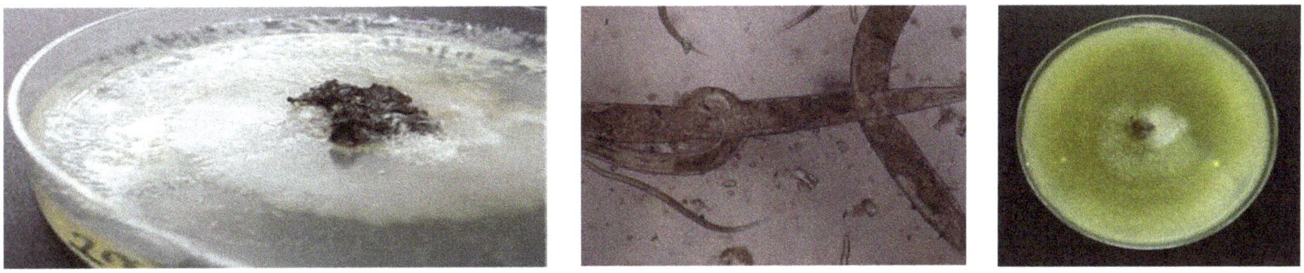

(A) (B) (C)

Figure 1. Identification of *S. stercoralis* larvae by agar plate culture and formalin sedimentation: (**A**) Bacterial growth on Mueller-Hinton agar in tracks made by helminth larvae; (**B**) *S. stercoralis* adults and filariform larvae in formalin sediment of agar culture; (**C**) Fungal overgrowth may have obscured larval tracks on some plates.

There were 28 blood spot samples for which a fecal sample had also been analyzed by agar plate culture at the same time point. Of these, 20 participants were negative for both methods, and five were positive by serology but negative by culture. It is unknown if these children had recent infections or if results were false positives, as children are rarely tested for *Strongyloides* in this setting. For three participants who were positive by agar plate culture and had blood spots collected, one was also positive by serology, but the other two were negative by serology. This indicates that this serological method may not detect some acute infections.

4. Discussion

This is one of the first NT studies to examine and compare helminth infections in a remote Aboriginal community using three different diagnostic methods. Aboriginal Australians are traditionally hunter-gatherer societies, and there has been a rapid and often problematic transition to permanent settlement since European colonization. Aboriginal Australians have a higher burden of disease compared with non-Aboriginal Australians, with the largest difference seen in remote communities [20]. In remote community settings in northern Australia, government programs concentrating on the provision of infrastructure alone have been shown to have limited impact on community-level crowding and hygiene [21] or common childhood infectious diseases [22,23].

The introduction of a deworming program using albendazole in 1995 [24] is likely to have contributed to the reduction in samples positive for *S. stercoralis* (not statistically significant), hookworm and *T. trichiura* between the two study periods. The observed low rate of hookworm in 2010–2011 is supported by a downward trend in hookworm infections seen in a hospital-based study conducted during the same time period, which reported 14 cases per 100,000 in 2002 and 2.2 cases per 100,000 in 2012 [25]. The percentage of fecal samples positive for *S. stercoralis* dropped from 13.1% in 1994–1996 to 4.7% in 2010–2011, which reflects an overall reduction in the NT [26]. The single-dose albendazole used in the NT deworming program may have had a partial effect despite being lower than the recommended dose for treating *S. stercoralis* infection [26]. Serology on blood spots was positive for 16.2% of children tested in 2010–2011, higher than for fecal detection methods. The community-wide mass drug administration at the time of this study was shown to reduce the rate of seropositivity in treated participants 12 months later [6]. The reduction in participants positive for *T. trichiura* between the 1994–1996 study and the 2010–2011 study is consistent with overall data for the NT [27]; however, the percentage of participants positive for *T. trichiura* remained high in 2010–2011 at 48.2%. This may be due to the fact that single-dose albendazole reduces egg counts but has a low cure rate for *T. trichiura* infection [28–30]. The prevalence of *R. nana* infection remained unchanged between the study periods, consistent with a recent analysis of infections in the NT, which showed that infections were predominantly in Aboriginal children aged under 5 years [31]. Single-dose albendazole does not appear to produce a significant cure rate for *R. nana* [28] and the recommended treatment, praziquantel [32], is rarely stocked in health services in rural and remote communities.

As *S. stercoralis* larval output is often low and intermittent in chronic cases [10], a limitation of this study is the examination of a single fecal specimen for diagnosis. Agar plate culture and formalin sedimentation yielded only a single additional *S. stercoralis* positive sample compared with the direct smear method in 2010–2011, and this method is reported to have greater sensitivity than both direct smear and formol-ether concentration [33]. Fungal growth on the agar culture plates was common, and may have hindered the identification of larval tracks. It is also possible, that in spite of the care taken to maintain the temperature of agar plates within the tolerance range of *S. stercoralis* larvae, some larval death may have occurred during transport. The sensitivity of the direct smear microscopy may have also been high due to large numbers of parasites present and/or an experienced microscopist.

As collection, processing and analysis of fecal samples presents a number of logistical challenges, we undertook three different methods for the diagnosis of *S. stercoralis* that might be more suited to studies in remote field sites. PCR on DNA extractions of ethanol-preserved fecal samples was at least as sensitive as agar plate culture and formalin sedimentation. PCR has the advantage of reducing the handling of fecal specimens in the field, and allowed samples to be batched for testing. This method could be modified to have greater utility in remote field settings. Alternative methods of fecal preservation that allow storage at room temperature [34] could be used, avoiding the need for cold storage. Methods utilizing loop-mediated isothermal amplification (LAMP) require only a single temperature incubation and have the possibility of incorporating visualization of positive results by color or turbidity change [35,36] that could be conducted in a field laboratory. Detection of multiple intestinal parasite species can also be achieved with PCR, using multi-parallel [37] or multiplexed reactions [38,39]. The sensitivity of DNA amplification methods may further be improved by targeting high copy number sequences identified by whole genome sequence analysis [40].

Serology was positive for 16.2% of samples in 2010–2011, higher than for the other diagnostic methods used, and consistent with previous reports [9,41]. In endemic areas, serology has a high positive predictive value due to the high prevalence of infection [8] but may not identify all acute infections, and may be of most use in monitoring the effect of treatment in an individual or population over time [6,19].

5. Conclusions

PCR of fecal samples and serological testing of dried blood spots were shown to be at least as sensitive as microscopy and culture for the diagnosis of *S. stercoralis* in this setting. These methods have considerable advantages for use in remote field studies and may be useful for the ongoing assessment of efforts to reduce the prevalence of *S. stercoralis* in remote communities.

Despite a reduction in the percentage of children aged <10 years positive for *S. stercoralis*, hookworm and *T. trichiura* in 2010–2011 compared to 1994–1996 in this remote Aboriginal community in Australia, the rates of *S. stercoralis* and *T. trichiura* remained high at 4.7% and 48.2% respectively. The percentage of children positive for *R. nana* was unchanged. The reduction is consistent with public health measures in the region to reduce intestinal helminths but requires further investigation to assess the impact that these infections are having on child health and development.

Acknowledgments: The 1994–1996 study was funded by a National Health and Medical Research Council grant through the Public Health Research and Development Committee. K.A. was supported by a Commonwealth Postgraduate Scholarship at the University of Queensland. The 2010–2011 study was funded by a National Health and Medical Research Council Project Grant (605804). We thank all of the study participants in both studies and Professor Ross Andrews and other investigators involved in these projects for their support.

Author Contributions: D.C.H., J.S., T.M.H., K.E.M., K.A., J.S.M., B.J.C. and T.M.K. conceived and designed the experiments; D.C.H., J.S., T.M.H., K.E.M., K.A., T.M.K. performed the experiments; D.C.H., J.S., T.M.H., K.E.M., K.A. and T.M.K analyzed the data; D.C.H., J.S., T.M.H., K.E.M., J.S.M., B.J.C. and T.M.K wrote the paper.

References

1. World Health Organization. Available online: http://www.who.int/mediacentre/factsheets/fs366/en/ (accessed on 17 July 2017).
2. Hopkins, R.M.; Gracey, M.S.; Hobbs, R.P.; Spargo, R.M.; Yates, M.; Thompson, R.C. The prevalence of hookworm infection, iron deficiency and anaemia in an aboriginal community in north-west Australia. *Med. J. Aust.* **1997**, *166*, 241–244. [PubMed]
3. Shield, J.; Aland, K.; Kearns, T.; Gongdjalk, G.; Holt, D.; Currie, B.; Prociv, P. Intestinal parasites of children and adults in a remote Aboriginal community of the Northern Territory, Australia, 1994–1996. *Western Pac. Surveill. Response J.* **2015**, *6*, 44–51. [CrossRef] [PubMed]
4. Fryar, D.; Hagan, S. Pilot screening program for intestinal parasites and anaemia in adults in a Top End Aboriginal community. *NT Comm Dis Bull.* **1997**, *4*, 20–21.
5. Johnston, F.H.; Morris, P.S.; Speare, R.; McCarthy, J.; Currie, B.; Ewald, D.; Page, W.; Dempsey, K. Strongyloidiasis: A review of the evidence for Australian practitioners. *Aust. J. Rural Health* **2005**, *13*, 247–254. [CrossRef] [PubMed]
6. Kearns, T.M.; Currie, B.J.; Cheng, A.C.; McCarthy, J.; Carapetis, J.R.; Holt, D.C.; Page, W.; Shield, J.; Gundjirryirr, R.; Mulholland, E.; et al. *Strongyloides* seroprevalence before and after an ivermectin mass drug administration in a remote Australian Aboriginal community. *PLoS Negl. Trop. Dis.* **2017**, *11*, e0005607. [CrossRef] [PubMed]
7. Siddiqui, A.A.; Berk, S.L. Diagnosis of *Strongyloides stercoralis* infection. *Clin. Infect. Dis.* **2001**, *33*, 1040–1047. [CrossRef] [PubMed]
8. Speare, R.; Durrheim, D.N. *Strongyloides* serology – useful for diagnosis and management of strongyloidiasis in rural Indigenous populations, but important gaps in knowledge remain. *Rural Remote Health* **2004**, *4*, 264. [PubMed]
9. Grove, D.I. Human strongyloidiasis. *Adv. Parasitol.* **1996**, *38*, 251–309. [PubMed]
10. Dreyer, G.; Fernandes-Silva, E.; Alves, S.; Rocha, A.; Albuquerque, R.; Addiss, D. Patterns of detection of *Strongyloides stercoralis* in stool specimens: Implications for diagnosis and clinical trials. *J. Clin. Microbiol.* **1996**, *34*, 2569–2571. [PubMed]
11. Tanaka, H. Experimental and epidemiological studies on strongyloidiasis of Amami Oshima island. *Jpn. J. Exp. Med.* **1958**, *28*, 159–182. [PubMed]
12. Kearns, T.M.; Speare, R.; Cheng, A.C.; McCarthy, J.; Carapetis, J.R.; Holt, D.C.; Currie, B.J.; Page, W.; Shield, J.; Gundjirryirr, R.; et al. Impact of an ivermectin mass drug administration on scabies prevalence in a remote Australian Aboriginal community. *PLoS Negl. Trop. Dis.* **2015**, *9*, e0004151. [CrossRef] [PubMed]
13. Australian Bureau of Statistics. Available online: http://www.censusdata.abs.gov.au/census_services/getproduct/census/2016/quickstat/SSC70106 (accessed on 31 August 2017).
14. VassarStats: Website for Statistical Computation. Available online: http://vassarstats.net/ (accessed on 30 September 2017).
15. Garcia, L. *Diagnostic Medical Parasitology*, 5th ed.; American Society for Microbiology Press: Washington DC, USA, 2007; pp. 837–840.
16. Sultana, Y.; Jeoffreys, N.; Watts, M.R.; Gilbert, G.L.; Lee, R. Real-time polymerase chain reaction for detection of *Strongyloides stercoralis* in stool. *Am. J. Trop. Med. Hyg.* **2013**, *88*, 1048–1051. [CrossRef] [PubMed]
17. Verweij, J.J.; Canales, M.; Polman, K.; Ziem, J.; Brienen, E.A.; Polderman, A.M.; van Lieshout, L. Molecular diagnosis of *Strongyloides stercoralis* in faecal samples using real-time PCR. *Trans. R. Soc. Trop. Med. Hyg.* **2009**, *103*, 342–346. [CrossRef] [PubMed]
18. Ravi, V.; Ramachandran, S.; Thompson, R.W.; Andersen, J.F.; Neva, F.A. Characterization of a recombinant immunodiagnostic antigen (NIE) from *Strongyloides stercoralis* L3-stage larvae. *Mol. Biochem. Parasitol.* **2002**, *125*, 73–81. [CrossRef]
19. Mounsey, K.; Kearns, T.; Rampton, M.; Llewellyn, S.; King, M.; Holt, D.; Currie, B.J.; Andrews, R.; Nutman, T.; McCarthy, J. Use of dried blood spots to define antibody response to the *Strongyloides stercoralis* recombinant antigen NIE. *Acta Trop.* **2014**, *138*, 78–82. [CrossRef] [PubMed]
20. Vos, T.; Barker, B.; Begg, S.; Stanley, L.; Lopez, A.D. Burden of disease and injury in Aboriginal and Torres Strait Islander Peoples: the Indigenous health gap. *Int. J. Epidemiol.* **2009**, *38*, 470–477. [CrossRef] [PubMed]

21. Bailie, R.S.; McDonald, E.L.; Stevens, M.; Guthridge, S.; Brewster, D.R. Evaluation of an Australian indigenous housing programme: Community level impact on crowding, infrastructure function and hygiene. *J. Epidemiol. Community Health* **2011**, *65*, 432–437. [CrossRef] [PubMed]
22. Bailie, R.S.; Stevens, M.; McDonald, E.L. The impact of housing improvement and socio-environmental factors on common childhood illnesses: A cohort study in Indigenous Australian communities. *J. Epidemiol. Community Health* **2012**, *66*, 821–831. [CrossRef] [PubMed]
23. McDonald, E.; Bailie, R. Hygiene improvement: Essential to improving child health in remote Aboriginal communities. *J. Paediatr. Child. Health* **2010**, *46*, 491–496. [CrossRef] [PubMed]
24. Central Australian Rural Practitioners Association. *CARPA Standard Treatment Manual*, 2nd ed.; Central Australian Rural Practitioners Association: Alice Springs, NT, Australia, 1994.
25. Davies, J.; Majumdar, S.S.; Forbes, R.T.; Smith, P.; Currie, B.J.; Baird, R.W. Hookworm in the Northern Territory: down but not out. *Med. J. Aust.* **2013**, *198*, 278–281. [CrossRef] [PubMed]
26. Mayer-Coverdale, J.K.; Crowe, A.; Smith, P.; Baird, R.W. Trends in *Strongyloides stercoralis* faecal larvae detections in the Northern Territory, Australia: 2002–2012. *Trop. Med. Infect. Dis.* **2017**, *2*, 18. [CrossRef]
27. Crowe, A.L.; Smith, P.; Ward, L.; Currie, B.J.; Baird, R. Decreasing prevalence of *Trichuris trichiura* (whipworm) in the Northern Territory from 2002 to 2012. *Med. J. Aust.* **2014**, *200*, 286–289. [CrossRef] [PubMed]
28. Horton, J. Albendazole: A review of anthelmintic efficacy and safety in humans. *Parasitology* **2000**, *121*, S113–S132. [CrossRef] [PubMed]
29. Keiser, J.; Utzinger, J. Efficacy of current drugs against soil-transmitted helminth infections: systematic review and meta-analysis. *J.A.M.A.* **2008**, *299*, 1937–1948. [CrossRef] [PubMed]
30. Steinmann, P.; Utzinger, J.; Du, Z.W.; Jiang, J.Y.; Chen, J.X.; Hattendorf, J.; Zhou, H.; Zhou, X.N. Efficacy of single-dose and triple-dose albendazole and mebendazole against soil-transmitted helminths and *Taenia* spp.: A randomized controlled trial. *PLoS One* **2011**, *6*, e25003. [CrossRef] [PubMed]
31. Willcocks, B.; McAuliffe, G.N.; Baird, R.W. Dwarf tapeworm (*Hymenolepis nana*): Characteristics in the Northern Territory 2002–2013. *J. Paediatr. Child. Health* **2015**, *51*, 982–987. [CrossRef] [PubMed]
32. Central Australian Rural Practitioners Association. *CARPA Standard Treatment Manual*, 5th ed.; Central Australian Rural Practitioners Association: Alice Springs, NT, Australia, 2014.
33. Sato, Y.; Kobayashi, J.; Toma, H.; Shiroma, Y. Efficacy of stool examination for detection of *Strongyloides* infection. *Am. J. Trop. Med. Hyg.* **1995**, *53*, 248–250. [CrossRef] [PubMed]
34. Beknazarova, M.; Millsteed, S.; Robertson, G.; Whiley, H.; Ross, K. Validation of DESS as a DNA preservation method for the detection of *Strongyloides* spp. in canine feces. *Int. J. Environ. Res. Public Health* **2017**, 14. [CrossRef]
35. Watts, M.R.; James, G.; Sultana, Y.; Ginn, A.N.; Outhred, A.C.; Kong, F.; Verweij, J.J.; Iredell, J.R.; Chen, S.C.; Lee, R. A loop-mediated isothermal amplification (LAMP) assay for *Strongyloides stercoralis* in stool that uses a visual detection method with SYTO-82 fluorescent dye. *Am. J. Trop. Med. Hyg.* **2014**, *90*, 306–311. [CrossRef] [PubMed]
36. Fernandez-Soto, P.; Sanchez-Hernandez, A.; Gandasegui, J.; Bajo Santos, C.; Lopez-Aban, J.; Saugar, J.M.; Rodriguez, E.; Vicente, B.; Muro, A. Strong-LAMP: A LAMP Assay for *Strongyloides* spp. detection in stool and urine samples. Towards the diagnosis of human strongyloidiasis starting from a rodent model. *PLoS Negl. Trop. Dis.* **2016**, *10*, e0004836. [CrossRef]
37. Mejia, R.; Vicuna, Y.; Broncano, N.; Sandoval, C.; Vaca, M.; Chico, M.; Cooper, P.J.; Nutman, T.B. A novel, multi-parallel, real-time polymerase chain reaction approach for eight gastrointestinal parasites provides improved diagnostic capabilities to resource-limited at-risk populations. *Am. J. Trop. Med. Hyg.* **2013**, *88*, 1041–1047. [CrossRef] [PubMed]
38. Basuni, M.; Muhi, J.; Othman, N.; Verweij, J.J.; Ahmad, M.; Miswan, N.; Rahumatullah, A.; Aziz, F.A.; Zainudin, N.S.; Noordin, R. A pentaplex real-time polymerase chain reaction assay for detection of four species of soil-transmitted helminths. *Am. J. Trop. Med. Hyg.* **2011**, *84*, 338–343. [CrossRef] [PubMed]
39. Llewellyn, S.; Inpankaew, T.; Nery, S.V.; Gray, D.J.; Verweij, J.J.; Clements, A.C.; Gomes, S.J.; Traub, R.; McCarthy, J.S. Application of a multiplex quantitative PCR to assess prevalence and intensity of intestinal parasite infections in a controlled clinical trial. *PLoS Negl. Trop. Dis.* **2016**, *10*, e0004380. [CrossRef] [PubMed]

40. Pilotte, N.; Papaiakovou, M.; Grant, J.R.; Bierwert, L.A.; Llewellyn, S.; McCarthy, J.S.; Williams, S.A. Improved PCR-based detection of soil transmitted helminth infections using a next-generation sequencing approach to assay design. *PLoS Negl. Trop. Dis.* **2016**, *10*, e0004578. [CrossRef] [PubMed]
41. Buonfrate, D.; Perandin, F.; Formenti, F.; Bisoffi, Z. A retrospective study comparing agar plate culture, indirect immunofluorescence and real-time PCR for the diagnosis of *Strongyloides stercoralis* infection. *Parasitology* **2017**, *144*, 812–816. [CrossRef] [PubMed]

14

Integrated Management of Skin NTDs—Lessons Learned from Existing Practice and Field Research

Rie R. Yotsu [1,2]

[1] School of Tropical Medicine and Global Health, Nagasaki University, Nagasaki 852-8102, Japan; ryotsu@nagasaki-u.ac.jp

[2] Department of Dermatology, National Center for Global Health and Medicine, Tokyo 162-8655, Japan

Abstract: Integration of neglected tropical diseases (NTDs) into the public health agenda has been a priority in global health for the last decade. Because a number of these diseases share not only the geographical distribution, but also a common feature which is skin involvement, bringing together a sub-group of 'skin NTDs' is one way forward to promote further integration among NTDs. With these diseases, which include leprosy, Buruli ulcer, yaws, mycetoma, lymphatic filariasis, and leishmaniasis, patients may be left with life-long deformities and disabilities when diagnosis and treatment are delayed. Stigma is another serious consequence of skin NTDs as it places a large barrier on the economic activities and social life of a patient. As a result, this creates a vicious cycle and obstructs a key goal of society, the elimination of poverty. Enhancement in surveillance systems as well as the further development of diagnostic methods, improvement in treatment and management, and identification of preventative measures for skin NTDs are therefore urgently needed. This article summarizes the existing practices and field research on skin NTDs and identifies potential synergies that could be achieved by adopting this integrated approach.

Keywords: case management; integration; mass drug administration; neglected tropical diseases; skin infections; skin NTDs; surveillance; training; tropical skin diseases

---

1. Introduction

Neglected tropical diseases (NTDs) are a group of infectious diseases that prevail in tropical and sub-tropical regions, affecting impoverished populations living in conditions of poor sanitation and in close contact with infectious vectors and livestock; such communities also have very limited access to adequate healthcare [1]. It is estimated that over one billion people in 149 countries are affected [2]. In May 2013, the World Health Assembly (WHA) adopted resolution WHA66.12, which calls on Member States to intensify and integrate measures against these NTDs to effectively and efficiently enhance the health and social well-being of the affected populations [2].

Successful integration of diagnostic and therapeutic interventions has happened for some NTDs, particularly among those that can be managed at community level by mass drug administration (MDA). This set of diseases forms the basis of a sub-group sometimes known as preventative chemotherapy and transmission control (PCT) NTDs, which includes such diseases as cysticercosis, foodborne trematode infections, lymphatic filariasis, onchocerciasis, schistosomiasis and soil-transmitted helminthiasis. Dracunculiasis (guinea-worm disease) is reaching close to eradication through transmission control; however, the recent transmission seen in dogs is hindering the last drive in Chad, which may show further spread [3]. In contrast, there are other NTDs where early diagnosis and management on an individual basis may be the only workable therapeutic measure, at least at present, and these are categorized as innovative and intensified disease management (IDM) NTDs. As IDM NTDs need considerable resources, including personnel with skills and financial support, and these measures do not produce a dramatic and immediately visible impact, which may lead to lower investment in research and development, the control of this set of diseases is lagging behind the PCT-NTDs [2].

Interestingly, a number of IDM-NTDs share a common feature, which is involvement of the skin, for example, in the forms of nodules, patches, edema, and ulceration (Figure 1). To assist in a breakthrough in the above-mentioned gap in the global health agenda, there is a move designed to improve integrated strategies to group these NTDs with skin manifestations under the banner of skin NTDs [4,5]. Among the skin NTDs are leprosy, Buruli ulcer, yaws, cutaneous and mucocutaneous leishmaniasis, chromoblastomycosis and mycetoma, and ectoparasites including scabies and tungiasis. Human African trypanosomiasis and post Kala-azar dermal leishmaniasis may present with skin signs, which although not the main symptom of the disease, may aid in early detection. Lymphatic filariasis and onchocerciasis are also skin NTDs, which are controlled by MDAs, but as control measures are rolled out across endemic areas there will be a residue of individual cases that have escaped detection or preemptive therapy with MDAs, whose recognition and treatment is essential in order to achieve effective control. Yaws and scabies are skin NTDs that are potentially controlled or eliminated through preventative chemotherapy, and the expansion of this approach on a larger scale is currently under study [6–10].

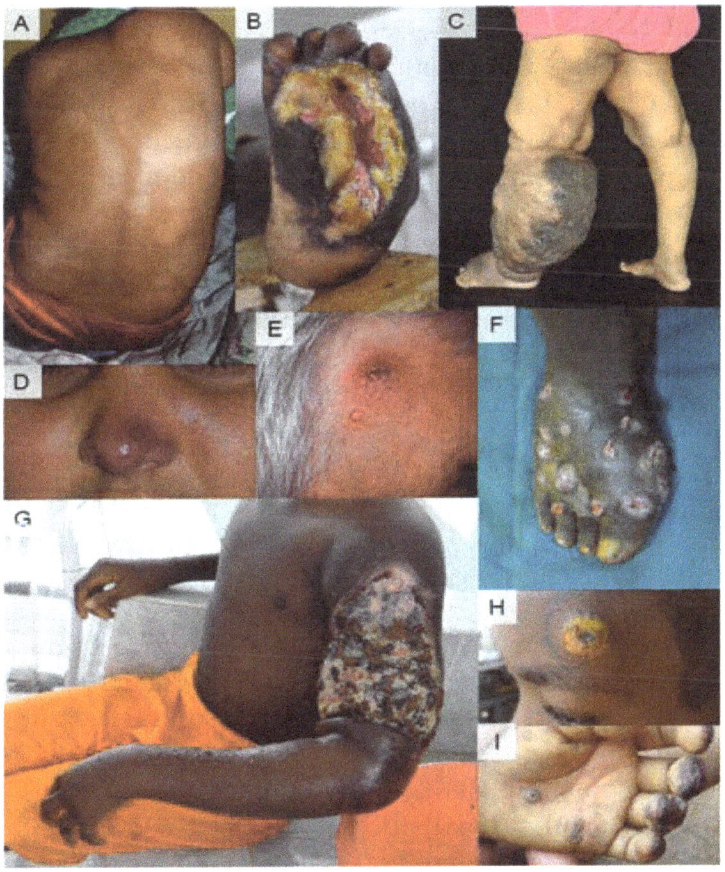

Figure 1. Clinical presentation of skin NTDs. (**A**) Leprosy (borderline tuberculoid leprosy). Ill-defined, multiple hypo-pigmented patches on the back. (**B**) Deformities of the feet and ulcer from peripheral neuropathy in leprosy. (**C**) Lymphatic filariasis. Unilateral lymphedema of the limb. (image: Saravu R. Narahari) (**D**) Mucocutaneous leishmaniasis. Redness and swelling of the nose. Inside: destruction of the nasal mucosa. Same patient as (**A**) (co-infection). (**E**) Cutaneous leishmaniasis. Infiltrated granulomatous lesion with central ulceration on the forehead. (**F**) Mycetoma. Multiple nodules with openings of draining sinuses discharging pus and blood. (image: Ahmed Fahal) (**G**) Buruli ulcer. Ulceration on the arm with extensive edema. Black and yellowish necrotic tissue on wound surface with some traditional remedies at first visit. (**H**) Yaws (primary yaws). Nodule with central ulceration with yellow crust on the forehead. (image: Kingsley Asiedu) (**I**) Tungiasis. Multiple small nodules with central black dot (body part of the adult flea) on the palm and on the finger tips.

In addition, there are other skin diseases that are not formally recognized by WHO as NTDs that contribute a huge disease burden in impoverished populations. These include podoconiosis (a geochemical, non-filarial elephantiasis due to long-term contact with irritant red clay soil), fungal and bacterial skin infections, and tropical ulcers [11,12]. These diseases should also be considered as neglected. However, their management as public health problems may also benefit from this skin NTDs integrative approach.

Surveillance and early detection, MDA, and case and morbidity management are potential areas for integrative initiatives for skin NTDs. This paper is not a systematic review of all skin NTDs, but rather it summarizes the current state of knowledge and lessons learned from existing practice and field research to aid in effective project implementation for managing skin NTDs.

2. Active Surveillance

There are several factors that hinder early detection and treatment of skin NTDs. Skin NTDs are often painless or accompanied by limited discomfort—this feature prevents patients and families from presenting to healthcare facilities at an early stage [13–15]. Low awareness of the disease among the populations at the highest risk also adds to the delay in seeking help, and this is compounded by the consequences of stigma and discrimination often associated with these diseases [13–16]. Many patients tend to seek treatment preferentially with traditional healers rather than at health care centers, as there is easier access and lower cost [15–17]. This health seeking behavior is also linked to the common perception that the diseases may result from mystical causes (witchcraft and curses) [15–17].

In the light of current perceptions among health authorities and communities, and given the lack of mass population measures or field-friendly diagnostic tests, active surveillance is still the most effective measure for early detection and thereby, treatment for most skin NTDs in order to prevent patients from developing disabilities, disfigurement, and comorbidities. Early detection and treatment are also key to cutting further transmission of the diseases, for instance, in leprosy, scabies, and yaws, and this underlines the importance of active surveillance.

As skin diseases can be detected by visual examination—a unique feature in this set of diseases—that if used effectively, for instance by organizing community skin surveys or treatment initiatives, is one simple approach for detection of skin NTDs that would otherwise remain hidden. Outreach skin surveys have been conducted with successful results in the case of leprosy in different parts of the world, for example, in India, Pacific Islands, Malawi, Cameroon, and recently in Brazil [18–25]. The Brazilian project led by the Ministry of Health targeted more than nine million schoolchildren aged between 5–14 years for skin screening of leprosy coupled with de-worming (albendazole for soil-transmitted helminthiases) [25]. In Japan where leprosy is no longer prevalent, school skin surveys played a considerable role in achieving a decline in cases during the 1970s in Okinawa, the most southern island of Japan, which remained as the last pocket during the endemic era [26]. Consecutive surveys at 3–5 year intervals were behind this success.

As part of promoting integration of skin NTDs, in line with the current global approach, there have been newer studies. An observational study in Cameroon reviewed the different means of detection of a total of 815 cases of yaws identified during the three-year period between 2012 and 2015 in one endemic region [27]. They reported that these cases were reported through the synergistic effect of five approaches: passive yaws detection at local clinics after training of local staff on NTDs, small community-based NTD case detection activities, community-based yaws screening immediately following Buruli ulcer outreach programs, school-based screening, and house-to-house searches. Rapid cure of yaws increased the uptake of, and confidence in, the treatment of Buruli ulcers, and thus led to a "win-win" situation for the two diseases.

In Côte d'Ivoire, another West African country, school skin surveys in areas identified as co-endemic for leprosy, Buruli ulcer, and yaws are also in the process of implementation [12]. The project is sometimes coupled with other activities, such as de-worming, if the timing coincides, to achieve resource mobilization as well as increased acceptance by the community. In this project, the latter is also enhanced by targeting all skin diseases, a strategy that also prevents creating unnecessary feelings of stigma and discrimination against skin NTDs. Targeting all skin diseases therefore appears to be a way forward. However, a careful strategy needs to be prepared as there is usually a high prevalence of skin diseases in such communities where skin NTDs are prevalent—ranging from infectious to inflammatory. This may pose a practical challenge in project implementation, i.e., cost of medications and ensuring referral pathways. In communities in African countries where skin NTDs are likely to be endemic, prevalence of skin diseases can range from 26% to 80% [12,28–33].

Key points in implementing integrated surveillance:

1. Selection of the intervention area: try to collect past data and develop mapping methods to identify co-distribution of cases of skin NTDs
2. Training of local healthcare workers both on skin NTDs and common skin diseases
3. Treatment: develop protocols on how to manage the different diseases anticipated; be prepared to treat or to refer
4. Look for opportunities for integration with other community- or school-based activities, e.g., de-worming, vitamin A and micronutrient supplementation, onchocerciasis and/or lymphatic filariasis control, to gain a synergic effect
5. Plan for repeat rounds/follow-up activities, decide on the appropriate intervals.

3. Mass Drug Administration and Prophylaxis

Lymphatic filariasis and onchocerciasis are already operationally covered by active MDA programs. In addition, several other skin NTDs are thought to be controllable using MDAs, and field research is ongoing.

Yaws comes first on that list, and recent studies have shown that high coverage with MDA consisting of single-dose azithromycin may be effective in control of the disease. A study conducted in an island off Papua New Guinea (16,092 residents) showed a rapid reduction in the prevalence of active yaws infection from 1.8% before mass treatment with azithromycin (30 mg/kg) to a minimum of 0.1% at 18 months, with 84% coverage [9,34]. However, with longer follow-up up to 42 months, a significant increase in cases to 0.4% was observed, indicating that a single round of drug administration may not be enough. These cases were mainly found in individuals who had not received the mass treatment or as new infection in residents. This finding suggests the need for repeated intervention to achieve elimination of yaws. In Ghana, a similar study to assess the effectiveness of this MDA strategy in endemic communities surrounded by other yaws-endemic communities is on-going, i.e., non-isolated communities in contrast to the work in Papua New Guinea. In the pilot study report, the prevalence of active and latent yaws in children reduced from 10.9% before mass treatment to 2.2% at 12 months, in 16,287 children with 89% coverage [7]. The best dosage regimen is also under investigation. An additional benefit would be that azithromycin MDA is also active against trachoma allowing for possible integration of the control of these two NTDs [8].

Scabies is also another disease that potentially may be targeted by MDAs, as oral ivermectin, one of the major drugs used in the control of a number of other NTDs, is also highly effective in scabies. Successful mapping and co-administration of mass treatment studies for scabies have been conducted in the Solomon Islands and integrated with existing programs for trachoma and yaws [10,35–37]. In Brazil, selective MDA by targeting communities heavily infected with ectoparasites and enteroparasites using ivermectin considerably reduced the prevalence of a range of coexisting parasitic skin infections, including scabies, pediculosis, cutaneous larva migrans and tungiasis [38]. Similarly, the African Program for Onchocerciasis [39] and the Global Programme to Eliminate Lymphatic Filariasis [40] reported a coincident effect in reducing the number of cases of scabies, an off-target disease. Further integrated activities are planned as part of the assessment of the impact of triple-drug treatment (ivermectin, albendazole, and diethylcarbamazine citrate) for lymphatic filariasis [41]. Use of ivermectin could increase community acceptance of the MDAs through the treatment of skin conditions, particularly if it benefits those severely affected by itching and sores.

Two countries with extensive experience in NTD control, Ethiopia and Fiji are currently developing comprehensive scabies control programs [42]. To further plan on the potential of MDAs for scabies, more studies on dosage and issues related to ivermectin use during pregnancy and in small children are needed. Furthermore, prevalence of scabies is likely to rise again after a certain period of time, and therefore, more operational research is needed to define the best intervals between rounds of MDA. The development of moxidectin, a macrocyclic lactone similar to ivermectin, but with a much longer half-life, for the treatment of human scabies may promote MDAs for scabies [43,44]. Recently in June 2018, the United States Food and Drug Administration (FDA) approved the use of moxidectin for onchocerciasis in patients aged 12 years and older [45].

Although not on the same massive scale as yaws or scabies, there have been attempts to prevent occurrence and interrupt transmission of leprosy using one-dose rifampicin chemoprophylaxis in contact cases (post-exposure prophylaxis). This intervention was tested in Bangladesh in a cluster-randomized controlled trial including 21,711 participants, with successful outcomes at 2-years with a 56.5% reduction in new cases in the intervention group [46]. This protective effect was seen only in the first two years. No additional protective effect was observed after 4 and 6 years, but the total impact of the intervention was still statistically significant after 6 years [47]. A similar result was reported from another study in Indonesia [48]. With the long latent period of leprosy—which can sometimes be more than several decades, long-term follow up is necessary to assess the true effect of interventions for this disease. In the past, chemoprophylaxis (1 to 2 doses of a combination of rifampicin, ofloxacin, and minocycline) has been tested in three Pacific Islands, namely Kiribati, the Federated States of Micronesia, and the Republic of the Marshall Islands, all small islands with a high level of leprosy endemicity [19–21]. Now two decades after this intervention, they remain among the countries with the highest new case detection rates for leprosy per population globally [49]. Short-term reduction in new cases of leprosy was observed during the first few years after the intervention, in which active case detection at baseline could have played a considerable role in enhancing the effect of treating some sub-clinical cases. In other words, chemoprophylaxis alone may not be effective unless it is coupled with well-planned active case finding, and the prophylaxis is delivered in the form of several rounds of medication at adequate intervals [26,50]. Currently, the Leprosy Post-Exposure Prophylaxis [51] study—a joint study between India, Indonesia, Myanmar, Nepal, Sri Lanka, and Tanzania using single dose rifampicin—was designed to accelerate the uptake of the evidence for post-exposure prophylaxis and introduce it into national leprosy programs [51]. Recently published interim analysis show that the program has enrolled 5941 index patients and identified a total of 123,331 contacts [52]. Efficacy results are awaited.

MDAs and prophylaxis may be effective in the control of several skin NTDs, but it is important to note that repeated dosing and other surveillance activities are often needed, as mentioned above. We should also be careful in implementing MDAs/prophylaxis as some drugs may not be safe for use in children, in pregnant women, and in individuals for whom they are contra-indicated. Monitoring for adverse reactions should be carefully done as their occurrence might have a negative impact on the campaigns. How to address these constraints should be elucidated before implementing the strategy on a larger scale. Furthermore, the funds necessary for implementation are not available at the moment, as there is limited interest from donors. Identification of the target populations is also very important not only for the success of the intervention, but also for minimizing cost.

Key points in implementing mass drug administration:

1. Careful identification of target populations or case definition
2. Identifying intervals between rounds and number of rounds; some diseases have long latent periods which may be difficult to assess

3. Obtaining strong, coordinated public-private partnerships, including pharmaceutical companies
4. Assessment of secondary effects on other diseases (e.g., leprosy vs. tuberculosis), including increasing the risk of drug resistance
5. Addressing the issues of stigma and discrimination if implementing for contact cases.

4. Current Status of Diagnosis and Treatment for Skin NTDs

Few skin NTDs can be confirmed with reliable point-of-care diagnostic tests, and therefore a clinical examination remains the cornerstone of diagnosis. This poses a major challenge, not just in case management of individual patients with skin NTDs, but also in understanding the true epidemiology and disease burden in endemic areas.

To take Buruli ulcer as an example, a study in Cameroon has shown that only 27% among the 327 patients with ulcerative lesions suspected as Buruli ulcer seen at one of their tertiary hospital were confirmed to be Buruli ulcer [53]. Other diagnosis ranged from vascular, bacterial infections, post-traumatic, fistulated osteomyelitis, as well as neoplasia. The team used a combination of Ziehl-Neelsen staining, PCR, and culture from either swab or fine-needle aspiration, skin biopsies, and several systemic tests for diagnostic confirmation [53]. In field settings, these tests are not easy to perform, and it is not difficult to imagine that some patients who have been given a diagnosis based solely on clinical appearance are treated unnecessarily or given the wrong drugs.

PCR targeting IS2404 is currently the test most used for confirming Buruli ulcer. However, access to PCR in many places in West Africa where Buruli ulcer is endemic is very limited. Moreover, adequate skills in sample taking and ensuring transportation of samples in good condition adds to the challenge. It sometimes may take weeks and months to reach the laboratory. It is very difficult to rule out the possibility of false negatives under such conditions. It is also noteworthy that some of the PCR positives with IS2404 include other mycobacterial diseases, for example, *M. marinum*, *M. chelonae*, and *M. smegmatis*, whose distribution in these countries is not yet well understood [54]. Some promising studies are underway in order to develop a rapid diagnostic tool for Buruli ulcer, including the loop-mediated isothermal amplification (LAMP) test [55,56], thin layer chromatography for the detection of mycolactone (lipid toxin produced by the causing bacteria of Buruli ulcer) [57], and antigen detection assays [58].

Table 1 provides the list of diagnostic tests and Table 2 provides treatments currently used for each skin NTD. As treatment of many skin NTDs is of long duration, it is important that diagnostic confirmation be made before initiating treatment. Furthermore, some skin NTDs are associated with considerable stigma and discrimination. Labeling a patient with a specific diagnosis unnecessarily is also another issue that needs to be addressed, and development of easier and more reliable diagnostic methods would also improve these important social aspects associated with skin NTDs. Recently, a point-of-care test for syphilis has been used for early detection of yaws, as they are both from the spirochete bacterium group, replacing the traditional laboratory methods such as rapid plasma reagin (RPR) and *Treponema pallidum* hemagglutination assay (TPHA) [59]. However, a positive test does not necessarily mean that the lesion is due to active yaws, as there are also other pathogenic species in this same group [59]. Further studies for the development of diagnostic tools and reliability checking are needed for all skin NTDs.

Treatments used for skin NTDs are also very limited and many are old drugs or combinations [60]. Integrated advocacy among the skin NTDs may aid in the development of better diagnostic tools and treatment options.

Table 1. Diagnostic methods and tools for skin NTDs.

	Pathogen	Rapid Diagnostic Test	PCR	Microscopy	Culture	Serology	Others
Buruli ulcer	*Mycobacterium ulcerans*	X	O	O	O	X	LAMP test, thin layer chromatography, antigen detection assays under development
Cutaneous leishmaniasis (CL)/mucocutaneous leishmaniasis (ML)	*Leishmania* species	X	O	O Skin smears	O	X	LAMP test, antigen detection assays under development (Montenegro skin test)
Lymphatic filariasis (LF)	Microfilaria (*Wuchereria bancrofti*, *Brugia malayi*, etc.)	O	O	O Blood smears	X	Δ Anti-filarial antibodies	Ultrasonography
Onchocerciasis	Microfilaria (*Onchocerca volvulus*)	O	O	O Skin snips	X	Δ Anti-filarial antibodies	Direct observation of adult worms from nodule(s), slit-lamp eye exam, serological and antigen tests under development
Leprosy	*Mycobacterium leprae*	X	O	O	X	Δ Anti-PGL-I antibody	Thickened nerves, loss of muscle strength, anesthetic skin lesion
Mycetoma	Fungal or bacterial species	X	O	Δ	O	X	X-rays, CT, ultrasonography, etc.
Podoconiosis	Irritant alkalic clay soils	N/A	N/A	N/A	N/A	N/A	Location, history, clinical findings; negative results for LF and other lymphedema-causing diseases; genetic susceptibility
Scabies	*Sarcoptes scabiei* var. *hominis*	X	Δ	O	X	X	Dermatoscopy, burrow ink test
Tungiasis	*Tunga penetrans* (sand fleas)	X	Δ	O	X	X	Direct observation of adult fleas and eggs from skin lesion(s), dermatoscopy
Yaws	*Treponema pallidum* subsp. *pertenue*	O	O	O	O	PRP, TPHA, FTA-ABS, etc.	Diagnostics for differentiation of *Treponema pallidum* species under development

O = available; Δ = available but not confirmatory or standardized; X = unavailable.

Table 2. Treatment and management for skin NTDs.

	Medical Treatment	Surgery	Wound or Lymphedema Management	Self-Morbidity Management	Prevention
Buruli ulcer	**Standard:** Oral rifampicin + clarithromycin for 8 weeks **Other tested regimens:** Oral rifampicin + either 1 or 2 of [ciprofloxacin, ethambutol, mofloxacin, amikacin, etc.]	Yes	Yes	Yes	Limited, route of transmission unknown (Stay away from contaminated water sources)
Cutaneous leishmaniasis (CL)/mucocutaneous leishmaniasis (ML)	Individualized treatment depending on species (no standard) Amphotericin B deoxycholate, pentavalent antimonials, fluconazole, ketoconazole, miltefosine, paromomycin ointment, etc. **Simple CL** lesion(s) with low ML-risk: natural healing may occur **Complex CL** lesion(s) with high-ML risk, severe lesion(s), immunocompromised persons, etc.: treat all cases	No	Yes	No	Limited (Avoid sand fly bites)
Lymphatic filariasis (LF)	Oral albendazole ± [diethylcarbamazine (DEC) or ivermectin] When long-term treatment is possible: Oral DEC (1–12 days) ± doxycycline for 4 to 6 weeks Note: DEC contraindicated in onchocerciasis endemic sites	Yes	Yes	Yes	Avoid mosquito bites, MDAs, vector control, etc.
Onchocerciasis	Oral ivermectin	Yes	No	No	Avoid blackfly bites, MDAs, vector control, etc.
Leprosy	**Multiple drug therapy (MDT):** Oral rifampicin + dapsone + clofazimine for 6 to 12 months	Yes	Yes	Yes	Contact tracing and early detection; prophylaxis with one-dose rifampicin in trial
Mycetoma	Antibiotics or antifungals depending on species for long-term	Yes	Yes	Yes	Footwear
Podoconiosis	N/A	Yes	Yes	Yes	Footwear
Scabies	Oral ivermectin, 1–2 doses 1 week apart	No	No	No	Early diagnosis and treatment of contacts, possible MDAs in endemic communities
Tungiasis	None (primary treatment: hygienic mechanical removal of fleas), antibiotics if secondary infection is indicated	No	Yes	No	Footwear
Yaws	Single oral azithromycin or injectable benzathine penicillin	No	Yes	No	Contact tracing and early detection, possible MDAs in endemic communities

Key points in diagnosis and treatment of skin NTDs:

1. Training of local healthcare workers on clinical diagnosis
2. Training of local healthcare workers on diagnostic tests, including sample taking; make a routine for performing diagnostic tests
3. Need for the development of new point-of-care diagnostic tools
4. Developments that enhance laboratory confirmation
5. Need for further investigation of new drugs and regimens for skin NTDs.

5. Wound and Lymphedema Management–Cross-Cutting Treatment

Despite the availability of different drugs for systemic treatment, the cross-cutting component in the management of a number of skin NTDs is wound (leprosy, Buruli ulcer, yaws, cutaneous leishmaniasis, tropical ulcers, etc.) and lymphedema (lymphatic filariasis and podoconiosis) management, which can be delivered potentially with the same knowledge, skills, and in the same settings. Integration of wound and lymphedema management for skin NTDs is already happening in the field. In many of the co-endemic areas, leprosy and Buruli ulcers are managed in the same facilities, as well as lymphatic filariasis and podoconiosis (Figure 2).

Wounds are among the most frequently encountered skin problems in rural settings in low- and middle-income countries, where skin NTDs are also endemic [53,61]. The causes can range from trauma, burns, bacterial infections as well as to non-communicable diseases such as diabetes and peripheral arterial diseases [53,61]. A large proportion of wounds are at risk of progressing to a chronic stage when not supported by proper diagnosis and wound care. Skills in evaluating the abnormal signs and symptoms, such as when to stop using topical antiseptics, when to suspect secondary infection, when to suspect malignant alteration, are skills that are lacking as there is limited training and the need for the expertise in wound care is not well recognized. A study conducted in Ghana and in Benin interviewing health care personnel dealing with the wound management of Buruli ulcer patients reported that standard of wound care differed greatly both between personnel and between institutions [62]. Limited accessibility to clean water can lead to prolonged secondary infection, as well as infrequent dressing changes due to poor availability of dressing materials and access to health facilities. Use of traditional medicines, and sometimes use of local folk treatments such as ash and toothpaste, hinder the normal wound healing process.

The most important component in wound management is achieving a clean wound bed with red granulation tissue, protected from infection and trauma [63,64]. Securing clean water to wash the wound surface regularly and thoroughly is the foremost priority; having normal saline solution is ideal, if not, tap water fit for drinking or cooled boiled water can be used for this purpose [65,66] (Figure 2). There is currently a wide range of wound dressing products designed for use in developed countries to keep the wound bed moist. They are often costly, although they may be useful if they shorten the wound healing time [67–70]. Nonetheless, there are good wound care techniques applicable in places where patients with ulcerative skin NTDs reside, using materials that are readily available, e.g., saline, vaseline [65]. The use of honey should not be dismissed although further assessment is needed [71]. Removal of necrotic tissue on the wound surface is another important component in wound management [63,64], which can be achieved through training of the local healthcare providers.

The main pillar in management of lymphedema is also based on hygiene—regular and thorough washing with soap and water—and skin care. A systematic review by Stocks et al., reported that participation in hygiene-based lymphedema management decreased the incidence of acute dermatolymphagioadenitis (ADLA) by one-third [72]. These inflammatory episodes, which are characterized by pain, fever, and swelling of the affected limb create a vicious cycle as they further erode lymphatic function stimulating more fibrosis and it is therefore important to prevent these [73]. Protecting the skin barrier function with simple emollients such as vaseline as well as limb exercise are also key to reducing inflammation and swelling [74,75].

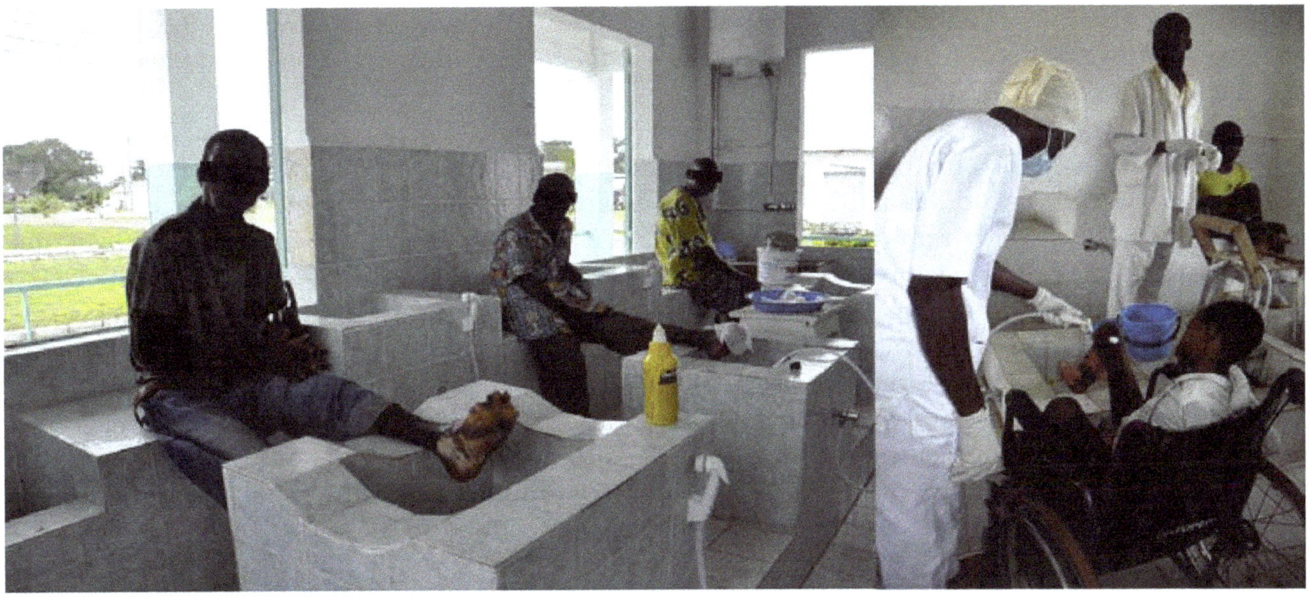

Figure 2. Wound care facility in Côte d'Ivoire for leprosy, Buruli ulcer, and other ulcers.

Studies investigating wound or lymphedema care in resource-limited settings are lacking. The severe impact a wound or a lymphedema can have on the quality of life of those affected is under-recognized [76–82]. Furthermore, findings from some cost analyses carried out in the developed world show a strikingly high cost burden [83,84], and this also needs to be assessed in resource-limited settings. There has been a recent study investigating the cost of wound care for cutaneous leishmaniasis in Afghanistan comparing different methods [85]. More studies of this kind will further improve the efficient management of skin NTDs. There are also other opportunities for integration between skin NTDs and chronic diseases, such as diabetes, in limb care or between other interventions such as clean water, better sanitation and hygiene (WASH) [77], which should be further explored.

Key points in wound and lymphedema management:

1. Implementation of a simple algorithm utilizing inexpensive and easily obtainable products for wound management/lymphedema management
2. Better use of those resources that are available in the local setting
3. Cost-analysis
4. Training and deployment of helpers including both local health care workers and "the expert patient".

6. Self-Morbidity Management to Improve Outcomes and Social Inclusion

Some skin NTDs, when diagnosed late, can lead to life-long disabilities and disfigurement. This may result from diseases with extensive ulceration or lymphedema as listed in the above section (Buruli ulcer, leprosy, tropical ulcers, lymphatic filariasis, podoconiosis, etc.) but there are other causes. For instance, ulceration, disabilities and deformities in a leprosy patient can also occur as a result of peripheral nerve damage—clawing toes, drop hands and feet, etc. Often patients with limb lesions from mycetoma are managed by amputation [80] as is the case with other severe forms of ulceration. Early identification and treatment can reduce this.

As outlined in the above section, the use of locally available methods and materials at low cost, which are also culturally accepted, are key in achieving a sustainable morbidity management program. A good example of this is a study by Narahari et al. in India, where the group developed an integrative treatment protocol for morbidity reduction of lymphatic filariasis by combining Ayurvedic exercises, compression therapy and modern dermatology drugs to treat bacterial entry points [77]. While the treatments for such conditions may include complex procedures such as lymphovascular shunts and debulking surgery, this integrative and non-invasive treatment, widely available in the local Indian settings was strikingly successful in reducing the volume of the limbs and also led to fewer episodes of ADLA.

In Ethiopia, integrated morbidity management for lymphatic filariasis and podoconiosis are in the process of implementation by the health ministry and partners, with some highly successful outcomes. Integration for leprosy and Buruli ulcer are already happening in the field, even in places where the national public health programs are still organized in a vertical pattern. As leprosy and Buruli ulcer share the same goal, which is prevention of disability (POD), the two diseases might be expected to benefit from synergies in management. It is of note that they also share similarities in diagnosis and treatment as the causative organisms come from the same mycobacterial disease group, and advocacy strategies have focused on more integration between the two [86].

As these skin NTDs are chronic, management of individual patients, including skin care and dressing or compression at home are critical in achieving success in treatment outcomes. A systematic review by Douglass et al., reported that intensity of training of patients in self-care practices and frequency of monitoring improved treatment outcomes [87], while similar findings were reported by Sathiaraj et al. for leprosy [88] (Figure 3).

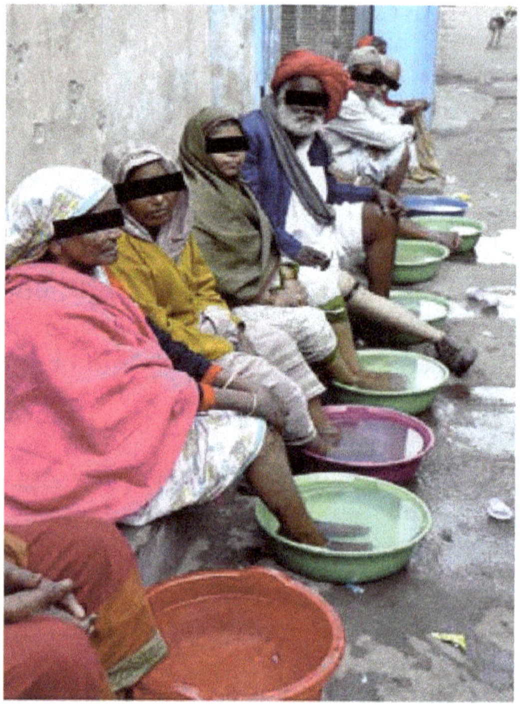

Figure 3. Education on self-skin care for prevention of disabilities (POD) for people affected by leprosy in a village in India.

Better treatment outcomes can be achieved when there is involvement of patients themselves and their carers. Self-care and carer assisted programs are also important in helping to reduce the work burden of local healthcare providers, as without these integrative techniques may even add to their work load. The success of Narahari et al. in their morbidity management for lymphatic filariasis was possible through recruiting patients accompanied by a family member willing to support self-care at home [77]. Carers must be willing and actively take part in the management of the family member, including support in dressing changes and skin care, relief of odor and pain, nourishment, helping with mobility, encouraging them to maintain adequate hygiene by bathing and, above all, making sure that they feel welcome in their society so that they can live full lives, marry, and achieve employment. [89]. As emphasized here, social inclusion is indeed another critical dimension in case management of skin NTDs, which can benefit from a synergized approach to skin NTD integration.

Key points in self-morbidity management to improve outcomes and social inclusion:

1. Use of locally available methods and materials at low cost
2. Patient training for self-care
3. Patient empowerment
4. Carer training
5. Interventions to promote social inclusion.

7. Training and Referrals

No disease control programs can be successful without good training of the local healthcare providers and workers, who are the closest to patients. This is certainly true for skin NTDs as clinical diagnosis remains the most readily available diagnostic measure and an important entry point for disease control of most skin NTDs. Most of the successful projects introduced here have been achieved through good and effective training. One of the major strategies deployed in the Ethiopian lymphatic filariasis-podoconiosis integrated program has been training, guideline development featuring a simple algorithm on clinical assessment, treatment and referral needs, and a defined care package [90]. This initiative also developed and rolled out a teaching video for healthcare workers on integrated morbidity management.

For integration, it is essential to provide suitable training for local healthcare providers on skin NTDs, as well as common skin diseases as these are more frequent and a better knowledge of these diseases will empower them. A well-trained healthcare provider who gains the confidence and acceptance of the population is key to achieving good results. In a study in Côte d'Ivoire during which we conducted screening of schoolchildren with skin NTDs, training was given with this consideration and it was effective in extending the program to a larger population with skilled local healthcare providers [12]. These healthcare providers perceived that the training was very helpful for their daily practices and their involvement in our project has been continuous. WHO and the expert panel group recently developed a training manual "Recognizing neglected tropical diseases through changes on the skin: a training guide for front-line health workers", which was developed with the vision to support such activities [91]. As the endemicity of diseases varies from one place to another, the document can be modified to be country/context-specific.

Along with capacity building at field level, clear referral pathways, e.g., for clinical consultation, referral for hospitalization, sending of samples to laboratories, etc. need to be established or strengthened to ensure better integrative management of skin NTDs, irrespective of disease type. We need to bear in mind that there is a wide range of skin diseases, other than skin NTDs, in which diagnosis are difficult, and some can even be fatal, e.g., acute infections, drug eruptions, and cutaneous malignancies. A study in Brazil where leprosy services have been decentralized has demonstrated the importance of referral centers in support of local health services in treating skin diseases [92].

With increasing availability and accessibility to mobile phones and internet, teledermatology is one way forward for establishing an adequate training, support and referral system. In a comprehensive project for mycetoma management in Sudan, a computer application on computer tablets or smartphones connected house-to-house survey medical teams, regional tertiary center, and experts at national level [80]. In Malawi and Ghana, a community-led SMS reporting tool for the rapid assessment of lymphatic filariasis morbidity burden was successful in involving community-based health surveillance workers/volunteers to participate in reporting and continuous monitoring of patients [93]. A similar approach could be established for other skin NTDs with respect to co-endemicity, and involvement of dermatologists will enable the approach. However, as there is a shortage of dermatologists in these settings, besides mobilization of local dermatologists, establishment of networks extending beyond the country may be necessary [94]. Two examples of such projects are described in this issue [95,96].

8. Next Steps

Integration of programs for skin NTDs is happening at national level. Some of the countries that have integrated their national public health programs for leprosy and Buruli ulcer include Benin, Cameroon, Congo Brazzaville, Gabon, Papua New Guinea and Togo; Nigeria combines leprosy, Buruli ulcer, and tuberculosis (TB). Some countries such as Côte d'Ivoire, Democratic Republic of Congo, and Ghana [86] still have separate control programs. However, these countries are also exploring integration of these skin NTDs, including yaws. Identifying the most appropriate combination of diseases, based on disease control measures and co-endemicity, is the key to successful integration.

Identifying opportunities beyond NTDs, such as integration with TB programs (DOTS), WASH, and non-communicable diseases (NCDs) may open a new door. Recent screening activities in Kiribati for NCDs and TB produced off-target results—identification of new leprosy cases. As the underlying risk factors for skin NTDs are poverty and poor hygiene, integration with poverty reduction programs should also be explored. A systematic review by Tomczyk et al. reported that access to footwear use significantly reduced the incidence of Buruli ulcer, cutaneous larva migrans, tungiasis, hookworm infection, soil-transmitted helminth infection, strongyloidiasis, and leptospirosis [97].

Whatever the case, attention needs to be paid to facilitating a reduction in the workload of front-line healthcare workers. Consideration is also needed as to how well any program can retain workers with skills needed in management of skin NTDs, to improve early detection and treatment outcomes, prevent or minimize disabilities, and ease the burden on governments and NGOs [86].

Establishment of expert working groups for guideline making, training materials, advocacy, etc. could facilitate this process. Recently, WHO and the working group on leprosy and yaws published guidelines for each disease [59,98]. An international alliance for the control of scabies (IACS) has been formed to advance collaboration [42,99]. Further research in the field demonstrating the burden of disease, and the effectiveness and synergies of control strategies, may increase the visibility of skin NTDs within the global health agenda and attract greater attention from international agencies and donors.

9. Conclusions

Many skin NTDs disproportionately affect the world's most disadvantaged people living in the low- and middle-income countries. They are often chronic in nature and may lead to chronic secondary conditions, including life-long disabilities and disfigurement, creating a vicious cycle for individuals, families, and society. Until recently, they were the most neglected among other NTDs as their disease control measures rely mostly on individual case management and any visible impact in the control achievements was limited. The present drive towards integration of skin NTDs together or with other programs has significant potential to reverse this limitation. There is a body of existing practice and field research for each disease among those interested in skin NTDs, which have the potential to further enhance the process of integration. There has also been new research on skin NTDs including approaches to integration that have had encouraging outcomes. It is essential that we build on these good practices and the lessons learned in order to formulate sound strategies for the shared goal of the fight against NTDs.

Acknowledgments: The author thanks the Côte d'Ivoire research team for our collaborative work which contributed to enrich the content of this article: National Leprosy Control Program Côte d'Ivoire, National Buruli Ulcer Control Program Côte d'Ivoire, Bamba Vagamon (Raoul Follereau Institute Côte d'Ivoire), Aubin Yao, Landry Koffi Kouadio (MAP International), Kouamé Kouadio, Aka N'Guetta, David Coulibaly N'Golo (Pasteur Institute Côte d'Ivoire), Julien Aké (Effect Hope), Konan N'Guessan (Sightsaver) and Amari Akpa. Thanks also goes to Daisuke Utsumi (Department of Dermatology, University of the Ryukyus, Okinawa, Japan) for his contribution in the wound management section through his experience in Kenya.

References

1. Hotez, P. *Forgotten People, Forgotten Diseases: The Neglected Tropical Diseaes and Their Impact on Global Health and Development*, 2nd ed.; ASM Press: Washington, DC, USA, 2013.
2. Department of Control of Neglected Tropical Diseases, WHO. *Neglected Tropical Diseases*; WHO: Geneva, Switzerland, 2018; Available online: http://www.who.int/neglected_diseases/diseases/en/ (accessed on 5 August 2018).
3. Eberhard, M.L.; Ruiz-Tiben, E.; Hopkins, D.R.; Farrell, C.; Toe, F.; Weiss, A.; Withers, P.C., Jr.; Jenks, M.H.; Thiele, E.A.; Cotton, J.A.; et al. The peculiar epidemiology of dracunculiasis in Chad. *Am. J. Trop. Med. Hyg.* **2014**, *90*, 61–70. [CrossRef] [PubMed]
4. Engelman, D.; Fuller, L.; Solomon, A.; McCarthy, J.; Hay, R.; Lammie, P.; Steer, A. Opportunities for integrated control of neglected tropical diseases that affect the skin. *Trends Parasitol.* **2016**, *32*, 843–854. [CrossRef] [PubMed]
5. Mitja, O.; Marks, M.; Bertran, L.; Kollie, K.; Argaw, D.; Fahal, A.H.; Fitzpatrick, C.; Fuller, L.C.; Garcia Izquierdo, B.; Hay, R.; et al. Integrated control and management of neglected tropical skin diseases. *PLoS Negl. Trop. Dis.* **2017**, *11*, e0005136. [CrossRef] [PubMed]
6. WHO. Eradication of yaws—The Morges strategy. *Wkly. Epidemiol. Rec.* **2012**, *87*, 189–194.
7. Abdulai, A.A.; Agana-Nsiire, P.; Biney, F.; Kwakye-Maclean, C.; Kyei-Faried, S.; Amponsa-Achiano, K.; Simpson, S.V.; Bonsu, G.; Ohene, S.A.; Ampofo, W.K.; et al. Community-based mass treatment with azithromycin for the elimination of yaws in Ghana-Results of a pilot study. *PLoS Negl. Trop. Dis.* **2018**, *12*, e0006303. [CrossRef] [PubMed]
8. Marks, M.; Mitja, O.; Bottomley, C.; Kwakye, C.; Houinei, W.; Bauri, M.; Adwere, P.; Abdulai, A.A.; Dua, F.; Boateng, L.; et al. Comparative efficacy of low-dose versus standard-dose azithromycin for patients with yaws: A randomised non-inferiority trial in Ghana and Papua New Guinea. *Lancet Glob. Health* **2018**, *6*, e401–e410. [CrossRef]
9. Mitja, O.; Godornes, C.; Houinei, W.; Kapa, A.; Paru, R.; Abel, H.; Gonzalez-Beiras, C.; Bieb, S.V.; Wangi, J.; Barry, A.E.; et al. Re-emergence of yaws after single mass azithromycin treatment followed by targeted treatment: A longitudinal study. *Lancet* **2018**, *391*, 1599–1607. [CrossRef]
10. Romani, L.; Whitfeld, M.J.; Koroivueta, J.; Kama, M.; Wand, H.; Tikoduadua, L.; Tuicakau, M.; Koroi, A.; Andrews, R.; Kaldor, J.M.; et al. Mass drug administration for scabies control in a population with endemic disease. *N. Engl. J. Med.* **2015**, *373*, 2305–2313. [CrossRef] [PubMed]
11. Elson, L.; Wright, K.; Swift, J.; Feldmeier, H. Control of tungiasis in absence of a roadmap: Grassroots and global approaches. *Trop. Med. Infect. Dis.* **2017**, *2*, 33. [CrossRef] [PubMed]
12. Yotsu, R.R.; Kouadio, K.; Vagamon, B.; N'Guessan, K.; Akpa, A.J.; Yao, A.; Ake, J.; Abbet Abbet, R.; Tchamba Agbor Agbor, B.; Bedimo, R.; et al. Skin disease prevalence study in schoolchildren in rural Cote d'Ivoire: Implications for integration of neglected skin diseases (skin NTDs). *PLoS Negl. Trop. Dis.* **2018**, *12*, e0006489. [CrossRef] [PubMed]
13. Atre, S.R.; Rangan, S.G.; Shetty, V.P.; Gaikwad, N.; Mistry, N.F. Perceptions, health seeking behaviour and access to diagnosis and treatment initiation among previously undetected leprosy cases in rural Maharashtra, India. *Lepr. Rev.* **2011**, *82*, 222–234. [PubMed]
14. Nicholls, P.G.; Chhina, N.; Bro, A.K.; Barkataki, P.; Kumar, R.; Withington, S.G.; Smith, W.C. Factors contributing to delay in diagnosis and start of treatment of leprosy: Analysis of help-seeking narratives in northern Bangladesh and in West Bengal, India. *Lepr. Rev.* **2005**, *76*, 35–47. [PubMed]
15. Mulder, A.A.; Boerma, R.P.; Barogui, Y.; Zinsou, C.; Johnson, R.C.; Gbovi, J.; van der Werf, T.S.; Stienstra, Y. Healthcare seeking behaviour for Buruli ulcer in Benin: A model to capture therapy choice of patients and healthy community members. *Trans. R. Soc. Trop. Med. Hyg.* **2008**, *102*, 912–920. [CrossRef] [PubMed]
16. Aujoulat, I.; Johnson, C.; Zinsou, C.; Guedenon, A.; Portaels, F. Psychosocial aspects of health seeking behaviours of patients with Buruli ulcer in southern Benin. *Trop. Med. Int. Health* **2003**, *8*, 750–759. [CrossRef] [PubMed]

17. Stienstra, Y.; van der Graaf, W.T.; Asamoa, K.; van der Werf, T.S. Beliefs and attitudes toward Buruli ulcer in Ghana. *Am. J. Trop. Med. Hyg.* **2002**, *67*, 207–213. [CrossRef] [PubMed]
18. Shetty, V.P.; Pandya, S.S.; Arora, S.; Capadia, G.D. Observations from a 'special selective drive' conducted under National Leprosy Elimination Programme in Karjat taluka and Gadchiroli district of Maharashtra. *Indian J. Lepr.* **2009**, *81*, 189–193. [PubMed]
19. Daulako, E.C. Population screening and mass chemoprophylaxis in Kiribati. *Int. J. Lepr. Mycobact. Dis.* **1999**, *67*, S23–S25.
20. Diletto, C. Elimination of leprosy in the federated states of micronesia by intensive case finding, treatment with WHO/MDT and administration of chemoprophylaxis. *Int. J. Lepr. Mycobact. Dis.* **1999**, *67*, S10–S13.
21. Tin, K. Population screening and chemoprophylaxis for household contacts of leprosy patients in the Republic of the Marshall Islands. *Int. J. Lepr. Mycobact. Dis.* **1999**, *67*, S26–S29.
22. Msyamboza, K.P.; Mawaya, L.R.; Kubwalo, H.W.; Ng'oma, D.; Liabunya, M.; Manjolo, S.; Msiska, P.P.; Somba, W.W. Burden of leprosy in Malawi: Community camp-based cross-sectional study. *BMC Int. Health Hum. Rights* **2012**, *12*, 12. [CrossRef] [PubMed]
23. Nsagha, D.S.; Bamgboye, E.A.; Yediran, A.B.O.O. Childhood leprosy in Essimbiland of Cameroon: Results of chart review and school survey. *Niger. Q. J. Hosp. Med.* **2009**, *19*, 214–219. [CrossRef]
24. Baretto, J.G.; Guimarães, L.D.S.; Frade, M.A.C.; Rosa, P.S.; Salgado, C.G. High rates of undiagnosed leprosy and subclinical infection amongst school children in the Amazon Region. *Mem. Inst. Oswaldo Cruz* **2012**, *107*, 60–67. [CrossRef]
25. WHO. Brazilian School-Based Deworming and Leprosy Case-Finding Campaign Targets More Than 9 Million Chilren. Available online: http://www.who.int/neglected_diseases/brazil_leprosy_sth_2013/en/ (accessed on 20 August 2018).
26. Saikawa, K. Epidemiological implications of school survey in Okinawa (in Japanese). *J. Health Welf. Stat.* **1978**, *25*, 6–23.
27. UmBoock, A.; Awah, P.K.; Mou, F.; Nichter, M. Yaws resurgence in Bankim, Cameroon: The relative effectiveness of different means of detection in rural communities. *PLoS Negl. Trop. Dis.* **2017**, *11*, e0005557. [CrossRef]
28. Ogunbiyi, A.O.; Owoaje, E.; Ndahi, A. Prevalence of skin disorders in school children in Ibadan, Nigeria. *Pediatr. Dermatol.* **2005**, *22*, 6–10. [CrossRef] [PubMed]
29. Hogewoning, A.; Amoah, A.; Bavinck, J.N.; Boakye, D.; Yazdanbakhsh, M.; Adegnika, A.; De Smedt, S.; Fonteyne, Y.; Willemze, R.; Lavrijsen, A. Skin diseases among schoolchildren in Ghana, Gabon, and Rwanda. *Int. J. Dermatol.* **2013**, *52*, 589–600. [CrossRef] [PubMed]
30. Mahe, A.; Prual, A.; Konate, M.; Bobin, P. Skin diseases of children in Mali: A public health problem. *Trans. R. Soc. Trop. Med. Hyg.* **1995**, *89*, 467–470. [CrossRef]
31. Komba, E.V.; Mgonda, Y.M. The spectrum of dermatological disorders among primary school children in Dar es Salaam. *BMC Public Health* **2010**, *10*, 765. [CrossRef] [PubMed]
32. Figueroa, J.I.; Fuller, L.C.; Abraha, A.; Hay, R.J. The prevalence of skin disease among school children in rural Ethiopia—A preliminary assessment of dermatologic needs. *Pediatr. Dermatol.* **1996**, *13*, 378–381. [CrossRef] [PubMed]
33. Murgia, V.; Bilcha, K.D.; Shibeshi, D. Community dermatology in Debre Markos: An attempt to define children's dermatological needs in a rural area of Ethiopia. *Int. J. Dermatol.* **2010**, *49*, 666–671. [CrossRef] [PubMed]
34. Mitja, O.; Houinei, W.; Moses, P.; Kapa, A.; Paru, R.; Hays, R.; Lukehart, S.; Godornes, C.; Bieb, S.V.; Grice, T.; et al. Mass treatment with single-dose azithromycin for yaws. *N. Engl. J. Med.* **2015**, *372*, 703–710. [CrossRef] [PubMed]
35. Lawrence, G.; Leafasia, J.; Sheridan, J.; Hills, S.; Wate, J.; Wate, C.; Montgomery, J.; Pandeya, N.; Purdie, D. Control of scabies, skin sores and haematuria in children in the Solomon Islands: Another role for ivermectin. *Bull. World Health Organ.* **2005**, *83*, 34–42.
36. Kearns, T.M.; Speare, R.; Cheng, A.C.; McCarthy, J.; Carapetis, J.R.; Holt, D.C.; Currie, B.J.; Page, W.; Shield, J.; Gundjirryirr, R.; et al. Impact of an ivermectin mass drug administration on scabies prevalence in a remote australian aboriginal community. *PLoS Negl. Trop. Dis.* **2015**, *9*, e0004151. [CrossRef] [PubMed]

37. Mason, D.S.; Marks, M.; Sokana, O.; Solomon, A.W.; Mabey, D.C.; Romani, L.; Kaldor, J.; Steer, A.C.; Engelman, D. The prevalence of scabies and impetigo in the Solomon islands: a population-based survey. *PLoS Negl. Trop. Dis.* **2016**, *10*, e0004803. [CrossRef] [PubMed]
38. Heukelbach, J.; Winter, B.; Wilcke, T.; Muehlen, M.; Albrecht, S.; de Oliveira, F.A.; Kerr-Pontes, L.R.; Liesenfeld, O.; Feldmeier, H. Selective mass treatment with ivermectin to control intestinal helminthiases and parasitic skin diseases in a severely affected population. *Bull. World Health Organ.* **2004**, *82*, 563–571.
39. Krotneva, S.P.; Coffeng, L.E.; Noma, M.; Zoure, H.G.; Bakone, L.; Amazigo, U.V.; de Vlas, S.J.; Stolk, W.A. African program for onchocerciasis control 1995–2010: Impact of annual ivermectin mass treatment on off-target infectious diseases. *PLoS Negl. Trop. Dis.* **2015**, *9*, e0004051. [CrossRef] [PubMed]
40. Ottesen, E.A.; Hooper, P.J.; Bradley, M.; Biswas, G. The global programme to eliminate lymphatic filariasis: Health impact after 8 years. *PLoS Negl. Trop. Dis.* **2008**, *2*, e317. [CrossRef] [PubMed]
41. Thomsen, E.K.; Sanuku, N.; Baea, M.; Satofan, S.; Maki, E.; Lombore, B.; Schmidt, M.S.; Siba, P.M.; Weil, G.J.; Kazura, J.W.; et al. Efficacy, safety, and pharmacokinetics of coadministered diethylcarbamazine, albendazole, and ivermectin for treatment of bancroftian filariasis. *Clin. Infect. Dis.* **2016**, *62*, 334–341. [CrossRef] [PubMed]
42. Engelman, D.; Kiang, K.; Chosidow, O.; McCarthy, J.; Fuller, C.; Lammie, P.; Hay, R.; Steer, A.; Members of the International Alliance for the Control of Scabies. Toward the global control of human scabies: Introducing the International Alliance for the Control of Scabies. *PLoS Negl. Trop. Dis.* **2013**, *7*, e2167. [CrossRef] [PubMed]
43. Mounsey, K.E.; Bernigaud, C.; Chosidow, O.; McCarthy, J.S. Prospects for moxidectin as a new oral treatment for human scabies. *PLoS Negl. Trop. Dis.* **2016**, *10*, e0004389. [CrossRef] [PubMed]
44. Mounsey, K.E.; Walton, S.F.; Innes, A.; Cash-Deans, S.; McCarthy, J.S. In vitro efficacy of moxidectin versus Ivermectin against *Sarcoptes scabiei*. *Antimicrob. Agents Chemother.* **2017**, *61*, e00381-17. [CrossRef] [PubMed]
45. Administration, U.S.F.A.D. Drugs@FDA: FDA Approved Drug Products. 2018. Available online: https://www.accessdata.fda.gov/scripts/cder/daf/index.cfm?event=BasicSearch.process (accessed on 31 August 2018).
46. Moet, F.J.; Pahan, D.; Oskam, L.; Richardus, J.H.; Group, C.S. Effectiveness of single dose rifampicin in preventing leprosy in close contacts of patients with newly diagnosed leprosy: Cluster randomised controlled trial. *BMJ* **2008**, *336*, 761–764. [CrossRef] [PubMed]
47. Feenstra, S.G.; Pahan, D.; Moet, F.J.; Oskam, L.; Richardus, J.H. Patient-related factors predicting the effectiveness of rifampicin chemoprophylaxis in contacts: 6 year follow up of the COLEP cohort in Bangladesh. *Lepr. Rev.* **2012**, *83*, 292–304. [PubMed]
48. Bakker, M.I.; Hatta, M.; Kwenang, A.; Van Benthem, B.H.; Van Beers, S.M.; Klatser, P.R.; Oskam, L. Prevention of leprosy using rifampicin as chemoprophylaxis. *Am. J. Trop. Med. Hyg.* **2005**, *72*, 443–448. [CrossRef] [PubMed]
49. WHO. Global leprosy update, 2016: Accelerating reduction of disease burden. *Wkly. Epidemiol. Rec.* **2017**, *35*, 501–520.
50. Tiwari, A.; Dandel, S.; Djupuri, R.; Mieras, L.; Richardus, J.H. Population-wide administration of single dose rifampicin for leprosy prevention in isolated communities: A three year follow-up feasibility study in Indonesia. *BMC Infect. Dis.* **2018**, *18*, 324. [CrossRef] [PubMed]
51. Barth-Jaeggi, T.; Steinmann, P.; Mieras, L.; van Brakel, W.; Richardus, J.H.; Tiwari, A.; Bratschi, M.; Cavaliero, A.; Vander Plaetse, B.; Mirza, F.; et al. Leprosy Post-Exposure Prophylaxis (LPEP) programme: Study protocol for evaluating the feasibility and impact on case detection rates of contact tracing and single dose rifampicin. *BMJ Open* **2016**, *6*, e013633. [CrossRef] [PubMed]
52. Steinmann, P.; Cavaliero, A.; Aerts, A.; Anand, S.; Arif, M.; Ay, S.S.; Aye, T.M.; Barth-Jaeggi, T.; Banstola, N.L.; Bhandari, C.M.; et al. The Leprosy Post-Exposure Prophylaxis (LPEP) programme: Update and interim analysis. *Lepr. Rev.* **2018**, *89*, 102–116.
53. Toutous Trellu, L.; Nkemenang, P.; Comte, E.; Ehounou, G.; Atangana, P.; Mboua, D.J.; Rusch, B.; Njih Tabah, E.; Etard, J.F.; Mueller, Y.K. Differential diagnosis of skin ulcers in a *Mycobacterium ulcerans* endemic area: Data from a prospective study in cameroon. *PLoS Negl. Trop. Dis.* **2016**, *10*, e0004385. [CrossRef] [PubMed]

54. Nguetta, A.; Coulibaly, N.D.; Kouamé-Elogne, N.C.; Acquah, K.J.R.; Christiane, A.A.; Kouamé, K.; N'Guessan, K.; Aboa, K.; Aubin, Y. Phenotypic and genotypic characterization of mycobacteria isolates from Buruli ulcer suspected patients reveals the involvement of several mycobacteria in chronic skin lesions. *Am. J. Microbiol. Res.* **2018**, *6*, 79–87. [CrossRef]
55. Ablordey, A.; Amissah, D.A.; Aboagye, I.F.; Hatano, B.; Yamazaki, T.; Sata, T.; Ishikawa, K.; Katano, H. Detection of *Mycobacterium ulcerans* by the loop mediated isothermal amplification method. *PLoS Negl. Trop. Dis.* **2012**, *6*, e1590. [CrossRef] [PubMed]
56. Beissner, M.; Phillips, R.O.; Battke, F.; Bauer, M.; Badziklou, K.; Sarfo, F.S.; Maman, I.; Rhomberg, A.; Piten, E.; Frimpong, M.; et al. Loop-mediated isothermal amplification for laboratory confirmation of buruli ulcer disease-towards a point-of-care test. *PLoS Negl. Trop. Dis.* **2015**, *9*, e0004219. [CrossRef] [PubMed]
57. Wadagni, A.; Frimpong, M.; Phanzu, D.M.; Ablordey, A.; Kacou, E.; Gbedevi, M.; Marion, E.; Xing, Y.; Babu, V.S.; Phillips, R.O.; et al. Simple, rapid *Mycobacterium ulcerans* disease diagnosis from clinical samples by fluorescence of mycolactone on thin layer chromatography. *PLoS Negl. Trop. Dis.* **2015**, *9*, e0004247. [CrossRef] [PubMed]
58. Dreyer, A.; Roltgen, K.; Dangy, J.P.; Ruf, M.T.; Scherr, N.; Bolz, M.; Tobias, N.J.; Moes, C.; Vettiger, A.; Stinear, T.P.; et al. Identification of the Mycobacterium ulcerans protein MUL_3720 as a promising target for the development of a diagnostic test for Buruli ulcer. *PLoS Negl. Trop. Dis.* **2015**, *9*, e0003477. [CrossRef] [PubMed]
59. WHO. *Eradication of Yaws: A Guide for Programme Managers*; WHO: Geneva, Switzerland, 2018.
60. Yotsu, R.; Richardson, M.; Ishii, N. *Drugs for Treating Buruli Ulcer*; Cochrane Systematic Review: London, UK, 2018.
61. Ryan, T.J. Public health dermatology: Regeneration and repair of the skin in the developed transitional and developing world. *Int. J. Dermatol.* **2006**, *45*, 1233–1237. [CrossRef] [PubMed]
62. Velding, K.; Klis, S.A.; Abass, K.M.; Tuah, W.; Stienstra, Y.; van der Werf, T. Wound care in Buruli ulcer disease in Ghana and Benin. *Am. J. Trop. Med. Hyg.* **2014**, *91*, 313–318. [CrossRef] [PubMed]
63. Attinger, C.E.; Janis, J.E.; Steinberg, J.; Schwartz, J.; Al-Attar, A.; Couch, K. Clinical approach to wounds: Debridement and wound bed preparation including the use of dressings and wound-healing adjuvants. *Plast. Reconstr. Surg.* **2006**, *117*, 72s–109s. [CrossRef] [PubMed]
64. Lee, J.C.; Kandula, S.; Sherber, N.S. Beyond wet-to-dry: A rational approach to treating chronic wounds. *Eplasty* **2009**, *9*, e14. [PubMed]
65. Fernandez, R.; Griffiths, R. Water for wound cleansing. *Cochrane Database Syst. Rev.* **2012**. [CrossRef] [PubMed]
66. Cooper, D.D.; Seupaul, R.A. Is water effective for wound cleansing? *Ann. Emerg. Med.* **2012**, *60*, 626–627. [CrossRef] [PubMed]
67. Anandan, V.; Jameela, W.A.; Saraswathy, P.; Sarankumar, S. Platelet rich plasma: Efficacy in treating trophic ulcers in leprosy. *J. Clin. Diagn. Res.* **2016**, *10*, WC06–WC09. [CrossRef] [PubMed]
68. Conde-Montero, E.; Horcajada-Reales, C.; Clavo, P.; Delgado-Sillero, I.; Suarez-Fernandez, R. Neuropathic ulcers in leprosy treated with intralesional platelet-rich plasma. *Int. Wound J.* **2016**, *13*, 726–728. [CrossRef] [PubMed]
69. Murase, C.; Kono, M.; Nakanaga, K.; Ishii, N.; Akiyama, M. Buruli ulcer successfully treated with negative-pressure wound therapy. *JAMA Dermatol.* **2015**, *151*, 1137–1139. [CrossRef] [PubMed]
70. Jebran, A.F.; Schleicher, U.; Steiner, R.; Wentker, P.; Mahfuz, F.; Stahl, H.C.; Amin, F.M.; Bogdan, C.; Stahl, K.W. Rapid healing of cutaneous leishmaniasis by high-frequency electrocauterization and hydrogel wound care with or without DAC N-055: A randomized controlled phase IIa trial in Kabul. *PLoS Negl. Trop. Dis.* **2014**, *8*, e2694. [CrossRef] [PubMed]
71. Jull, A.B.; Walker, N.; Deshpande, S. Honey as a topical treatment for wounds. *Cochrane Database Syst. Rev.* **2013**. [CrossRef]
72. Stocks, M.E.; Freeman, M.C.; Addiss, D.G. The effect of hygiene-based lymphedema management in lymphatic filariasis-endemic areas: A systematic review and meta-analysis. *PLoS Negl. Trop. Dis.* **2015**, *9*, e0004171. [CrossRef] [PubMed]
73. Dreyer, G.; Medeiros, Z.; Netto, M.J.; Leal, N.C.; de Castro, L.G.; Piessens, W.F. Acute attacks in the extremities of persons living in an area endemic for bancroftian filariasis: Differentiation of two syndromes. *Trans. Roy. Soc. Trop. Med. Hyg.* **1999**, *93*, 413–417. [CrossRef]

74. Brooks, J.; Ersser, S.J.; Cowdell, F.; Gardiner, E.; Mengistu, A.; Matts, P.J. A randomized controlled trial to evaluate the effect of a new skincare regimen on skin barrier function in those with podoconiosis in Ethiopia. *Br. J. Dermatol.* **2017**, *177*, 1422–1431. [CrossRef] [PubMed]
75. Negussie, H.; Molla, M.; Ngari, M.; Berkley, J.A.; Kivaya, E.; Njuguna, P.; Fegan, G.; Tamiru, A.; Kelemework, A.; Lang, T.; et al. Lymphoedema management to prevent acute dermatolymphangioadenitis in podoconiosis in northern Ethiopia (GoLBeT): A pragmatic randomised controlled trial. *Lancet Glob. Health* **2018**, *6*, e795–e803. [CrossRef]
76. Effah, A.; Ersser, S.J.; Hemingway, A. Support needs of people living with *Mycobacterium ulcerans* (Buruli ulcer) disease in a Ghana rural community: A grounded theory study. *Int. J. Dermatol.* **2017**, *56*, 1432–1437. [CrossRef] [PubMed]
77. Narahari, S.R.; Bose, K.S.; Aggithaya, M.G.; Swamy, G.K.; Ryan, T.J.; Unnikrishnan, B.; Washington, R.G.; Rao, B.P.; Rajagopala, S.; Manjula, K.; et al. Community level morbidity control of lymphoedema using self care and integrative treatment in two lymphatic filariasis endemic districts of South India: A non randomized interventional study. *Trans. R. Soc. Trop. Med. Hyg.* **2013**, *107*, 566–577. [CrossRef] [PubMed]
78. Bartlett, J.; Deribe, K.; Tamiru, A.; Amberbir, T.; Medhin, G.; Malik, M.; Hanlon, C.; Davey, G. Depression and disability in people with podoconiosis: A comparative cross-sectional study in rural Northern Ethiopia. *Int. Health* **2016**, *8*, 124–131. [CrossRef] [PubMed]
79. Bennis, I.; De Brouwere, V.; Belrhiti, Z.; Sahibi, H.; Boelaert, M. Psychosocial burden of localised cutaneous Leishmaniasis: A scoping review. *BMC Public Health* **2018**, *18*, 358. [CrossRef] [PubMed]
80. Bakhiet, S.M.; Fahal, A.H.; Musa, A.M.; Mohamed, E.S.W.; Omer, R.F.; Ahmed, E.S.; El Nour, M.; Mustafa, E.R.M.; Sheikh, A.R.M.E.; Suliman, S.H.; et al. A holistic approach to the mycetoma management. *PLoS Negl. Trop. Dis.* **2018**, *12*, e0006391. [CrossRef] [PubMed]
81. Wiese, S.; Elson, L.; Feldmeier, H. Tungiasis-related life quality impairment in children living in rural Kenya. *PLoS Negl. Trop. Dis.* **2018**, *12*, e0005939. [CrossRef] [PubMed]
82. Walker, S.L.; Lebas, E.; De Sario, V.; Deyasso, Z.; Doni, S.N.; Marks, M.; Roberts, C.H.; Lambert, S.M. The prevalence and association with health-related quality of life of tungiasis and scabies in schoolchildren in southern Ethiopia. *PLoS Negl. Trop. Dis.* **2017**, *11*, e0005808. [CrossRef] [PubMed]
83. Guest, J.F.; Ayoub, N.; McIlwraith, T.; Uchegbu, I.; Gerrish, A.; Weidlich, D.; Vowden, K.; Vowden, P. Health economic burden that different wound types impose on the UK's National Health Service. *Int. Wound J.* **2017**, *14*, 322–330. [CrossRef] [PubMed]
84. Tchero, H.; Kangambega, P.; Lin, L.; Mukisi-Mukaza, M.; Brunet-Houdard, S.; Briatte, C.; Retali, G.R.; Rusch, E. Cost of diabetic foot in France, Spain, Italy, Germany and United Kingdom: A systematic review. *Ann. Endocrinol.* **2018**, *79*, 67–74. [CrossRef] [PubMed]
85. Stahl, H.C.; Ahmadi, F.; Nahzat, S.M.; Dong, H.J.; Stahl, K.W.; Sauerborn, R. Health economic evaluation of moist wound care in chronic cutaneous leishmaniasis ulcers in Afghanistan. *Infect. Dis. Poverty* **2018**, *7*, 12. [CrossRef] [PubMed]
86. Walsh, D.S.; De Jong, B.C.; Meyers, W.M.; Portaels, F. Leprosy and Buruli ulcer: Similarities suggest combining control and prevention of disability strategies in countries endemic for both diseases. *Lepr. Rev.* **2015**, *86*, 1–5. [PubMed]
87. Douglass, J.; Graves, P.; Gordon, S. Self-care for management of secondary lymphedema: A systematic review. *PLoS Negl. Trop. Dis.* **2016**, *10*, e0004740. [CrossRef] [PubMed]
88. Sathiaraj, Y.; Norman, G.; Richard, J. Long term sustainability and efficacy of self-care education on knowledge and practice of wound prevention and management among leprosy patients. *Indian J. Lepr.* **2010**, *82*, 79–83. [PubMed]
89. Ryan, T. Wound healing in the developing world. *Dermatol. Clin.* **1993**, *11*, 791–800. [CrossRef]
90. Deribe, K.; Kebede, B.; Tamiru, M.; Mengistu, B.; Kebede, F.; Martindale, S.; Sime, H.; Mulugeta, A.; Kebede, B.; Sileshi, M.; et al. Integrated morbidity management for lymphatic filariasis and podoconiosis, Ethiopia. *Bull. World Health Organ.* **2017**, *95*, 652–656. [CrossRef] [PubMed]
91. WHO. *Recognizing Neglected Tropical Diseases through Changes on the Skin: A Training Guide for Front-Line Health Workers*; WHO: Geneva, Switzerland, 2018.
92. Barbieri, R.R.; Sales, A.M.; Hacker, M.A.; Nery, J.A.; Duppre, N.C.; Machado, A.M.; Moraes, M.O.; Sarno, E.N. Impact of a reference center on leprosy control under a decentralized public health care policy in Brazil. *PLoS Negl. Trop. Dis.* **2016**, *10*, e0005059. [CrossRef] [PubMed]

93. Stanton, M.C.; Mkwanda, S.Z.; Debrah, A.Y.; Batsa, L.; Biritwum, N.K.; Hoerauf, A.; Cliffe, M.; Best, A.; Molineux, A.; Kelly-Hope, L.A. Developing a community-led SMS reporting tool for the rapid assessment of lymphatic filariasis morbidity burden: Case studies from Malawi and Ghana. *BMC Infect. Dis.* **2015**, *15*, 214. [CrossRef] [PubMed]
94. Hay, R.; Estrada, R.; Grossmann, H. Managing skin disease in resource-poor environments—The role of community-oriented training and control programs. *Int. J. Dermatol.* **2011**, *50*, 558–563. [CrossRef] [PubMed]
95. Faye, O.; Bagayoko, C.O.; Dicko, A.; Ciseé, L.; Berthé, S.; Traoré, B.; Fofana, Y.; Niang, M.; Traoré, S.T.; Karabinta, Y.; et al. A teledermatology pilot programme for the management of skin diseases in primary health care centres: Experiences from a Resource-Limited Country (Mali, West Africa). *Trop. Med. Infect. Dis.* **2018**, *3*, 88. [CrossRef] [PubMed]
96. Mieras, L.F.; Taal, A.T.; Post, E.B.; Ndeve, A.G.Z.; van Hees, C.L.M. The development of a mobile application to support peripheral health workers to diagnose and treat people with skin diseases in resource-poor settings. *Trop. Med. Infect. Dis.* **2018**, *3*, 102. [CrossRef] [PubMed]
97. Tomczyk, S.; Deribe, K.; Brooker, S.J.; Clark, H.; Rafique, K.; Knopp, S.; Utzinger, J.; Davey, G. Association between footwear use and neglected tropical diseases: A systematic review and meta-analysis. *PLoS Negl. Trop. Dis.* **2014**, *8*, e3285. [CrossRef] [PubMed]
98. WHO. *Guidelines for the Diagnosis, Treatment and Prevention of Leprosy*; WHO, Regional Office for South-East Asia: New Delhi, India, 2018.
99. Engelman, D.; Fuller, L.C.; Steer, A.C.; International Alliance for the Control of Scabies. Consensus criteria for the diagnosis of scabies: A Delphi study of international experts. *PLoS Negl. Trop. Dis.* **2018**, *12*, e0006549. [CrossRef] [PubMed]

15

Preliminary Characterization of Triatomine Bug Blood Meals on the Island of Trinidad Reveals Opportunistic Feeding Behavior on Both Human and Animal Hosts

Alexandra Hylton [1,2,3], Daniel M. Fitzpatrick [2], Rod Suepaul [4], Andrew P. Dobson [1], Roxanne A. Charles [4] and Jennifer K. Peterson [1,5,*]

1 Department of Ecology and Evolutionary Biology, Princeton University, Princeton, NJ 08544, USA; aeeakes@gmail.com (A.H.); dobson@princeton.edu (A.P.D.)
2 Department of Pathobiology, School of Veterinary Medicine, St. George's University, True Blue, Grenada; dfitzpat@sgu.edu
3 College of Medicine, University of Oklahoma, Oklahoma City, OK 73117, USA
4 Department of Basic Veterinary Sciences, School of Veterinary Medicine, Faculty of Medical Sciences, The University of the West Indies, Trinidad and Tobago, West Indies; Rod.Suepaul@sta.uwi.edu (R.S.); Roxanne.Charles@sta.uwi.edu (R.A.C.)
5 University Honors College, Portland State University, Portland, OR 97207-075, USA
* Correspondence: jenni.peterson@gmail.com

Abstract: Chagas disease is a neglected tropical disease caused by infection with *Trypanosoma cruzi*. The parasite is endemic to the Americas, including the Caribbean, where it is vectored by triatomine bugs. Although Chagas disease is not considered a public health concern in the Caribbean islands, studies in Trinidad have found *T. cruzi*-seropositive humans and *T. cruzi*-infected triatomine bugs. However, little is known about triatomine bug host preferences in Trinidad, making it difficult to evaluate local risk of vector-borne *T. cruzi* transmission to humans. To investigate this question, we collected triatomine bugs in Trinidad and diagnosed each one for *T. cruzi* infection (microscopy and PCR). We then carried out a blood meal analysis using DNA extracted from each bug (PCR and sequencing). Fifty-five adult bugs (54 *Panstrongylus geniculatus* and one *Rhodnius pictipes*) were collected from five of 21 sample sites. All successful collection sites were residential. Forty-six out of the 55 bugs (83.6%) were infected with *T. cruzi*. Fifty-three blood meal hosts were successfully analyzed (one per bug), which consisted of wild birds (7% of all blood meals), wild mammals (17%), chickens (19%), and humans (57%). Of the 30 bugs with human blood meals, 26 (87%) were from bugs infected with *T. cruzi*. Although preliminary, our results align with previous work in which *P. geniculatus* in Trinidad had high levels of *T. cruzi* infection. Furthermore, our findings suggest that *P. geniculatus* moves between human and animal environments in Trinidad, feeding opportunistically on a wide range of species. Our findings highlight a critical need for further studies of Chagas disease in Trinidad in order to estimate the public health risk and implement necessary preventative and control measures.

Keywords: chagas disease; *Trypanosoma cruzi*; triatomine bugs; *Panstrongylus geniculatus*; *Rhodnius pictipes*; Trinidad and Tobago; West Indies; vector host-feeding preferences; blood meal analysis

---

1. Introduction

Chagas disease (American trypanosomiasis) is a neglected tropical disease (NTD) caused by infection with the protozoan parasite *Trypanosoma cruzi*. Symptoms of the disease include cardiac, gastrointestinal, and/or neurological alterations. An estimated six million people are currently infected with *T. cruzi*, with 25 million more at risk [1].

T. cruzi is endemic to the Americas, where it cycles between mammalian hosts and triatomine bug vectors. Vector-borne *T. cruzi* transmission to humans can occur via contact with infected triatomine excrement during or after the bug takes a blood meal, or orally, through ingestion of *T. cruzi*-contaminated food or beverages [2–5]. Food or beverage contamination with *T. cruzi* can occur in a number of ways, but most commonly an infected bug either falls into or defecates on the food. Other human *T. cruzi* infection routes include contaminated blood transfusions or organ transplants, transplacental transmission, and laboratory accidents [1].

Triatomine bugs acquire *T. cruzi* infection by taking blood meals from infected mammals in sylvatic or domestic/peridomestic transmission cycles. These transmission cycles can be connected, especially in disturbed or fragmented habitats [6], by triatomines that forage opportunistically in both their sylvatic habitats and nearby residential areas, including human homes [7,8]. Due to the existence of distinct *T. cruzi* transmission cycles, the presence of triatomine bugs in a region does not necessarily mean that the region is Chagas-endemic. Such is the case in the Caribbean islands, where triatomine bugs are widely distributed [9], but believed to be primarily sylvatic, making infrequent contact with humans [9–11]. Although *T. cruzi*-positive serology in humans has been reported in at least three Caribbean islands (Curacao, Jamaica, and Trinidad [9,12–14]), there have been few diagnosed clinical cases. As such, Chagas disease is not recognized by major public or global health organizations as endemic to any Caribbean island [10,15].

Of particular interest for Chagas disease in the Caribbean is the island of Trinidad, of the dual-island Republic of Trinidad and Tobago. Trinidad has geological origins on the continental shelf of South America [16], and shares much of its flora and fauna with Chagas-endemic, neighboring Venezuela (located just eight miles west of Trinidad, Figure 1). Included in the fauna found in both Trinidad and Venezuela are six triatomine bug species: *Eratyrus mucronatus*, *Microtriatoma trinidadensis*, *Rhodnius pictipes*, *Panstrongylus geniculatus*, *Panstrongylus rufotuberculatus*, and *Triatoma rubrofasciata* [17–19]. All species are competent vectors of *T. cruzi* [11], but *P. geniculatus* is believed to be the most abundant [17], and of the highest epidemiological importance [3,20–24].

Although there are only a few studies of Chagas disease in Trinidad, they provide compelling evidence that *T. cruzi* may not be strictly enzootic on the island. Cardiologist Boris Fistein first suspected that Chagas disease was endemic to the island in the early 1960s, when he observed the clinical picture of the disease in several patients with congestive heart failure not attributable to common causes [12,13]. Fistein found that some of these patients were seropositive for *T. cruzi* [12,13,25], and a follow-up study of the vector yielded 79 triatomine bugs collected in and around the patients' homes. Of 69 bugs examined, 35 (50.72%) were infected with *T. cruzi* [25]. A later study of sera collected from venereal disease clinics and antenatal clinics (meant to represent the general population) found a *T. cruzi* seroprevalence of 0.45% [12]. Several years later, a larger study of triatomines in Trinidad yielded the same species infected with *T. cruzi* distributed widely throughout the island [17]. Finally, in a 1992 serological survey of 192 cardiac patients in south Trinidad, 72 (37.50%) tested positive for *T. cruzi* antibodies [26]. The authors report that 49 of the 72 patients (68.06%) had *T. cruzi* trypomastigotes in peripheral blood, although this number seems unusually high.

While these findings provide mounting evidence of a vector-borne Chagas disease transmission cycle existing in Trinidad, there are no known published data demonstrating the species on which *T. cruzi*-infected triatomine bugs are feeding, other than a single wild rat found infected with *T. cruzi* in 1963 [27]. Identification of the host species with which triatomines come into contact by taking a blood meal can give us a sense of the frequency with which the bugs invade domestic environments, and in turn, the risk of vector-borne Chagas disease. For example, a diet of primarily wild animal hosts would suggest that there is little risk of the disease on the island, while a diet involving domestic animals and/or humans would imply that Chagas disease may be of local epidemiologic importance. As such, we asked, from which species are *T. cruzi*-infected triatomines in Trinidad taking blood meals?

We aimed to use our findings to further characterize the current *T. cruzi* transmission cycle in Trinidad, and in turn, better understand the risk of Chagas disease transmission on the island.

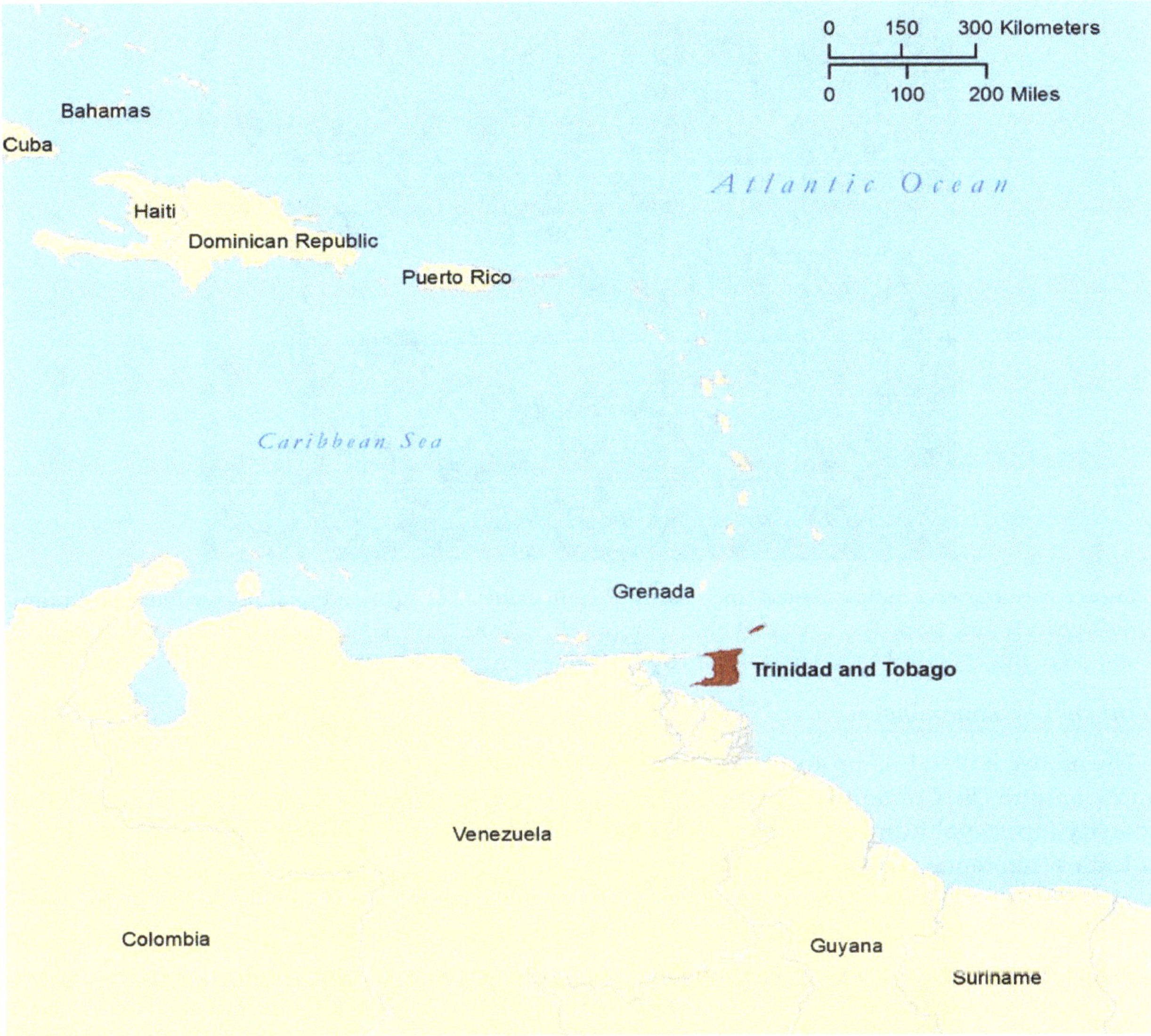

Figure 1. Location of Trinidad and Tobago relative to South America, Venezuela, and other Caribbean islands. Map created with the assistance of T. W. Shawa, Princeton Geographic Information Systems Librarian.

2. Materials and Methods

2.1. Overview

Triatomine bugs were sampled on the island of Trinidad between May and August, 2016. Bugs were collected using mouse-baited traps placed near animal resting/nesting sites and artificial light sources (Figure 2), in addition to manual collection when a bug was found resting on a wall or other surface. Public submissions were also accepted. Upon collection, bugs were examined for *T. cruzi* infection before undergoing blood meal analysis to identify a species on which each bug had recently taken a blood meal.

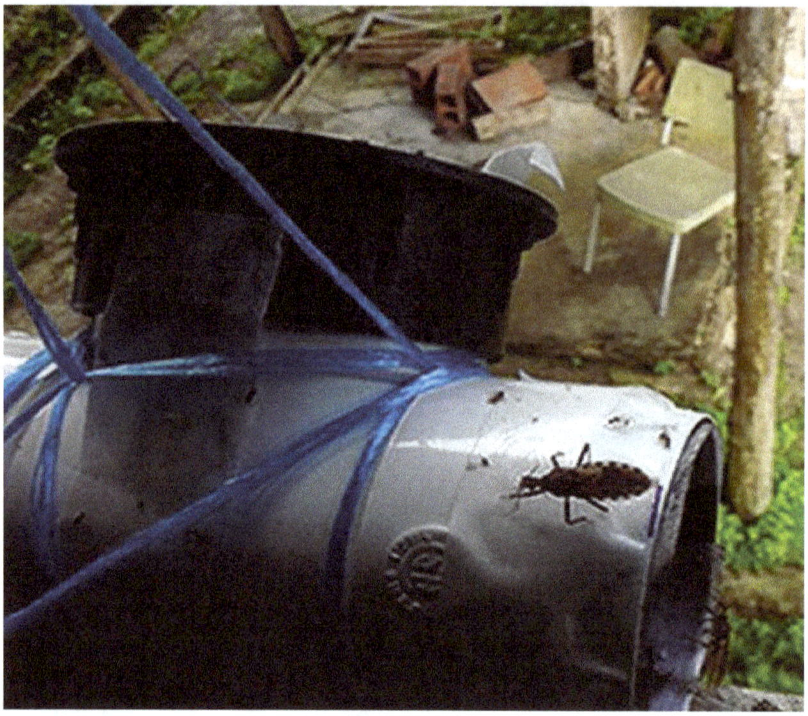

Figure 2. Successful mouse-baited trap. Adult *P. geniculatus* is caught on the adhesive material lining the outside of the trap. The trap is set on a windowsill, near an artificial light on the exterior of a ranger station in the village of Mt. Harris. Photo by J. K. Peterson.

2.2. *Animal Use Ethics Statement*

The mouse-baited trap protocol used in this study was reviewed and approved by The Institutional Animal Care and Use Committee (IACUC) of Princeton University (protocol # 2065F-16) and St. George's University (approval number 16010-R), and the Campus Ethics Committee at the University of the West Indies (reference number CEC172/04/16).

2.3. *Study Sites*

A total of 21 sites were sampled across 11 villages concentrated mostly in northern and central Trinidad (site-specific details in Table S1, Supplementary Materials). All sites except one were residential or very close to human disturbance (i.e., residential, farm, logging, alongside a road, etc.). Within each site, particular attention was paid to *Attalea maripa* palms known locally as 'cocorite,' which are known habitat for local fauna. We sampled for one night per location, with repeat sampling of a site occurring after a successful collection.

2.4. *Triatomine Bug Collection*

We used three methods to collect triatomine bugs: mouse-baited traps, manual trapping, and community collection. Mouse-baited traps (Figure 2, [28]) were placed in animal resting sites, as triatomines tend to live near their food source. These sites included rat nests, opossum nests, bat-infested structures, and 18 *A. maripa* palms (details for each site in Table S1). In residential areas, we placed traps near light sources in building exteriors.

Mouse-baited traps consisted of a 'T-shaped' PVC pipe (3″ diameter) covered in Duck® Brand Indoor Heavy Traffic Carpet Tape, which is a double-sided adhesive material (Figure 2). A Swiss albino mouse was placed inside the trap just before use, along with shredded paper for bedding and a piece of potato or fruit that served as a food and water source. Trap openings were closed by a two-inch section of PVC pipe covered in chicken wire and fine mesh. Traps were placed at dusk (5:00 p.m.–8:00 p.m.) and retrieved the next day in the morning (7:00 a.m.–9:00 a.m.). After each use, the mouse was removed from the trap and returned to its cage. Traps were cleaned and disinfected, and the water source, bedding, and tape were changed before reusing the trap. Each mouse was used in a trap only once per week. Mice were obtained from the laboratory animal rearing facility of the University of the West Indies Veterinary School.

In addition to trapping, we collected bugs opportunistically when found resting on exterior walls near artificial lights. We also accepted public submissions, as described in [29]. Chagas disease information pamphlets with pictures of local bug species were distributed (Figure S1) to those residing near positive collection sites.

2.5. Specimen Processing and Molecular Analyses

All protocols were performed under carefully controlled laboratory conditions. DNA extraction and blood meal analyses were carried out in separate laboratories to minimize cross-contamination risk. Bugs were processed in the Pathology and Parasitology Laboratory at the School of Veterinary Medicine of the University of the West Indies (UWI), St. Augustine, Trinidad. Triatomine species were determined using taxonomic keys and images from Lent and Wygodzinsky [30], Carcavallo et al. [31], and Patterson et al. [32]. *T. cruzi* infection in live bugs was diagnosed through direct microscopy observation (DMO) and staining of bug excrement and stomach contents (Figure 3), while *T. cruzi* infection in dead bugs was diagnosed using PCR. For DMO, 10 μL of Phosphate Buffer Solution (PBS) was mixed with 10 μL of excrement from each bug. A 5 μL aliquot of the solution was examined microscopically at 40× magnification. Trypanosomes were identified by their movement and morphology. Bugs were stored in 70% ethanol (EtOH) for approximately one to three days, until molecular analysis was carried out.

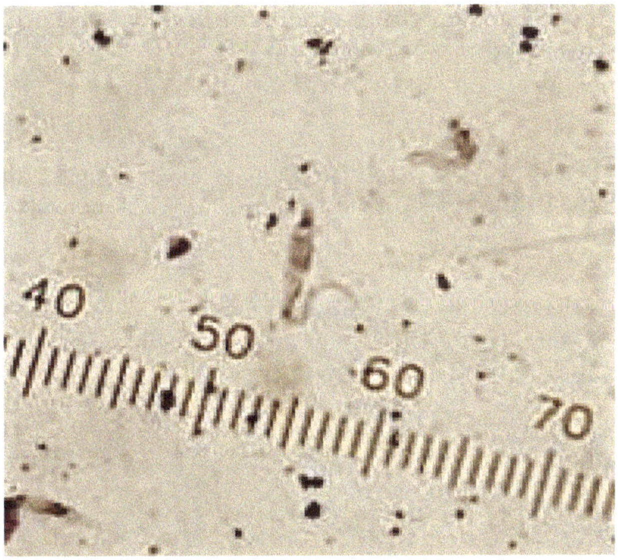

Figure 3. Giemsa stain of *T. cruzi* isolated from *P. geniculatus* collected in this study. Scale shown is in μm. Photo: J. K. Peterson.

DNA was isolated from each bug using the Qiagen DNeasy® Blood and Tissue DNA isolation kit, using a modified protocol for tissue extraction (described in [33]). PCR diagnosis of *T. cruzi* was performed for all bugs using the TcZF/R primer (5′-GCTCTTGCCCACAAGGGTGC-3′ and 5′-CCAAGCAGCGGATAGTTCAGG-3′, [34]), which targets a 182 bp sequence of *T. cruzi* satellite DNA. Following optimization, the final recipe consisted of 1.25 μL of each TcZ-F/R, 1 μL DNA, 21.5 μL dH_2O, and one GE Healthcare illustra PuReTaq Ready-To-Go PCR bead. PCR conditions were as follows: 94 °C for 5 min, followed by 40 cycles of 94 °C for 20 s, 57 °C for 10 s, 72 °C for 30 s, with a final extension of 72 °C for 7 min, and held at 4 °C. All samples were visualized in a 1.5% agarose gel to confirm amplicon size. To confirm that the amplified PCR product was indeed *T. cruzi*, we extracted three of the 182 bp bands from the agarose gel following PCR using the Qiagen QIAEX II Gel Extraction Kit, and sent the bands for Sanger sequencing at the Plant-Microbe Genomics Facility at The Ohio State University. We edited sequences with Chromas Lite 2.6.4, and compared them to known sequences in NIH-NCBI GenBank using the Basic Local Alignment Search Tool (BLAST). These analyses confirmed the DNA sequence amplified was from *T. cruzi*.

2.6. Blood Meal Analyses

Blood meal analyses were performed in the Molecular Biology Lab at the St. George's University School of Veterinary Medicine in True Blue, Grenada. We amplified a 360–380 bp fragment of the vertebrate cytochrome b (cytb) gene from the DNA of each bug using the L14841 primer (5′-CCCCTCAGAATGATATTTGTCCTCA-3′) and the H15149 primer (5′-CCATCCAACA TCTCAGCATGATGAAA-3′) [35]. These primers are vertebrate-specific, and are used frequently to preferentially amplify host DNA from blood meals in hematophagous insects [35]. After optimization, the final recipe used was: 1.25 μL of each primer, 2 μL of $MgCl_2$, 3 μL of bug DNA, 17.5 μL of dH_2O, and one GE Healthcare illustra PuReTaq Ready-To-Go PCR bead. All PCRs included appropriate controls. Each sample was run under the following thermal cycling conditions: preheat at 95 °C for 5 min, then 50 cycles of 95 °C for 30 s, 50 °C for 45 s, 72 °C for 90 s, followed by 72 °C for 7 min, then hold at 4 °C. All samples were electrophoresed, extracted from gels, sequenced, edited, and compared to known GenBank entries, as described above. The cut off for accepting an identity match in BLAST was ≥90%, and an e-value below 1e−10. (The e-value describes the number of hits one can expect by chance, given database size.) In instances where more than one species had an identity match in BLAST over >90%, the GenBank sequence entry with highest e-value was called. Overlapping, short, or messy sequences were re-run using the same blood meal analysis protocol but with avian-specific and mammal-specific primers that amplified a 508 and 772 bp fragment of the cytb gene, respectively [36]. Sequence data are found in File S1.

3. Results

A total of 55 adult triatomine bugs were collected (54 *Panstrongylus geniculatus* and one *Rhodnius pictipes*) in five of the 11 villages sampled (Table 1). All successful collection spots were in or around human dwellings.

Table 1. Triatomine Bug Collection Site Descriptions with *T. cruzi* Infection Status of Bugs Collected from Each Site, and Human Blood Meals Taken by the Bugs. Only Successful Collection Site Details Are Listed. Details for Every Sample Site Are in Table S1.

Site Name	Location	Site Description	Bugs Collected [1,2]			Human Blood Meals		
			Infected	Uninfected	Total	Infected [3]	Uninfected [3]	Total
Blanchisseuse	Northern coast	Coastal human home adjacent to secondary forest	1 (100%)	0	1	1 (100%)	0	1
Coal Mine	Central range [4]	Scattered human homes adjacent to secondary forest	40 (87%)	6 (13%)	46	22 (92%)	2 (8%)	24
Matura	Northeast coast	Rural human home surrounded by secondary forest	1 (50%)	1 (50%)	2	0	1 (100%)	1
Mt Harris	Central range [4]	Rural neighborhood in close proximity to secondary forest	3 (60%)	2 (40%)	5	2 (67%)	1 (33%)	3
Santa Cruz	Northern range [4]	Laundry area of peri-urban human home	1 (100%)	0	1	1 (100%)	0	1

[1] All bugs collected were *Panstrongylus geniculatus*, except for one *Rhodnius pictipes* male infected with *T. cruzi*. The *R. pictipes* individual was collected manually from the exterior wall of a house in Coal Mine. [2] Sites where just one bug was collected were public submissions, and not sites that were actively sampled. [3] Infection status refers to the bug with the blood meal, not the human.[4] Central and northern ranges are the names of the east-west mountain ranges found in central and northern Trinidad.

No bugs were collected in traps placed in or near animal nesting sites. The majority of bugs (46 of 55; 83.6%) were collected from a single rural area with scattered human dwellings located adjacent to secondary forest. All triatomines collected were in the adult stage; 18 were female and 37 were male.

3.1. *T. cruzi* Infection

T. cruzi DNA was amplified from 46 out of the 55 bugs collected (83.6%). Of these bugs, six were also diagnosed through microscopy (Figure 3; 12 bugs in total were alive upon arrival to the lab). Bugs diagnosed microscopically (in addition to PCR diagnosis) were from Coal Mine (N = 4), Matura (N = 1), and Mt. Harris (N = 1). All successful collection villages (N = 5, Table 1) yielded at least one bug infected with *T. cruzi* (Tables 1 and 2).

Table 2. Blood Meal Species Identified in Triatomine Bugs Collected, and *T. cruzi* Infection Status of the Bug or Bugs Corresponding to Each Species. All Data Are Available in File S1, Including Accession Numbers and Sequences.

Blood Meal Hosts [1]			Triatomine Bugs [2]		Collection Sites [5]	BLAST Results [3]	
Class	Genus/Species	Common Name	Blood Meals [1]	*T. cruzi*-Positive Bugs [4]		% Identity Match	E-Value
Mammalia	*Homo sapiens*	Human	30	26 (87%)	All	99%	1×10^{-58}
	Alouatta seniculus	Red howler monkey	2	2 (100%)	CM, MH	98%	5×10^{-134}
	Dasyprocta leporina	Red-rumped agouti	2	2 (100%)	CM, MT	100%	2×10^{-128}
	Coendou prehensilis	Brazilian porcupine	1	1 (100%)	CM	100%	1×10^{-144}
	Herpestes javanicus	Javan mongoose	1	1 (100%)	CM	100%	8×10^{-116}
	Metachirus nudicaudatus	Brown four-eyed opossum	1	0 (0%)	CM	99%	8×10^{-136}
	Nectomys [6]	Water rat	1	1 (100%)	CM	98%	9×10^{-138}
	Proechimys trinitatis	Trinidad spiny rat	1	0 (0%)	MH	100%	3×10^{-64}
Aves	*Gallus gallus*	Chicken	10	9 (10%)	CM	99%	3×10^{-106}
	Pionus menstruus	Blue-headed parrot	2	1 (50%)	CM	90%	2.5×10^{-77}
	Dryocopus lineatus	Lineated woodpecker	1	1 (100%)	CM	99%	1×10^{-92}
	Pulsatrix perspicillata	Spectacled owl	1	0 (0%)	CM	98%	0 *

[1] One blood meal host was identified per bug. [2] All bugs were *P. geniculatus* except for one *R. pictipes* collected in Coal Mine, which was *T. cruzi* positive and contained a human blood meal. [3] Cut off for accepting an identity match in BLAST was ≥ 90%, and an e-value below 1×10^{-10}. (The e-value describes the number of hits one can expect by chance, given database size.) Average % match and average e-value is shown for species found in more than one blood meal. [4] Positive *T. cruzi* infection in the bug does not mean positive host infection (and birds are not competent for *T. cruzi* infection). [5] CM = Coal Mine, MH = Mount Harris, MT = Matura. Site descriptions in Table 1. [6] BLAST hit corresponded to *Nectomys rattus*, which is not found in Trinidad. The cytb gene sequence for the congeneric species native to Trinidad (*Nectomys palmipes*) is not currently in the Genbank database. * E-values approaching 0 are rounded to 0 in BLAST.

3.2. Blood Meal Analyses

We identified a recent blood meal host species for 53 of the 55 bugs (96.4%; Figure 4, Table 2). Thirty bugs (56.6%) fed on humans, of which 26 (86.7%) were infected with *T. cruzi*, including the single *R. pictipes* individual. The second most common blood meal hosts were chickens (10 bugs; 18.9%), followed by red howler monkeys (2 bugs, 4.0%), red-rumped agoutis (2 bugs, 4.0%), and blue-headed parrots (2 bugs, 4.0%). One blood meal each was identified from a porcupine, mongoose, opossum, water rat, spiny rat, woodpecker, and owl (detailed in Table 2). Overall, nine bugs (17.0%) fed on wild mammals and four bugs (7.5%) fed on wild birds. Each site yielded at least one bug with a human blood meal, and four of the five sites had at least one *T. cruzi*-infected bug with a human blood meal.

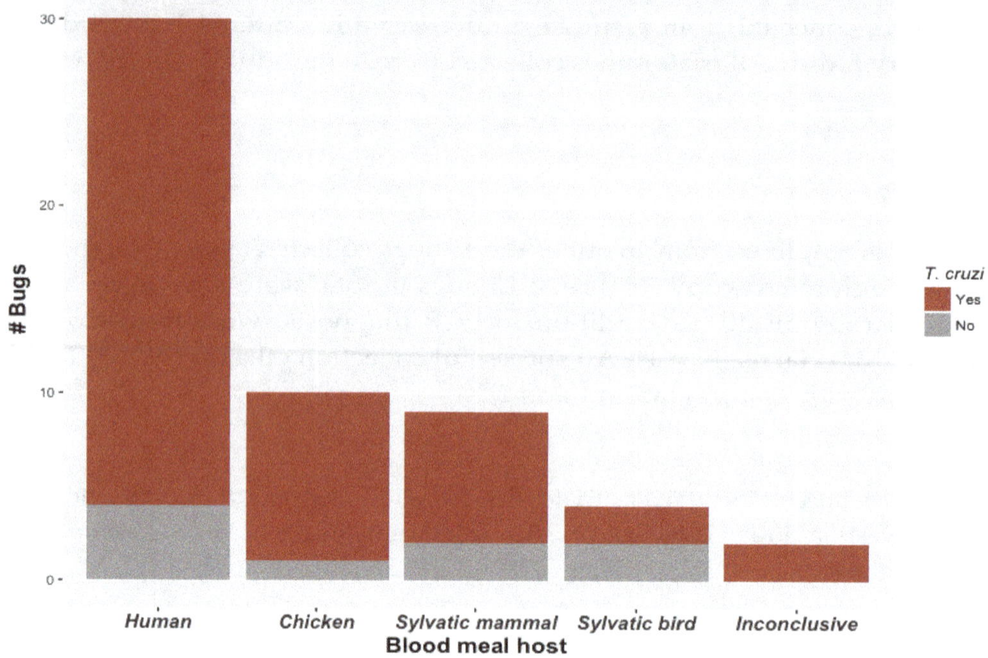

Figure 4. Number of bugs (i.e., blood meals) by blood meal host category and *T. cruzi* infection status of triatomine bug. Data were pooled across sites. One blood meal host was identified per bug. All triatomine species were adult *P. geniculatus* except for one adult male *R. pictipes*, which was infected with *T. cruzi*, and contained a human blood meal. Blood meal host species information is found in Table 2.

4. Discussion

In this study, we aimed to better understand the potential for vector-borne Chagas disease in Trinidad by characterizing the feeding preferences of *T. cruzi* vectors on the island. We found that at least one triatomine bug species on the island, *Panstrongylus geniculatus*, feeds on humans, chickens, and wild animals. While previous studies have found *T. cruzi* infection in humans [12,26] and triatomine bugs [17,25] in Trinidad, our study is the first to demonstrate that the bug feeds opportunistically across a wide range of host species, including humans, on the island.

4.1. P. geniculatus Breeding Habitat Remains Cryptic

All bugs in our study were adults collected from residential areas, despite efforts to sample a wide range of animal resting sites where the bugs might breed (i.e., cocorite palms, opossum nests, bat colonies, etc., Table S1). Still, approximately one-quarter of identified blood meals came from wild animals. Prior studies of *P. geniculatus* in Trinidad found nymphs only in caves and burrows of the nine-banded armadillo (*Dasypus novemcinctus*) [12,17], while in Venezuela, *P. geniculatus* was also associated with the common or black-eared opossum (*Didelphis marsupialis*) [37]. While our blood meal analyses did not reveal either of these host species, we did identify blood meals from several other nesting animals in addition to arboreal species, both of which could provide suitable habitats for the bugs. Thus, it is possible that *P. geniculatus* in Trinidad select breeding sites in a similar manner to how they feed—opportunistically, across a range of species.

Our failure to find juvenile triatomine bugs in residential areas suggests that the bugs forage, but do not breed, in domestic settings. Nonetheless, it important to note that almost one-fifth of identified blood meals in this study were from chickens in residential settings. Although birds are not competent *T. cruzi* hosts, they are a common food source for triatomines, which may in turn amplify *T. cruzi* transmission by increasing carrying capacity of vector populations [38]. Moreover, chicken coops are often found infested with triatomine bugs in other regions, and have even been used as sentinels for Chagas disease [39]. Thus, it will be of critical importance to sample more widely across residential settings in Trinidad in order to understand the potential for triatomines to breed in domestic settings, especially those with chickens.

4.2. Are Wildlife Population Declines Driving *P. geniculatus* Host Shifts?

Although we did not find blood meals from nine-banded armadillos in this study, carcasses with *T. cruzi* amastigotes are occasionally brought by hunters to the Veterinary Pathology lab at the University of the West Indies. A larger study would likely yield blood meals from armadillos and possibly *Didelphis* opossums as well, although it is unclear if either species would carry the same importance for *P. geniculatus* as they did 40 years ago (when triatomines were last studied in Trinidad, [17]). Nine-banded armadillos and *Didelphis* opossums are regularly hunted in Trinidad as bushmeat, for which there is high demand; an opossum carcass in Trinidad currently sells for TT$ 300–500 (USD $40–$70). Thus, it is possible that these species are now less abundant, which could be driving *P. geniculatus* into new areas to nest and forage, a phenomenon observed in *P. geniculatus* in the Amazon basin [40,41]. Further studies of wildlife population decline in Trinidad would help identify if reduced wild host species abundance is causing the bugs to leave their nesting sites to feed on humans and domestic animals.

4.3. *P. geniculatus*: A Cosmopolitan Species of Emerging Importance

P. geniculatus is highly adaptive in both its feeding and habitat preferences. The species is widely distributed in Latin America across a multitude of landscapes [32]. Though historically associated with enzootic *T. cruzi* transmission, the species is increasingly reported in human homes and with human blood meals [21–23]. While once considered to be incapable of domiciliation, the species is now considered to be domiciliated or in the process of domiciliation in several regions [20,21,42], which is reviewed in [43]. Additionally, *P. geniculatus* is no longer limited to forested areas; in the Metropolitan district of Caracas, Venezuela, thousands of *P. geniculatus* were found in both poor and wealthy areas of 31 out of 32 parishes, with nymphs found in 14 of the parishes. The species has also been reported in urban centers in Brazil (Sao Paulo [44] and Rio de Janeiro [45]) and Bolivia (Cochabamba [24]).

4.4. Multiple Paths to *T. cruzi* Exposure in Trinidad

In addition, it is important to highlight that several different *T. cruzi* transmission routes could pose a risk to humans in Trinidad. The presence of *P. geniculatus* in areas of human use presents a risk for oral transmission of *T. cruzi*. Between 2007 and 2009, there were three oral Chagas disease outbreaks at schools in Venezuela [46,47]. Subsequent analysis implicated *P. geniculatus* contamination of food or drinks in all three outbreaks [23,46,47]. Oral contamination does not require insect domiciliation or colonization of a residence; rather, it can occur merely by triatomines attracted to areas of food preparation by artificial lights. Handling of *T. cruzi*-infected wild animal carcasses by both hunters and researchers in Trinidad presents a *T. cruzi* transmission risk as well [48]. Transmission may also be possible by consuming undercooked, *T. cruzi*-infected bushmeat, although this is yet to be confirmed [49]. Considering the popularity of bushmeat in Trinidad, these transmission routes merit further investigation. Taken together, the multiple possible means of *T. cruzi* exposure in Trinidad suggest that *P. geniculatus* should be taken seriously on the island as a vector species of emerging epidemiologic importance.

4.5. Chagas Disease in Trinidad: Official Endemicity Would Bring Critical Resources

In our experience with community collection, we observed that community members wanted to know more about Chagas disease and its vectors. We were unable to find a local resource to reference, so we created the informational pamphlet (Figure S1 in Supplementary Materials). However, a pamphlet cannot compensate for the resources that are missing due to the country not being officially designated as 'Chagas endemic' by major global health organizations [10,15,50]. With official

Chagas disease endemic status comes numerous resources [50], such as donated medications [51], blood bank monitoring support data coordination [52], and a framework for increasing *T. cruzi* screening in pregnant women [53,54]. Furthermore, endemicity provides the opportunity to participate in subregional intergovernmental Chagas disease control initiatives such as the Southern Cone Initiative (INCOSUR, [55]) and the Initiative for Chagas Disease Control in Central America and Mexico (IPCAM, [56]). Countries in these groups set joint regional goals, and annual meetings to share progress and challenges serve as a source of motivation and accountability. All of the aforementioned resources are available to 'endemic' countries with *T. cruzi* seroprevalences that are likely comparable to Trinidad, such as Costa Rica and Belize, and would be useful in Trinidad, where heart disease was the leading cause of death in 2015 [57].

4.6. Study Limitations

Our results are preliminary, with a small sample size that was limited in geographic distribution and duration. We hope to conduct a larger study in order to define the scope of *T. cruzi* transmission between humans and animals on the island, and determine whether our results are representative of the island as a whole. Additionally, seasonality may have contributed to our failure to find bugs in animal resting sites. Due to logistical constraints, the field work portion of this study took place during the rainy season, when palms, burrows, or other animal nests can be vacated due to humidity or inundation. Indeed, Fistein [12] found that the number of triatomines found inside houses was inversely proportional to both relative humidity and monthly rainfall. Accordingly, follow-up studies should be carried out in the rainy and dry seasons to accurately characterize *P. geniculatus* breeding sites in Trinidad.

Finally, it must be kept in mind that a 'bite' (i.e., blood meal) from a *T. cruzi*-infected triatomine does not guarantee *T. cruzi* transmission, since the parasite is transmitted in vector excrement and not saliva. Thus, our finding of human blood meals in *T. cruzi*-infected bugs does not mean that the bugs transmitted *T. cruzi* to those humans. There is one published study of *P. geniculatus* defecation timing, and the authors found that the bugs do, on average, defecate while feeding [42], which is a key characteristic of epidemiologically important Chagas disease vector species. It is also important to mention that oral transmission is a risk simply with vector presence, regardless of whether or not the bug feeds or defecates on a human host.

5. Conclusions and Future Directions

Although our findings are preliminary, our study is an important first step in furthering our understanding of *T. cruzi* dynamics in Trinidad. The results of our blood meal analysis suggest that *T. cruzi* in Trinidad may not be strictly enzootic, but rather could be a parasite of humans, domestic animals, and wild animals. Our findings support those of prior studies suggesting that Chagas disease in Trinidad needs to be more comprehensively studied, and perhaps re-considered in terms of its public health importance on the island.

Future studies would benefit from taking a One Health approach entailing multidisciplinary research and outreach work focused on interactions between humans, domestic and wild animal populations, triatomine bugs, and the environment. Open questions include triatomine bug seasonality, regional variation, breeding habitats, and juvenile *T. cruzi* infection rates. Identifying mammalian hosts serving as *T. cruzi* infection sources for the bugs and measuring *T. cruzi* infection prevalence in wild and domestic animals will form a more complete picture of the *T. cruzi* transmission cycle on the island. Connections between human land use and *T. cruzi* transmission must be investigated. Epidemiologic surveys are needed to estimate baseline *T. cruzi* prevalence in humans in Trinidad, and it will be of critical importance to determine whether *T. cruzi* infection contributes to the high rates of heart disease on the island. If after further study, it is confirmed that Chagas disease is indeed a public health concern in Trinidad, a holistic prevention approach that integrates an awareness of animal hosts, human hosts, and the environment may be necessary in order to effectively address all aspects of this zoonotic NTD.

Author Contributions: Conceptualization, J.K.P. and A.H.; methodology, J.K.P., A.H., D.M.F., R.S. and R.A.C.; formal analysis, A.H., J.K.P. and D.M.F.; investigation, J.K.P., A.H., D.M.F., R.S. and R.A.C.; resources, J.K.P., A.H., D.M.F., R.S. and R.A.C.; data curation, A.H., J.K.P. and D.M.F.; writing—original draft preparation, J.K.P. and A.H.; writing—review and editing, J.K.P., A.H., D.M.F., R.S., R.A.C. and A.P.D.; visualization, J.K.P. and A.H.; supervision, J.K.P.; project administration, J.K.P.; funding acquisition, A.H., D.M.F., R.S. and A.P.D. All authors have read and agreed to the published version of the manuscript.

Acknowledgments: The authors extend their gratitude to Ravindra Sharma of St. George's University for logistical support and assistance, the University of the West Indies School of Veterinary Medicine (UWI SVM) for providing materials and other resources, and Chris Oura of the UWI SVM for use of his laboratory. Mice were provided by the UWI SVM Laboratory Animal Facility.

References

1. World Health Organization. Chagas disease in Latin America: An epidemiological update based on 2010 estimates. *Wkly. Epidemiol. Rec.* **2015**, 33–44. [CrossRef]
2. Shikanai-Yasuda, M.A.; Carvalho, N.B. Oral transmission of chagas disease. *Clin. Infect. Dis.* **2012**, *54*, 845–852. [CrossRef] [PubMed]
3. Miles, M. Orally acquired Chagas disease: Lessons from an urban school outbreak. *J. Infect. Dis.* **2010**, *201*, 1282–1284. [CrossRef] [PubMed]
4. Filigheddu, M.T.; Górgolas, M.; Ramos, J.M. Orally-transmitted Chagas disease. *Med. Clín. (Engl. Ed.)* **2017**, *148*, 125–131. [CrossRef]
5. Nóbrega, A.A.; Garcia, M.H.; Tatto, E.; Obara, M.T.; Costa, E.; Sobel, J.; Araujo, W.N. Oral transmission of chagas disease by consumption of Acai palm fruit, Brazil. *Emerg. Infect. Dis.* **2009**, *15*, 653–655. [CrossRef] [PubMed]
6. Gottdenker, N.L.; Chaves, L.F.; Calzada, J.E.; Saldaña, A.; Carroll, C.R. host life history strategy, species diversity, and habitat influence *Trypanosoma cruzi* vector infection in changing landscapes. *PLoS Negl. Trop. Dis.* **2012**, *6*, e1884. [CrossRef] [PubMed]
7. Guhl, F.; Pinto, N.; Aguilera, G. Sylvatic triatominae: A new challenge in vector control transmission. *Mem. Do Inst. Oswaldo Cruz* **2009**, *104*, 71–75. [CrossRef]
8. Rabinovich, J.E.; Kitron, U.D.; Obed, Y.; Yoshioka, M.; Gottdenker, N.; Chaves, L.F. Ecological patterns of blood-feeding by kissing-bugs (Hemiptera: Reduviidae: Triatominae). *Memórias Do Inst. Oswaldo Cruz* **2011**, *106*, 479–494. [CrossRef]
9. Petana, W.B. American trypanosomiasis (Chagas' disease) in the Caribbean. *Bull. Panam. Health Organ.* **1978**, *12*, 45–51.
10. Centers for Disease Control and Prevention. Parasites-American Trypanosomiasis (also known as Chagas Disease). Available online: https://www.cdc.gov/parasites/chagas/gen_info/detailed.html (accessed on 31 May 2020).
11. Armed Forces Pest Management Board. *Regional Disease Vector Ecology Profile: Caribbean*; Walter Reed Army Medical Center: Washington, DC, USA, 2002.
12. Fistein, B. A review of Chagas disease in Trinidad. *Caribb. Med. J.* **1981**, *42*, 17–28.
13. Fistein, B.; Sutton, R.N.P. Chagas disease in the West Indies. *Lancet* **1963**, *281*, 330–331. [CrossRef]
14. Fistein, B. Aetiology of Jamaican cardiomyopathy. *Lancet* **1966**, *288*, 386. [CrossRef]

15. World Health Organization. *Working to Overcome the Global Impact of Neglected Tropical Diseases First WHO Report on Neglected Tropical Diseases*; No. WHO/HTM/NTD/2010.1.; World Health Organization: Geneva, Switzerland, 2010.
16. Erlich, R.N.; Barrett, S.F. Cenozoic Plate tectonic history of the northern Venezuela-Trinidad Area. *Tectonics* **1990**, *9*, 161–184. [CrossRef]
17. Omah-Maharaj, I. Studies on vectors of *Trypanosoma cruzi* in Trinidad. *Med. Vet. Entomol.* **1992**, *6*, 115–120. [CrossRef]
18. Ryckman, R.E. The Triatominae of South America: A checklist with synonymy (Hemiptera: Reduviidae: Triatominae). *Bull. Soc. Vector Ecol.* **1986**, *11*, 199–208.
19. Cazorla-Perfetti, D. Revisión de los vectores de la enfermedad de Chagas en Venezuela (Hemiptera-Heteroptera, Reduviidae, Triatominae). *Saber Univ. De Orient Venez.* **2016**, *28*, 387–470.
20. Reyes-Lugo, M.; Rodriguez-Acosta, A. Domiciliation of the sylvatic Chagas disease vector *Panstrongylus geniculatus* Latreille, 1811 (Triatominae: Reduviidae) in Venezuela. *Trans. R. Soc. Trop. Med. Hyg.* **2000**, *94*, 508. [CrossRef]
21. Feliciangeli, M.D.; Carrasco, H.; Patterson, J.S.; Suarez, B.; Martínez, C.; Medina, M. Mixed domestic infestation by *Rhodnius prolixus* StäL, 1859 and *Panstrongylus geniculatus* Latreille, 1811, vector incrimination, and seroprevalence for *Trypanosoma cruzi* among inhabitants in El Guamito, Lara State, Venezuela. *Am. J. Trop. Med. Hyg.* **2004**, *71*, 501–505. [CrossRef]
22. Carrasco, H.J.; Torrellas, A.; García, C.; Segovia, M.; Feliciangeli, M.D. Risk of *Trypanosoma cruzi* I (Kinetoplastida: Trypanosomatidae) transmission by *Panstrongylus geniculatus* (Hemiptera: Reduviidae) in Caracas (Metropolitan District) and neighboring States, Venezuela. *Int. J. Parasitol.* **2005**, *35*, 1379–1384. [CrossRef]
23. Carrasco, H.J.; Segovia, M.; Londoño, J.C.; Ortegoza, J.; Rodríguez, M.; Martínez, C.E. *Panstrongylus geniculatus* and four other species of triatomine bug involved in the *Trypanosoma cruzi* enzootic cycle: High risk factors for Chagas' disease transmission in the Metropolitan District of Caracas, Venezuela. *Parasites Vectors* **2014**, *7*, 1003–1028. [CrossRef]
24. Rojas-Cortez, M.; Pinazo, M.J.; Garcia, L.; Arteaga, M.; Uriona, L.; Gamboa, S.; Mejía, C.; Lozano, D.; Gascon, J.; Torrico, F.; et al. *Trypanosoma cruzi*-infected *Panstrongylus geniculatus* and *Rhodnius robustus* adults invade households in the Tropics of Cochabamba region of Bolivia. *Parasites Vectors* **2016**, *9*, 1–6. [CrossRef]
25. Fistein, B. *Trypanosoma cruzi* infection in blood-sucking Reduviid bugs in Trinidad. *Trans. R. Soc. Trop. Med. Hyg.* **1966**, *60*, 536–538. [CrossRef]
26. Aziz, E.S.; Parsad, K.R. *Trypanosoma cruzi* infection associated with Chagas' heart disease in humans in South Trinidad. *West. Indian Med. J.* **1993**, *42*, 18.
27. Downs, W.G. The presence of *Trypanosoma cruzi* in the island of Trinidad, W.I. *J. Parasitol.* **1963**, *49*, 50. [CrossRef]
28. Abad-Franch, F.; Noireau, F.; Paucar, A.C.; Aguilar, H.M.V.; Carpio, C.C.; Racines, J.V. The use of live-bait traps for the study of sylvatic *Rhodnius* populations (Hemiptera: Reduviidae) in palm trees. *Trans. R. Soc. Trop. Med. Hyg.* **2000**, *94*, 629–630. [CrossRef]
29. Curtis-Robles, R.; Wozniak, E.J.; Auckland, L.D.; Hamer, G.L.; Hamer, S.A. Combining public health education and disease ecology research: Using citizen science to assess Chagas disease entomological risk in Texas. *PLoS Negl. Trop. Dis.* **2015**, *9*, e0004235. [CrossRef]
30. Lent, H.; Wygodzinsky, Z. Revision of the Triatominae (Hemiptera, Reduviidae), and their significance as vectors of Chagas' disease. *Bull. Am. Mus. Nat. Hist.* **1979**, *163*, 1–520.
31. Carcavallo, R.U.; Galindez Giron, I.; Jurberg, J.; Lent, H. *Atlas of Chagas Disease Vectors in the Americas*; Editora Fiocruz: Rio de Janeiro, Brazil, 1998.
32. Patterson, J.S.; Barbosa, S.E.; Feliciangeli, M.D. On the genus *Panstrongylus* Berg 1879: Evolution, ecology and epidemiological significance. *Acta Trop.* **2009**, *110*, 187–199. [CrossRef]
33. Peterson, J.K.; Graham, A.L.; Dobson, A.P.; Chavez, O.T. *Rhodnius prolixus* life history outcomes differ when Infected with different *Trypanosoma cruzi* I strains. *Am. J. Trop. Med. Hyg.* **2015**, *93*, 564–572. [CrossRef]
34. Combs, T.P.; Nagajyothi; Mukherjee, S.; de Almeida, C.J.G.; Jelicks, L.A.; Schubert, W.; Lin, Y.; Jayabalan, D.S.; Zhao, D.; Braunstein, V.L.; et al. The adipocyte as an important target cell for *Trypanosoma cruzi* infection. *J. Biol. Chem.* **2005**, *280*, 24085–24094. [CrossRef]

35. Boakye, D.A.; Tang, J.; Truc, P.; Merriweather, A.; Unnasch, T.R. Identification of bloodmeals in haematophagous Diptera by cytochrome B heteroduplex analysis. *Med. Vet. Entomol.* **1999**, *13*, 282–287. [CrossRef]
36. Ngo, K.A.; Kramer, L.D. Identification of mosquito bloodmeals using polymerase chain reaction (PCR) with order-specific primers. *J. Med. Entomol.* **2003**, *40*, 215–222. [CrossRef]
37. Pifano, F. El potencial enzootico silvestre del complejo ecológico Schizotrypanum cruzi—Didelphis marsupialis—Panstrongylus geniculatus y sus incursiones a la vivienda humana del valle de Caracas. *Bol Acad Cien Fis Mat. Nat. (Caracas)* **1986**, *XLVI*, 9–37.
38. Peterson, J.K.; Bartsch, S.M.; Lee, B.Y.; Dobson, A.P. Broad patterns in domestic vector-borne *Trypanosoma cruzi* transmission dynamics: Synanthropic animals and vector control. *Parasites Vectors* **2015**, *8*, 537. [CrossRef]
39. Martínez-Ibarra, J.A.; Martínez-Grant, J.A.; Verdugo-Cervantes, M.R.; Bustos-Saldaña, R.; Nogueda-Torres, B. Monitoring triatomid bug (Hemiptera: Reduviidae) presence by sentinel chicken coops in Southern Jalisco State, México. *Biomed. Rev. Del Inst. Nac. De Salud* **2010**, *30*, 140–145.
40. Valente, V.D.C. Potential for domestication of *Panstrongylus geniculatus* (Latreille 1811) (Hemiptera, Reduviidae, Triatominae) in the municipality of Muaná, Marajó Island, Pará State, Brazil. *Mem. Do Inst. Oswaldo Cruz* **1999**, *94*, 399–400. [CrossRef] [PubMed]
41. Valente, V.C.; Valente, S.A.S.; Noireau, F.; Carrasco, H.J.; Miles, M.A. Chagas disease in the Amazon basin: Associaion of *Panstrongylus geniculatus* (Hemiptera: Reduviidae) with domestic pigs. *J. Med. Entomol.* **1998**, *35*, 5. [CrossRef]
42. Wolff, M.; Castillo, D. Evidencias de domesticación y aspectos biológicos de panstrongylus de *Panstrongylus geniculatus* (Latreille 1811) (Hemiptera: Reduviidae). *Acta Entomol. Chil.* **2000**, *24*, 77–83.
43. Rabinovich, J.E.; Feliciangeli, M.D. Vital statistics of Triatominae (Hemiptera: Reduviidae) under laboratory conditions: IV. *Panstrongylus Geniculatus. J. Med. Entomol.* **2015**, *52*, 797–805. [CrossRef]
44. Ceretti-Junior, W.; Vendrami, D.P.; de Matos-Junior, M.O.; Rimoldi-Ribeiro, A.; Alvarez, J.V.; Marques, S.; Duarte, A.N.; da Silva, R.A.; da Rosa, J.A.; Marrelli, M.T. Occurrences of triatomines (Hemiptera: Reduviidae) and first reports of *Panstrongylus geniculatus* in urban environments in the city of Sao Paulo, Brazil. *Rev. Inst. Med. Trop. S. Paulo* **2018**, 60. [CrossRef] [PubMed]
45. 45. Peixoto, S.R.; da Silva Rocha, D.; Dale, C.; Galvão, C. *Panstrongylus geniculatus* (Latreille, 1811) (Hemiptera, Reduviidae, Triatominae): First record on Ilha Grande, Rio de Janeiro, Brazil. *Check List* **2020**, *16*, 391–394. [CrossRef]
46. Segovia, M.; Carrasco, H.J.; Martínez, C.E.; Messenger, L.A.; Nessi, A.; Londoño, J.C.; Espinosa, R.; Martínez, C.; Alfredo, M.; Bonfante-Cabarcas, R.; et al. Molecular epidemiologic source tracking of orally transmitted chagas disease, Venezuela. *Emerg. Infect. Dis.* **2013**, *19*, 1098–1101. [CrossRef]
47. Alarcón de Noya, B.; Díaz-Bello, Z.; Colmenares, C.; Ruiz-Guevara, R.; Mauriello, L.; Zavala-Jaspe, R.; Suarez, J.A.; Abate, T.; Naranjo, L.; Paiva, M.; et al. Large urban outbreak of orally acquired acute Chagas disease at a school in Caracas, Venezuela. *J. Infect. Dis.* **2010**, *201*, 1308–1315. [CrossRef]
48. Brenière, S.F.; Waleckx, E.; Aznar, C. Other forms of transmission. In *American Trypanosomiasis Chagas Disease*; Elsevier: Amsterdam, The Netherlands, 2017; pp. 561–578. ISBN 978-0-12-801029-7.
49. de Noya, B.A.; Díaz-Bello, Z.; Colmenares, C.; Ruiz-Guevara, R.; Mauriello, L.; Muñoz-Calderón, A.; Noya, O. Update on oral Chagas disease outbreaks in Venezuela: Epidemiological, clinical and diagnostic approaches. *Mem. Inst. Oswaldo Cruz* **2015**, *110*, 377–386. [CrossRef]
50. Pan American Health Organization. *Chagas Disease*; Pan American Health Organization: Washington, DC, USA, 2017.
51. Manne, J.; Snively, C.S.; Levy, M.Z.; Reich, M.R. Supply chain problems for Chagas disease treatment. *Lancet Infect. Dis.* **2012**, *12*, 173–175. [CrossRef]
52. Pan American Health Organization. *Supply of Blood for Transfusion in Latin American and Caribbean Countries, 2014 and 2015*; Pan American Health Organization: Washington, DC, USA, 2017.
53. Peterson, J.K.; Yoshioka, K.; Hashimoto, K.; Caranci, A.; Gottdenker, N.; Monroy, C.; Saldaña, A.; Rodriguez, S.; Dorn, P.; Zúniga, C. Chagas disease epidemiology in Central America: An update. *Curr. Trop. Med. Rep.* **2019**, *6*, 92–105. [CrossRef]
54. Pan American Health Organization. EMTCT Plus. In *Framework for Elimination of Mother-to-Child Transmission of HIV, Syphilis, Hepatitis B, and Chagas*; Pan American Health Organization: Washington, DC, USA, 2017.
55. Schofield, C.J.; Dias, J.C.P. The southern cone initiative against Chagas disease. *Adv. Parasitol.* **1999**, *42*, 1–27.

56. Iniciativa de los Países de América Central, Para la Interrupción de la Transmisión Vectorial y Transfusional de la Enfermedad de Chagas (IPCA). Historia de 12 años de una Iniciativa Subregional 1998-2010. Representación de la OPS/OMS en Honduras; 2011; 89p, ISBN 978-99926-742-5-3.
57. Pan American Health Organization. *2017–2021 PAHO/WHO Country Cooperation Strategy Report Trinidad and Tobago*; Pan American Health Organization: Washington, DC, USA, 2018.

16

Diagnosis and Management of Fungal Neglected Tropical Diseases In Community Settings—Mycetoma and Sporotrichosis

Roberto Estrada-Castañón [1], Guadalupe Estrada-Chávez [2] and María de Guadalupe Chávez-López [3,*]

[1] Community Dermatology Mexico C.A.; Health Secretary Guerrero, 39355 Acapulco, Guerrero, Mexico; restrada_13@hotmail.com

[2] Department of Dermatology and Dermato-Oncology, Instituto Estatal de Cancerología "Dr. Arturo Beltrán Ortega", Health Secretary Guerrero, Faculty of Medicine, Universidad Autónoma de Guerrero Mexico, Community Dermatology Mexico C.A., 39850 Acapulco, Guerrero, Mexico; estradaguadalupe@hotmail.com

[3] Department of Dermatology and Mycology Acapulco General Hospital, Health Secretary Guerrero, Community Dermatology Mexico C.A., 39355 Acapulco, Guerrero, Mexico

* Correspondence: chavezg13@live.com.mx;

Abstract: Background: This is a retrospective, analytic observational study where we describe cases of sporotrichosis and mycetoma from Acapulco General Hospital and Community Dermatology Mexico C.A. over 25 years. Analysis of environmental features that favour the development of such diseases has been made, as well as the limitations in the study and treatment of such diseases in resource poor settings. Methods: We reviewed the information on 76 sporotrichosis and 113 mycetoma patients out of a total of 14,000 consultations at Acapulco General Hospital and from Community Dermatology clinics. We analysed the epidemiological and mycological characteristics and the investigations used for diagnosis such as direct examination, culture, intradermal test reactions, and biopsy. Results: In total 91 confirmed cases of actinomycetoma, 22 of eumycetoma and 76 of sporotrichosis have been identified including diagnostic studies for both diseases and their treatment. Discussion: The results obtained have been analysed and interpreted in patients with mycetoma and sporotrichosis in the state of Guerrero, México, along with limitations in their management in areas with limited economic and logistical resources. The prevalence of mycetoma in our setting is compared with other centres where patients from all over the country are seen. The possible causes for variations in prevalence in specific areas has been looked for, in one of the poorest states of the Mexican Republic.

Keywords: subcutaneous mycosis; actinomycetoma; eumycetoma; sporotrichosis Community dermatology

---

1. Introduction

Mycetoma and sporotrichosis are two of the most widely distributed implantation (subcutaneous) mycoses worldwide. Mycetoma is a chronic infectious disease, which can be caused by different species of fungus (eumycetoma) or by aerobic filamentous bacteria (actinomycetoma). Clinical characteristics include, local swelling, and draining sinuses with serosanguinous or purulent exudates (Figure 1), which contains the infective forms known as "grains" (Figure 2) Climatic and geographic conditions have been described previously and the main endemic zone identified as between the Tropic of Cancer at lattitudes 15° south and 30° north; this has been referred to as the "Mycetoma belt" by the World Health Organisation (WHO). It includes countries like Chad, Ethiopia, India, Mauritania, Senegal, Somalia, Sudan, Yemen, and in the Americas: Mexico and Venezuela [1].

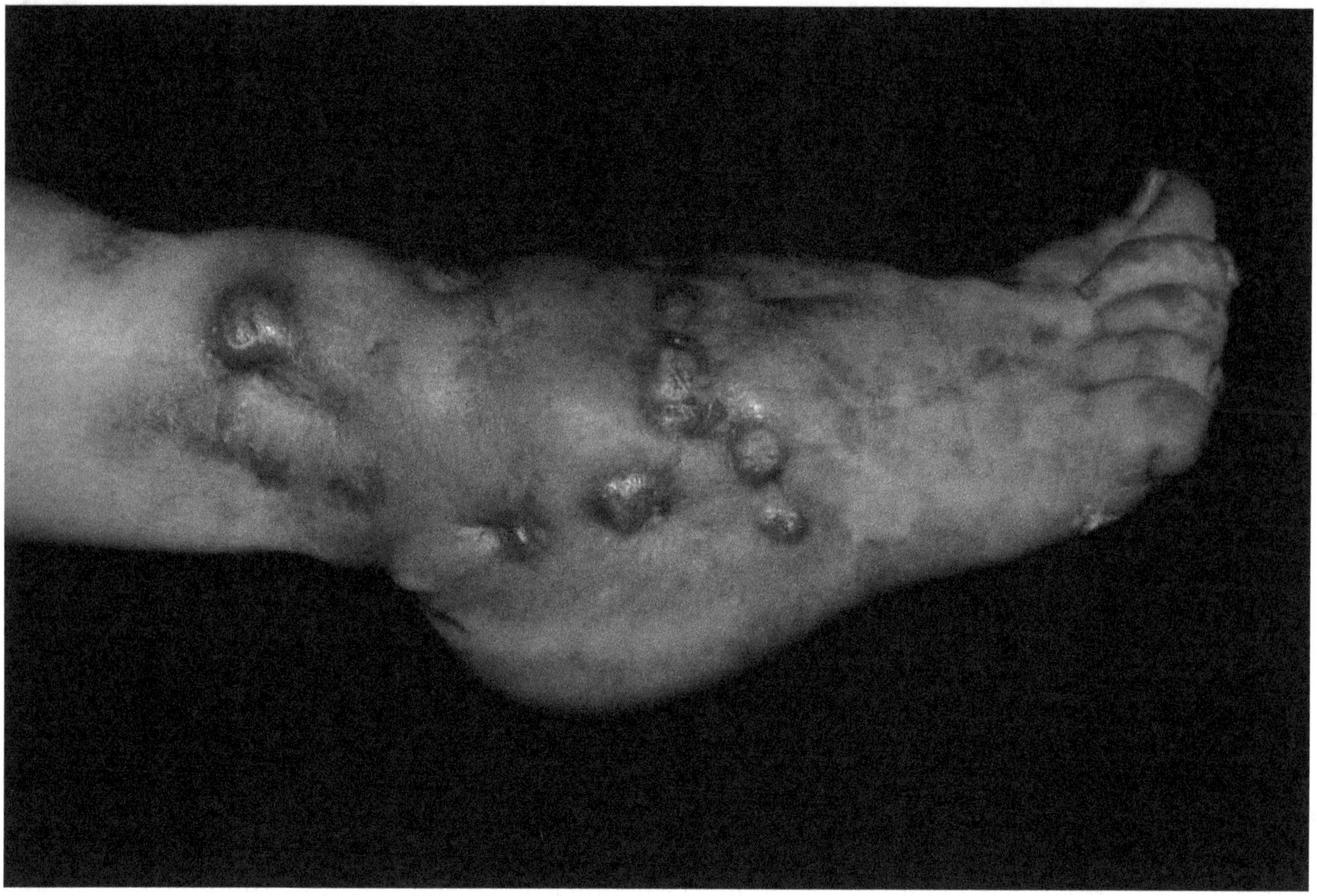

Figure 1. Eumycetoma of the foot.

Mexico has been identified as the country with the highest incidence of mycetoma in Latin America [2] and one of the most endemic countries around the world [3]. Mycetoma has been recognised by the WHO, as a neglected tropical disease (NTD) in 2016 in a WHA 69.21 resolution [4].

Even though sporotrichosis does not have the same morbidity patterns, except in disseminated or systemic forms, as mycetoma, because of its capacity for dissemination, its severity and neglect; it accounts for significant disability, morbidity, and reduction in the quality of life of affected individuals, who are mostly peasants; these are mainly farmers living in remote areas where diagnosis and treatment is frequently delayed due to lack of experience of local health personal working in the communities. Sporotrichosis is a chronic granulomatous implantation mycosis, caused by a group of dimorphic fungi belonging to the genus, *Sporothrix* . It affects either humans or some animal species [5] It is considered, in some cases, to be an occupational disease, not only in farmers, but also in florists, carpenters, and workers using hay for packing or building. Latin America has reported a high incidence of the infection, particularly in Brazil and Mexico [6], although in the former most cases, in the most recent outbreak, are caused by the zoonotic species *Sporothrix brasiliensis*, spread by cats, unlike the disease in Mexico.

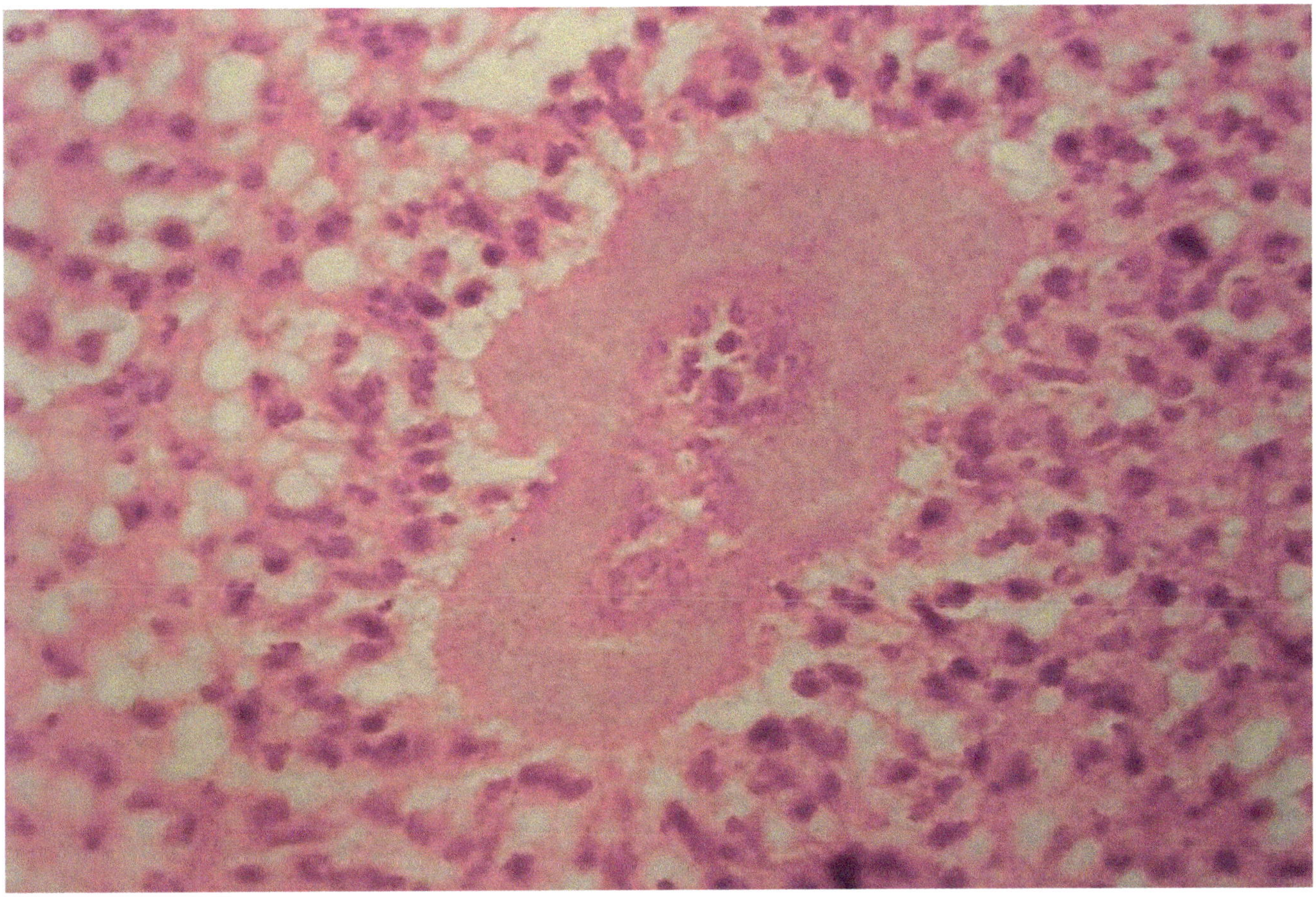

Figure 2. Grain histopathology (actinomycetoma) Haematoxylin and Eosin 100X.

Guerrero State in Mexico, is located at the south west of the Mexican Republic, on the coast of the Pacific Ocean between the coordinates 17°36′47″N 99°57′00″O with a territory of 63,794 km^2; to the West it is crossed by the mountain chain, the Sierra Madre del Sur, which provides very wide climatic and environmental diversity, with valleys and hills suitable for the development of different deep and subcutaneous mycoses. It is divided into seven natural regions, which determined its political division (Figure 3): The North and Mountain areas "Norte" and "Montaña" are arid and with difficult terrain, rich in mining and caves that are frequently visited by cave explorers and tourists, in whom cases of histoplasmosis have been reported [7], the "Tierra Caliente" (warm earth) area, has a wide valley crossed by the Balsas river and very high daily temperatures which provides the name to the region, cases of coccidioidomycosis [8] have been reported from there. A mountain chain divides the central region "Centro" into the other two regions, which are the small and big coastal areas, "Costa chica" and "Costa Grande", these are rich in vegetation, with coffee and palm plantations, where cases of paracoccidioidomycosis [9] and chromoblastomycosis [10] have been reported. Nevertheless, as in other areas of the world, mycetoma and sporotrichosis are the most frequent subcutaneous mycoses in Mexico [3] and in Guerrero State [11], making it the country with second or third highest prevalence of these disesases [1,2].

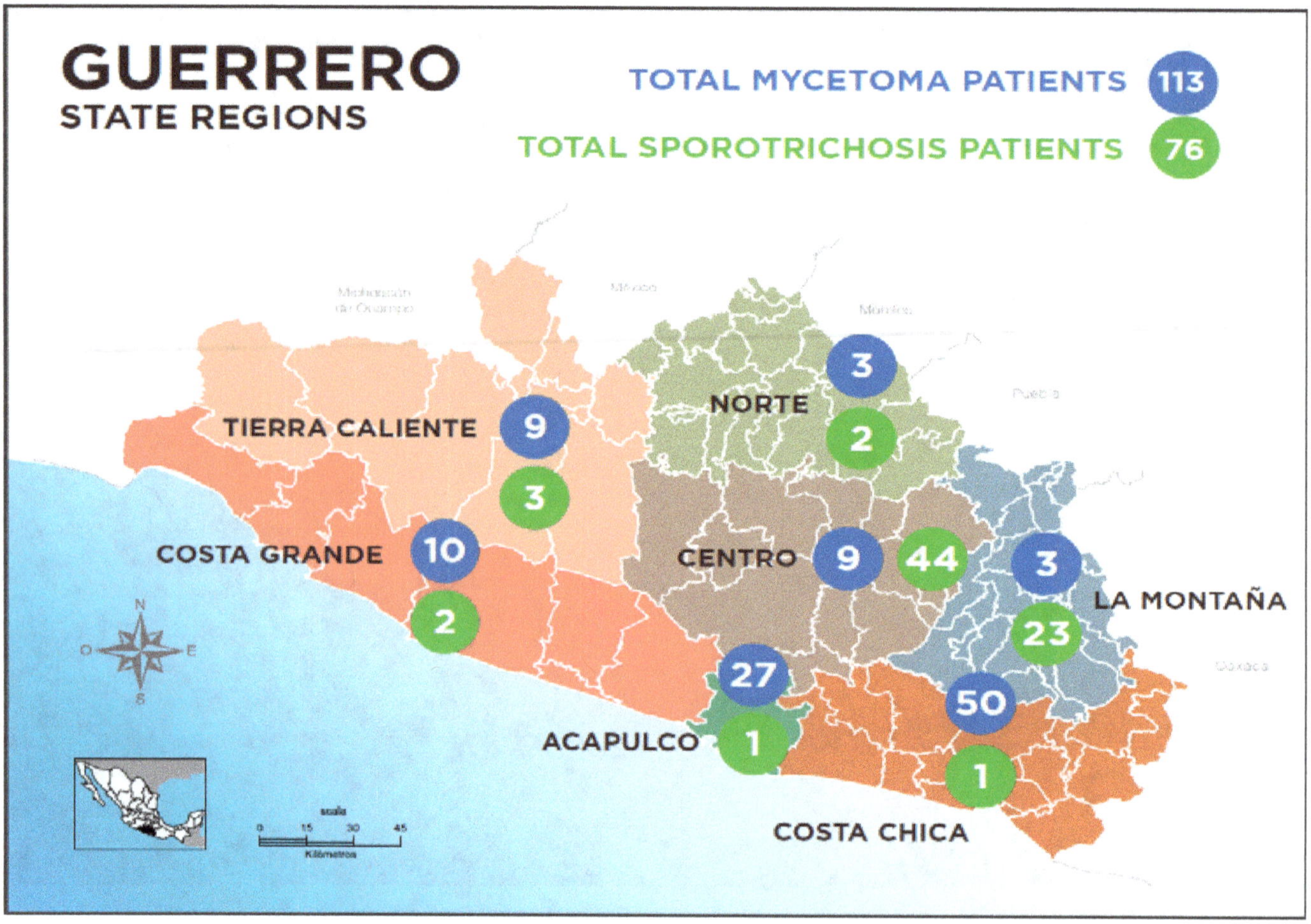

Figure 3. Map of Guerrero State showing cases of mycetoma and sporotrichosis.

Mycetoma is more frequent in the Coastal and Tierra Caliente areas. Sporotrichosis is more frequent in the Mountain and Central areas (Figure 3). Affected farmers live in conditions of poverty that can be severe in isolated regions.

Community Dermatology Mexico (CDM) is a 28 year old programme whose goal is to assist people in need or without access to specialized dermatological care, by teaching basic dermatology to health workers working in remote areas where there is less opportunity for continuous medical education and to identify, refer, and/or treat patients with both simple and complicated dermatological problems and to carry out research [12,13], the reason for this communication.

2. Methods

We report an analytical, retrospective, observational study in which we reviewed 14,000 consultations at the Acapulco General Hospital and records of the Community Dermatology program over the last 20 years. The information obtained in the communities was the result of visits to the areas with a high marginality index amongst the seven regions of Guerrero state, with the support of the State health programme called Desarollo Integral de la Familia or DIF and the Secretary of Health. Of the mycetoma and sporotrichosis cases that were identified clinically, all were referred to our Dermatology Department at the Acapulco General Hospital for further studies and treatment.

Due to limitations associated with field work and the logistics needed for transportation of basic material and equipment, the studies, that were feasible, were restricted to mycological scrapings for direct examination, punch biopsies, and occasionally the inoculation of samples of lesional exudate onto media for subsequent culture, which were subsequently completed in the mycology facility in our institution. All organisms that were speciated in this study were identified by culture.

In order to facilitate and assist the management of affected patients, we provided financial support for transportation and food during their trip to Acapulco city, where after having any ancillary studies such as imaging including Computer Assisted Tomography (CAT) scans in specific cases, culture, or further mycological studies, free treatment for their specific health conditions was provided after evaluation; this included: Trimethoprim sulfamethoxazole and dapsone (DDS) for patients with actinomycetoma, itraconazole (100–200mg daily), and terbinafine (250 mg daily) for eumycetoma patients and potassium iodide for sporotrichosis; the use of the latter medication is due to cost constraints.

Despite the support given to the patients, 38% did not attend subsequent consultations because of economic, language, personal reasons or sometimes because family members or friends, raised the spectre of unnecessary amputation. Distance and poverty were constant barriers to consent, study, and treatment.

In order to review cases we developed a basic recording format including, patient information, in Excel and graphics were made with statistics analysis SPSS.9

3. Results

Table 1 shows the results from 113 confirmed mycetomas studied. For logistical reasons not all mycological studies could be carried out on all patients. There were more actinomycetomas than eumycetomas with scattered anatomical distributions

Table 1. Mycetoma Patients.

VARIABLE	VALUES	
GENDER	Male	= 85 (75.2%)
	Female	= 28 (24.8%)
AGE	Adults > 18a	= 104 (92.0%)
	Children < 18a	= 9 (8.0%)
OCCUPATION	Farmers	= 53 (48.6%)
	Housewives	= 23 (21.1%)
	Others	= 37 (30.3%)
AFFECTED AREA	Feet	= 34 (30.1%)
	Legs	= 11 (9.7%)
	Upper limbs	= 22 (19.5%)
	Pelvic area	= 19 (16.8%)
	Abdomen	= 6 (5.3%)
	Trunk	= 17 (15.1%)
	Cervical column	= 4 (3.5%)
MYCOLOGY	Cultures (+)	= 82
	Direct Exam (+)	= 101
	Biopsy	= 79
	X ray	= 75
	CT	= 7
TYPE OF MYCETOMA	Actinomycetoma	= 81 (78.6%)
	Eumycetoma	= 22 (21.4%)
ACTINOMYCETES	*Nocardia brasiliensis*	= 64 (70.4%)
	Nocardia spp	= 19 (20.9%)
	Actinomadura madurae	= 6 (6.6%)
	N. otitidis caviarum	= 2 (2.1%)
FUNGI	*Madurella mycetomatis*	= 16 (72.8%)
	Trematosphaeria grisea	= 3 (13.7%)
	Scedosporium boydii	= 2 (9.0%)
	Phomopsis longicola	= 1 (4.5%)
EVOLUTION	<five years	= 84 (74.3%)
	>five years	= 29 (25.7%)
REGION	Costa Chica	= 50 (44.2%)
	Acapulco	= 27 (23.9%)
	Costa Grande	= 10 (8.8%)
	Tierra Caliente	= 9 (8.0%)
	Centro	= 9 (8.0%)
	Norte	= 5 (4.4%)
	Montaña	= 3 (2.7%)

Studies made for confirmation of the diagnosis were: Biopsy in 79 cases, direct examination in 101 and culture in 82 cases. Actinomycetoma cases were caused by *Nocardia brasiliensis* in 64 cases, *Nocardia sp* 19 cases, *Actinomadura madurae* 6, *Nocardia otitidis caviarum* 2. The causative agents in eumycetomas were in most of the cases *Madurella mycetomatis* 16, *Trematosphaeria grisea* 3, *Scedosporium apiospermum* 2, and *Phomopsis longicolla* 1 case.

Table 2 shows the 76 cases of sporotrichosis studied, of which 43 were of the lymphangitic clinical pattern, fixed type 24 and cutaneous disseminated 8.35 were male, 40 female; 39 adults and 36 children. Most of these patients were farmers; men, women or children work, or are partially involved, in field activities.

Table 2. Sporotrichosis Patients.

VARIABLE	VALUES	
GENDER	Male	= 35 (46.0%)
	Female	= 41 (54.0%)
AGE	Adults > 18	= 39 (51.3%)
	Children < 18	= 37 (48.7%)
OCCUPATION	Farmers	= 62 (81.6%)
	Students	= 2 (2.6%)
	Children not working	= 12 (15.8%)
AFFECTED AREA	Upper limbs	= 32 (42.1%)
	Lower limbs	= 16 (21.1%)
	Face	= 16 (21.1%)
	Trunk	= 4 (5.3%)
	Other	= 8 (10.4%)
MYCOLOGY	Cultures	= 52 (+)
	IDR (Skin Test) [1]	= 45 (+)
	Biopsy	= 31
CLINICAL FORM	Lymphangitic	= 43 (56.8%)
	Fixed	= 24 (32.2%)
	Disseminated	= 8 (11.0%)
EVOLUTION	<1 year	= 18 (23.7%)
	<5 years	= 41 (53.9%)
	>5 years	= 17 (22.4%)
REGION	Centre	= 44 (57.9%)
	High Mountain	= 23 (30.3%)
	Others	= 9 (11.8%)
TREATMENT	Treated	= 56 (73.7%)
	Not treated	= 20 (26.3%)

The sporotrichin used was prepared by the Laboratory of Basic Mycology, Universidad Nacional Autonoma de Mexico.

The most commonly affected area was the upper limb in 32 cases, 16 in lower limbs, 16 on the face, 4 on the thorax and 3 in other localizations. All cases studied included auxiliary laboratory methods such as culture 52 cases, biopsy in 31 cases, intradermal skin test reaction with mycelial sporotrichin of which 45 cases had positive reactions (one was negative). Of diagnosed cases 56 received treatment with saturated solution of potassium iodide (at full dose 4–6 mls three times daily) with complete healing of the clinical lesions. The rest of the patients did not attend consultation for treatment. Almost 60% of cases occurred in patients in the "Central area" adjacent to the "Mountain area" - for this reason often referred to as the "low mountain" zone—but the other 30% were in the "high Mountain" zone; the remaining 11% were from other areas of the state.

4. Discussion

Neglected diseases in developing countries are usually located in remote, isolated areas with limited access, and communication. This means that health systems are limited, and there is a high level of ignorance and malnutrition all of which are reasons why these diseases develop without intervention and reach extremes of severity, leading to severe morbidity and even death amongst affected patients. One of the main and persistent obstacles to care and further research is the lack of properly trained health personnel to identify patients or to perform studies [14]. Additionally personal safety of staff is a further obstacle to investigation and care, imposing a risk in visits to isolated communities. Even though, encounters with criminal groups have been few and without severe consequences during work in the communities, the potential risk for personnel, has now forced us to adapt our working methods to include the use of teledermatology and telemedicine in order to continue the work of teaching, research, and advice for the health personnel based in remote areas [15].

In 1988, Lavalle and Padilla described in a communication [16] that Guerrero was the second commonest source in the country of mycetoma cases attending the "Centro Dermatológico Pascua" (CDP), which is a referral centre for treatment of dermatological problems. In another review of mycetomas by Bonifaz et al., Guerrero was rated 3rd in incidence (1). In comparing our data with that of Lavalle and Bonifaz for patients coming from Guerrero, but diagnosed and treated in the Department of Mycology at the Hospital General de Mexico (HGM), patient parameters were similar: male predominance in 70%, mostly middle aged, foot involvement, though in our studies uncommon areas such as the perianal region [17] or the neck, a source of considerable morbidity, have also been seen to be involved [18]. Causal agents reported in these other studies are also similar with a predominance of actinomycetes in 97% (Lavalle), 82% (Bonifaz), and 81% (Current study). It is worth mentioning that both centres in Mexico city are among the main primary mycology referral laboratories where patients are seen from every part of the country.

Our studies have also found that there are regional variations in disease prevalence for both mycoses in our environment. Eumycetomas are predominantly found in the Costa Chica area where they account for a much higher proportion of cases (30%) compared with the 2–3% reported nationally. Most sporotrichosis cases originate from the Central and Montaña regions (Figure 3). In explanation, besides the environmental characteristics–in the Costa Chica there is pastureland and cattle farming in commo—it is possible that there is a higher genetic predisposition, related to a high proportion of indigenous Mexican groups, for some mycoses. In the Costa Chica there is also a well established population of individuals of African Mexican origin. It has also been suggested in cases of sporotrichosis, in patients of indigenous origin in the Central Mountain areas carry alleles of Class II [19].

Madurella mycetomatis is the most important causal agent found in our series which is similar to studies reported in patients from other areas with high endemicity [20–22]; these isolates have not been subject to molecular identification, therefore the presence of other *Madurella* species is possible. Mycetomas per se have a low mortality, except those cases with neck and dorsal spine involvement [18], nevertheless they do have severe morbidity, which has a serious impact on the earning capacity of the affected patients as they are usually farmers with reduced economic resources and depend directly on their ability to work in the fields. The high cost of the treatment and the long term course of the disease, have a critical impact on the family's health and financial well-being [21].

Histopathological studies are a very valuable diagnostic auxiliary method used to differentiate the actinomycetomas and eumycetomas, for which treatment is completely different. Samples can be easily obtained even in remote areas and together with direct examination and culture can be accessible in areas where resources are extremely limited. Molecular diagnostic techniques are usually out of the reach of decentralized institutions where mycetoma patients are studied and treated [22] and even though simple imaging studies and ultrasound are accessible in order to identify bone involvement, other studies like CAT scan or MRI, can be unaffordable for patients of low income, which represent most of the patients studied in our group [23].

We firmly believe that mycetoma treatment should be as integrated or "holistic" [24]. In our opinion this should include (1) training of the local health personnel, providing the basic knowledge to identify and refer mycetoma cases to centres where they can be properly diagnosed, studied and treated, (2) facilitating the means for patients to attend for consultation, (3) provide appropriate tests for identification of causal agents, together with estimation of the severity index in order to determine the best available treatment for each case, (4) provide free medications throughout treatment duration, and (5) register of every case in order to contribute with information on the epidemiology of mycetoma worldwide (6) establishing a robust system for early detection, and ultimately, prevention of cases in collaboration with local health workers. In the case of sporotrichosis further work needs to be carried out, in order to establish the specific molecular identification of the causative *Sporothrix* species and the reasons for small outbreaks in specific areas, although feline sources of infection are not suspected. As with mycetoma, improving early case recognition is an important goal.

We should point out that even though the number of suspected mycetoma cases diagnosed in Community Dermatology over the last 28 years of work exceeds 240 patients, the diagnosis in many cases has been mainly determined on clinical grounds with some laboratory tests, as discussed previously; in these patients other essential laboratory studies could not be done in order to establish the causal species. Hence, the clinically diagnosed cases have not been included in the analysis.

Finally it is important to mention that 2019 is the year when the Community Dermatology Centre "Dr. Ramon Ruiz Maldonado" (CDM) has been opened in Acapulco in order to treat patients of low and very low incomes from the urban, and especially, rural areas where access to specialized attention is limited or absent.

Author Contributions: All participated in reviewing patients, planning the study and writing the manuscript.

Acknowledgments: We would like to mention our sincere appreciation to Alexandro Bonifaz MSc for the data from the laboratory of mycology regarding patients from Guerrero State. As well we would like to acknowledge Roderick Hay for the very valuable help, orientation and his participation during the activities of Community Dermatology Mexico and constant encouragement for this communication. To the Secretary of State Health and the DIF Guerrero for the support given to the activities of Community Dermatology Mexico through which fundamental information for this study was obtained. Also to the International Foundation for Dermatology, the American Academy of Dermatology, Galderma Skin Pact Awards and Vaseline Direct Relief for their contributions in order to purchase medicaments and for providing resources to mycetoma and sporotrichosis patients for their study and treatment.

References

1. Bonifaz, A.; Tirado Sánchez, A.; Calderón, L.; Saul, A.; Araiza, J.; Hernández, M.; González, G.M.; Ponce, R.M. Mycetoma: Experience of 482 cases in a single center in Mexico. *PLoS Negl. Trop. Dis.* **2014**, *8*. [CrossRef] [PubMed]
2. Lopez-Mtnez, R.; Mendez-Tovar, L.J.; Bonifaz, A.; Arenas, R.; Mayorga, J.; Welsh, O.; Vera-Cabrera, L.; Padilla-Desgarennes, M.C.; Contreras Pérez, C.; Chávez, G. Update on the epidemiology of Mycetoma in Mexico. A review of 3933 cases. *Gac. Med. Mex.* **2013**, *149*, 586–592.
3. Van de Sande, W. Global burden of human mycetoma: A systemic review and metanalisis. *PLoS Negl. Trop. Dis.* **2013**, *7*. [CrossRef]
4. WHO. Available online: https://www.who.int/neglected_diseases/mediacentre/WHA_69.21_Eng.pdf?ua=1 (accessed on 2 February 2019).
5. Werner, A.; Werner, B. Sporotrichosis in man and animals. *Int. J. Dermatol.* **1994**, *33*, 692–700. [CrossRef] [PubMed]
6. Conti, A.D. Sporotrichosis in Latin America. *Mycopath* **1989**, *108*, 113–116.
7. Corcho-Berdugo, A.; Muñoz Hndez, B.; Palma-Cortes, G.; Ramirez Hndez, A.; Martínez-Rivera, M.; Frías-de León, M.; Reyes-Montes, M.; Martínez-Valadez, E.; Manjarrez-Zavala, M.; Alfaro-Ramos, L.; et al. Brote inusual de histoplasmosis en residentes del estado de México. *Gaceta Med. Mex.* **2011**, *5*, 377–384.

8. Mayorga, P.; Epinoza, H. Coccidioidomycosis in México and Central America. *Mycopathol. Mycol. Appl.* **1970**, *41*, 13–23. [CrossRef] [PubMed]
9. Lopez-Martinez, R.; Hernandez-Hernandez, F.; Mendez-Tovar, LJ.; Manzano-Gayosso, P.; Bonifaz, A.; Arenas, R.; Padilla-Desgarennes Mdel, C.; Estrada, R.; Chávez, G. Paracoccidioidomycosis en Mexico. Clinical and epidemiological data from 93 new cases (1972–2012). *Mycoses* **2014**, *57*, 525–530. [CrossRef]
10. Chavez, L.G.; Estrada, C.R.; Estrada, C.G.; Moreno, C.G. Cromoblastomicosis y micetoma. Informe de un caso por presentación simultanea de Fonseca pedrosoi y Nocardia brasiliensis. *Dermatol. Cosm. Med. Quir.* **2014**, *12*, 268–271.
11. Estrada, C.R.; Chavez, L.G.; Estrada, C.G.; Bonifaz, A. Report of 73 cases of cutaneous sporotrichosis in Mexico. *An. Bras. Dermatol.* **2018**, *93*, 907–909. [CrossRef]
12. Estrada, C.R.; Chavez-Lopez, M.G.; Estrada-Chavez, G.; Paredes-Solis, S. Specialized dermatological care for marginalized populations and education at primary care level: Is community dermatology a feasible proposal? *Int. J. Dermatol.* **2012**, *51*, 1345–1350. [CrossRef]
13. Hay, R.J.; Estrada, C.R.; Grossmann, H. Managing skin disease in resource-poor environments- the role of community oriented training and control programs. *Int. J. Dermatol.* **2011**, *50*, 558–563. [CrossRef]
14. El-Safi, S.; Chappuis, F.; Boelaert, M. The Challenges of Conducting Clinical Research on neglected tropical diseases in remote endemic áreas of Sudan. *PLoS Negl. Trop. Dis.* **2016**, *10*. [CrossRef] [PubMed]
15. Chávez, L.G.; Estrada, C.G.; Orozco, F.M.; Solis, R.A.; Solchaga-Rosas, J.; Armendariz-Valle, F.; Estrada-Castañón, R.A. Teledermatología, un modelo de enseñanza y asistencia en atención primaria a la salud. *Gac. Med. Mex.* **2018**, *154*, 1–5.
16. Lavalle, P.; Padilla, M.C.; Perez, J.; Reynoso, S. Contribución al conocimiento de los micetomas en el estado de Guerrero, México. Origen disctribución geográfica y evolución de 100 casos de micetomas. *Dermatol. Rev. Mex.* **1988**, *42*, 232–238.
17. Chávez, G.; Estrada, R.; Bonifaz, A. Perianal actinomycetoma, experience of 20 cases. *Int. J. Dermatol.* **2002**, *41*, 491–493. [CrossRef] [PubMed]
18. Estrada-Chavez, G.; Estrada, R.; Fernandez, R.; Arenas, R.; Reyes, A.; Guevara, C.; Chávez-López, G. Cervical and middle actinomycetomas from Guerrero State, Mexico. *Int. J. Dermatol.* **2017**, *56*, 1146–1149. [CrossRef] [PubMed]
19. Estrada-Chavez, G.; Estrada, R.; Chavez, G.; Vega Memije, M.; Guzmán, R.; García-Lechuga, M.; Granados, J.; Rangel-Gamboa, L. HLA Class II alleles in human sporotrichosis in Mexican Amerindians. *Asia-Pacif. J. Blood Types Genes* **2018**, *2*, 183–190.
20. Ahmed, A.O.; Van-Leeuwen, W.; Fahal, A.; Van de Sande, W. Mycetoma caused by Madurella mycetomatis: A neglected infectious burden. *Lancet Infect. Dis.* **2004**, *4*, 566–574. [CrossRef]
21. Torres, G.E.; Niebla, M.A. *Mycetoma. Clinical and Microbiological Monograph*; Scholar Press: Brivibas gatve, Riga, 2015.
22. Mehantappa, H.; Sruthi, P.; Kusuma, V.; Niveditha, S.R.; Kumar, S.A. Cytological diagnosis of actinomycosis. and eumycetoma. A report of two cases. *Diagn. Cytopathol.* **2010**, *38*, 918–920.
23. Fahal, A.H.; Sjeikh, H.E.; Lider, M.A.; Homeida, M.A.; El Arabi, Y.E.; Mahgoub, E.S. Ultrasonic imaging in mycetoma. *Br. J. Surg.* **1997**, *78*, 765–766.
24. Mubarak, B.S.; Fahal, A.H.; Mudawi, M.A.; El Samani, W.M.; Fathelrahman, R.O.; Eiman, S.A.; El Nour, M.; El Rayah, M.M.; El Sheikh Rahman, M.A.; Suliman, H.S.; et al. A holistic approach to the mycetoma management. *PLoS Negl. Trop. Dis.* **2018**, *12*. [CrossRef]

Permissions

All chapters in this book were first published by MDPI; hereby published with permission under the Creative Commons Attribution License or equivalent. Every chapter published in this book has been scrutinized by our experts. Their significance has been extensively debated. The topics covered herein carry significant findings which will fuel the growth of the discipline. They may even be implemented as practical applications or may be referred to as a beginning point for another development.

The contributors of this book come from diverse backgrounds, making this book a truly international effort. This book will bring forth new frontiers with its revolutionizing research information and detailed analysis of the nascent developments around the world.

We would like to thank all the contributing authors for lending their expertise to make the book truly unique. They have played a crucial role in the development of this book. Without their invaluable contributions this book wouldn't have been possible. They have made vital efforts to compile up to date information on the varied aspects of this subject to make this book a valuable addition to the collection of many professionals and students.

This book was conceptualized with the vision of imparting up-to-date information and advanced data in this field. To ensure the same, a matchless editorial board was set up. Every individual on the board went through rigorous rounds of assessment to prove their worth. After which they invested a large part of their time researching and compiling the most relevant data for our readers.

The editorial board has been involved in producing this book since its inception. They have spent rigorous hours researching and exploring the diverse topics which have resulted in the successful publishing of this book. They have passed on their knowledge of decades through this book. To expedite this challenging task, the publisher supported the team at every step. A small team of assistant editors was also appointed to further simplify the editing procedure and attain best results for the readers.

Apart from the editorial board, the designing team has also invested a significant amount of their time in understanding the subject and creating the most relevant covers. They scrutinized every image to scout for the most suitable representation of the subject and create an appropriate cover for the book.

The publishing team has been an ardent support to the editorial, designing and production team. Their endless efforts to recruit the best for this project, has resulted in the accomplishment of this book. They are a veteran in the field of academics and their pool of knowledge is as vast as their experience in printing. Their expertise and guidance has proved useful at every step. Their uncompromising quality standards have made this book an exceptional effort. Their encouragement from time to time has been an inspiration for everyone.

The publisher and the editorial board hope that this book will prove to be a valuable piece of knowledge for researchers, students, practitioners and scholars across the globe.

List of Contributors

Jesse Masson, Jan Douglass, Maureen Roineau, Jeffrey Warner and Patricia M. Graves
College of Public Health, Medical and Veterinary Sciences, James Cook University, Cairns, QLD 4870, Australia

Khin Saw Aye and Kyi May Htwe
Department of Medical Research, Myanmar Ministry of Health and Sports, Nay Pyi Taw, Myanmar

Wendemagegn Enbiale
Dermatology and Venerology, Bahir Dar University, Bahir Dar, Ethiopia

Ashenafi Ayalew
Amhara Regional Health Bureau, Amhara, Ethiopia

Adam Stewart and Mark Armstrong
Department of Infectious Diseases, Royal Brisbane and Women's Hospital, Butterfield St & Bowen Bridge Rd, Herston, Queensland 4029, Australia

Stephen Graves
Australian Rickettsial Reference Laboratory, Barwon Health, Geelong Hospital, Bellerine Street, Geelong, Victoria 3220, Australia

Krispin Hajkowicz
Department of Infectious Diseases, Royal Brisbane and Women's Hospital, Butterfield St & Bowen Bridge Rd, Herston, Queensland 4029, Australia
School of Medicine, University of Queensland, St Lucia, Queensland 4072, Australia

Liesbeth F. Mieras and Anna T. Taal
Technical Department, Netherlands Leprosy Relief, 1090 HA Amsterdam, The Netherlands

Erik B. Post
Challenge TB, KNCV Tuberculosis Foundation, Jakarta 12870, Indonesia

Alcino G. Z. Ndeve
Technical Department, Netherlands Leprosy Relief, Maputo, Mozambique

Colette L. M. van Hees
Department of Dermatology, Erasmus Medical Centre, 3000 CA Rotterdam, The Netherlands

Rajashree Chowdhury, Prakash Ghosh, Md. Anik Ashfaq Khan, Faria Hossain, Khaledul Faisal, Rupen Nath, James Baker, Debashis Ghosh, Md. Utba Bin Rashid and Dinesh Mondal
Nutrition and Clinical Service Division (NCSD), International Centre for Diarrhoeal Disease Research, Bangladesh

Ahmed Abd El Wahed
Institute of Animal Hygiene and Veterinary Public Health, University of Leipzig, D-04103 Leipzig, Germany

Shomik Maruf
Nutrition and Clinical Service Division (NCSD), International Centre for Diarrhoeal Disease Research, Bangladesh
London School of Hygiene and Tropical Medicine, University of London, London WC1E 7HT, UK

Progganananda Nath
Infection and Tropical Medicine, Mymensingh Medical College and Hospital (MMCH), Mymensingh 2200, Bangladesh

Md. Masud-Ur-Rashid
Department of Cardiovascular and Thoracic Surgery, National Heart Foundation Hospital and Research Institute, Dhaka 1216, Bangladesh

Malcolm S. Duthie
Host Directed Therapeutics (HDT) Bio Corp, Seattle, WA 98102, USA

Ousmane Faye, Adama Dicko, Lamissa Cissé, Siritio Berthé, Bekaye Traoré, Youssouf Fofana, Yamoussa Karabinta, Mamadou Gassama, Binta Guindo, Alimata Keita, Koreissi Tall and Somita Keita
Department of Dermatology, Faculty of Medicine and Odontostomatology, Bamako, Mali

Cheick Oumar Bagayoko, Mahamoudan Niang and Seydou Tidiane Traoré
CERTES, Bamako, Mali

Antoine Mahé
Service de Dermatologie, Hôpital Pasteur, Colmar 68000, France

Antoine Geissbuhler
Département de Radiologie et Informatique médicale, Université de Genève, Genaven 1211, Switzerland

Matthew R. Boyce, Ellen P. Carlin, Jordan Schermerhorn and Claire J. Standley
Center for Global Health Science & Security, Georgetown University, Washington, DC 20057, USA

Benjamin F. R. Dickson and William J. McBride
College of Medicine & Dentistry, James Cook University, Cairns, QLD 4870, Australia

Catherine A. Gordon and Donald P. McManus
QIMR Berghofer Medical Research Institute, Molecular Parasitology Laboratory, Queensland 4006, Australia

Johanna Kurscheid and Darren J. Gray
Australian National University, Department of Global Health, Research School of Population Health, Australian Capital Territory 2601, Australia

Malcolm K. Jones
School of Veterinary Science, University of Queensland, Brisbane, QLD 4067, Australia

Avishek Singh and William John Hannan McBride
Cairns Clinical School, College of Medicine and Dentistry, James Cook University, Cairns City, QLD 4870, Australia

Brenda Govan
College of Public Health, Medical & Vet Sciences, James Cook University, Townsville, QLD 4811, Australia

Mark Pearson
Australian Institute of Tropical Health & Medicine, James Cook University, Smithfield, QLD 4878, Australia

Narayan Gyawali
School of Health, Medical & Applied Sciences, Central Queensland University, Rockhampton, QLD 4702, Australia
Institute of Health & Biomedical Innovation, Queensland University of Technology, Brisbane, QLD 4059, Australia

Andrew W. Taylor-Robinson
School of Health, Medical & Applied Sciences, Central Queensland University, Brisbane, QLD 4000, Australia

Victoria Williams and Carrie Kovarik
Department of Dermatology, Perelman School of Medicine, University of Pennsylvania, Philadelphia, PA 19104, USA

Deborah C. Holt, Tegan M. Harris, Bart J. Currie and Therese M. Kearns
Menzies School of Health Research, Charles Darwin University, Darwin NT 0811, Australia

Jennifer Shield
Menzies School of Health Research, Charles Darwin University, Darwin NT 0811, Australia
Department of Pharmacy and Applied Science, La Trobe University, Bendigo VIC 3550, Australia

Kate E. Mounsey
School of Health and Sports Science, University of the Sunshine Coast, Maroochydore QLD 4558, Australia

Kieran Aland
Queensland Museum, South Brisbane QLD 4101, Australia

James S. McCarthy
QIMR Berghofer Medical Research Institute, Herston QLD 4006, Australia
School of Medicine, University of Queensland, Brisbane QLD 4072, Australia

Rie R. Yotsu
School of Tropical Medicine and Global Health, Nagasaki University, Nagasaki 852-8102, Japan
Department of Dermatology, National Center for Global Health and Medicine, Tokyo 162-8655, Japan

Andrew P. Dobson
Department of Ecology and Evolutionary Biology, Princeton University, Princeton, NJ 08544, USA

Alexandra Hylton
Department of Ecology and Evolutionary Biology, Princeton University, Princeton, NJ 08544, USA
Department of Pathobiology, School of Veterinary Medicine, St. George's University, True Blue, Grenada
College of Medicine, University of Oklahoma, Oklahoma City, OK 73117, USA

Daniel M. Fitzpatrick
Department of Pathobiology, School of Veterinary Medicine, St. George's University, True Blue, Grenada

Rod Suepaul and Roxanne A. Charles
Department of Basic Veterinary Sciences, School of Veterinary Medicine, Faculty of Medical Sciences, The University of the West Indies, Trinidad and Tobago, West Indies

Jennifer K. Peterson
Department of Ecology and Evolutionary Biology, Princeton University, Princeton, NJ 08544, USA
University Honors College, Portland State University, Portland, OR 97207-075, USA

Guadalupe Estrada-Chávez
Department of Dermatology and Dermato-Oncology, Instituto Estatal de Cancerología "Dr. Arturo Beltrán Ortega", Health Secretary Guerrero, Faculty of Medicine, Universidad Autónoma de Guerrero Mexico, Community Dermatology Mexico C.A., 39850 Acapulco, Guerrero, Mexico

María de Guadalupe Chávez-López
Department of Dermatology and Mycology Acapulco General Hospital, Health Secretary Guerrero, Community Dermatology Mexico C.A., 39355 Acapulco, Guerrero, Mexico

Roberto Estrada-Castañón
Community Dermatology Mexico C.A.; Health Secretary Guerrero, 39355 Acapulco, Guerrero, Mexico

Index

www.ingramcontent.com/pod-product-compliance
Lightning Source LLC
LaVergne TN
LVHW082222200926
848484LV00008B/2290
* 9 7 9 8 8 8 7 4 0 2 9 6 3 *